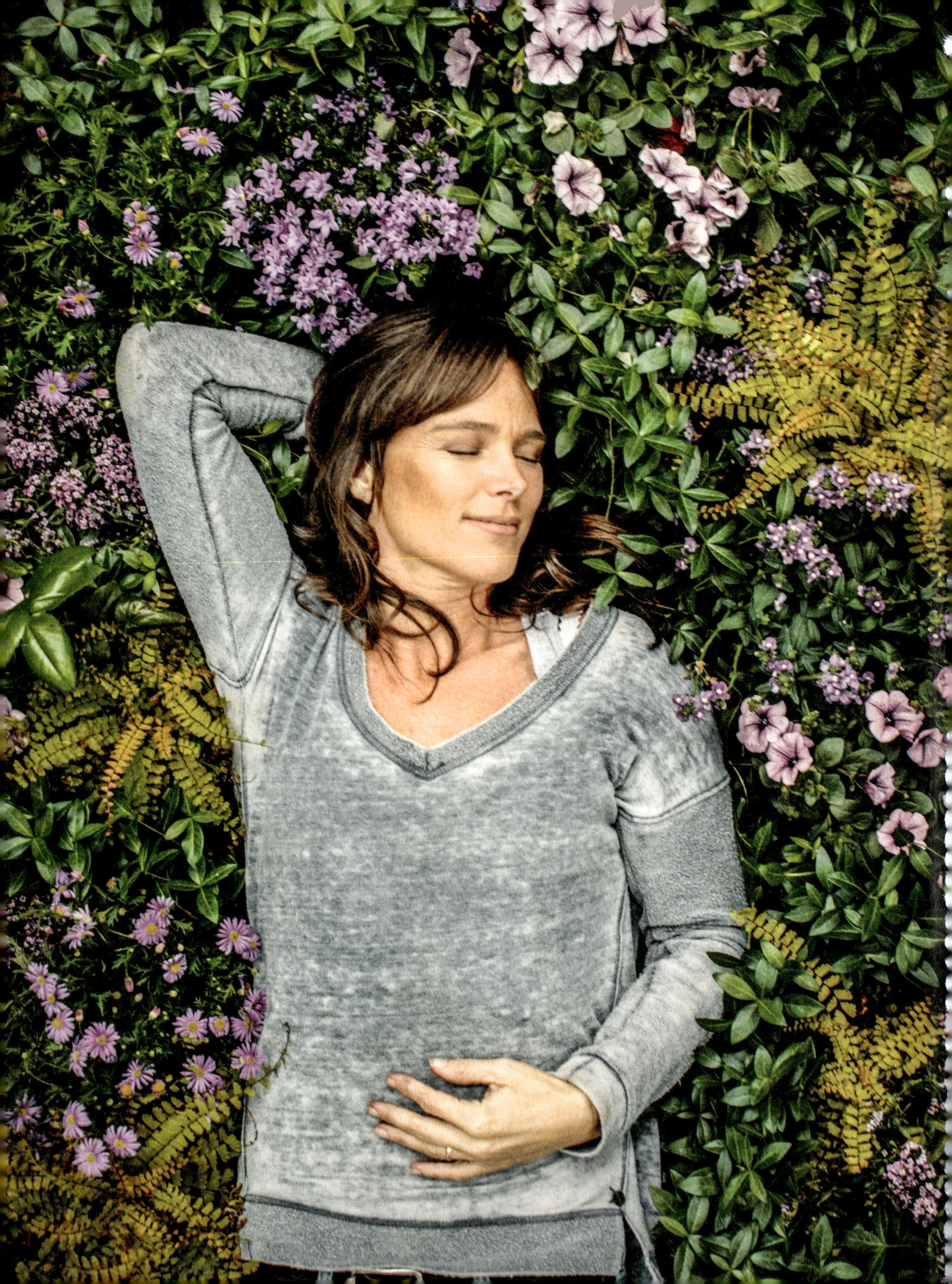

It is better to be grass.
People mow it, tend it,
And it grows wild again,
never the same.

Hugo Claus

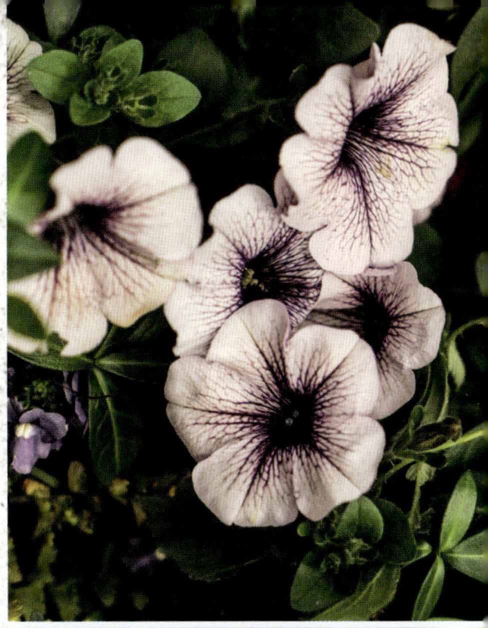

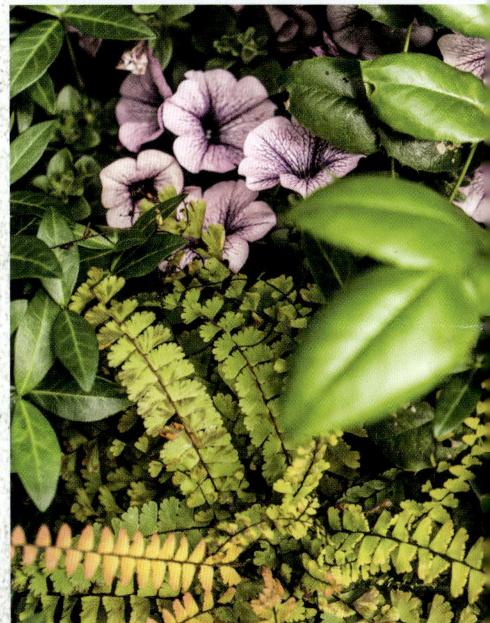

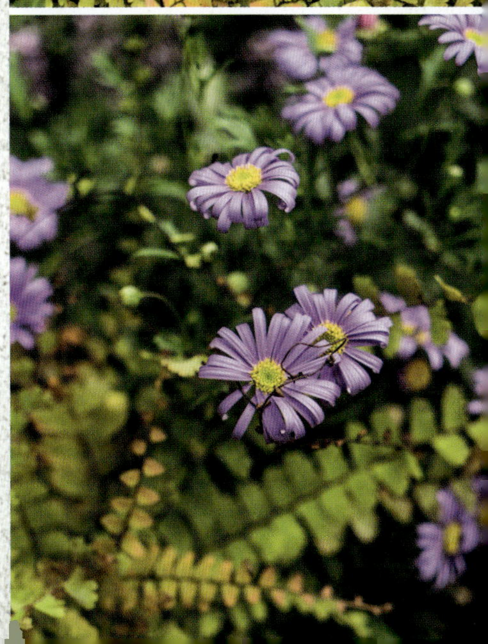

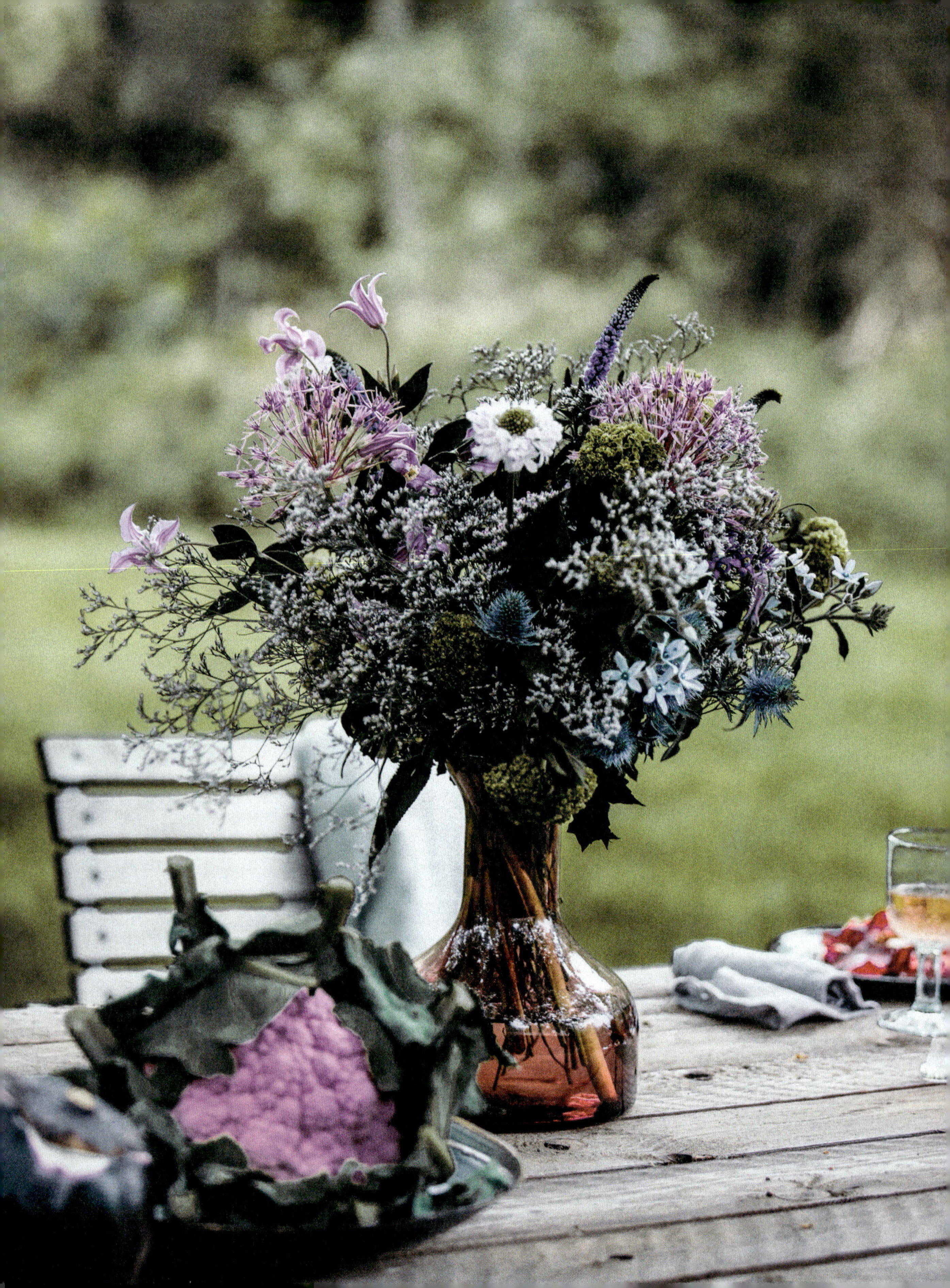

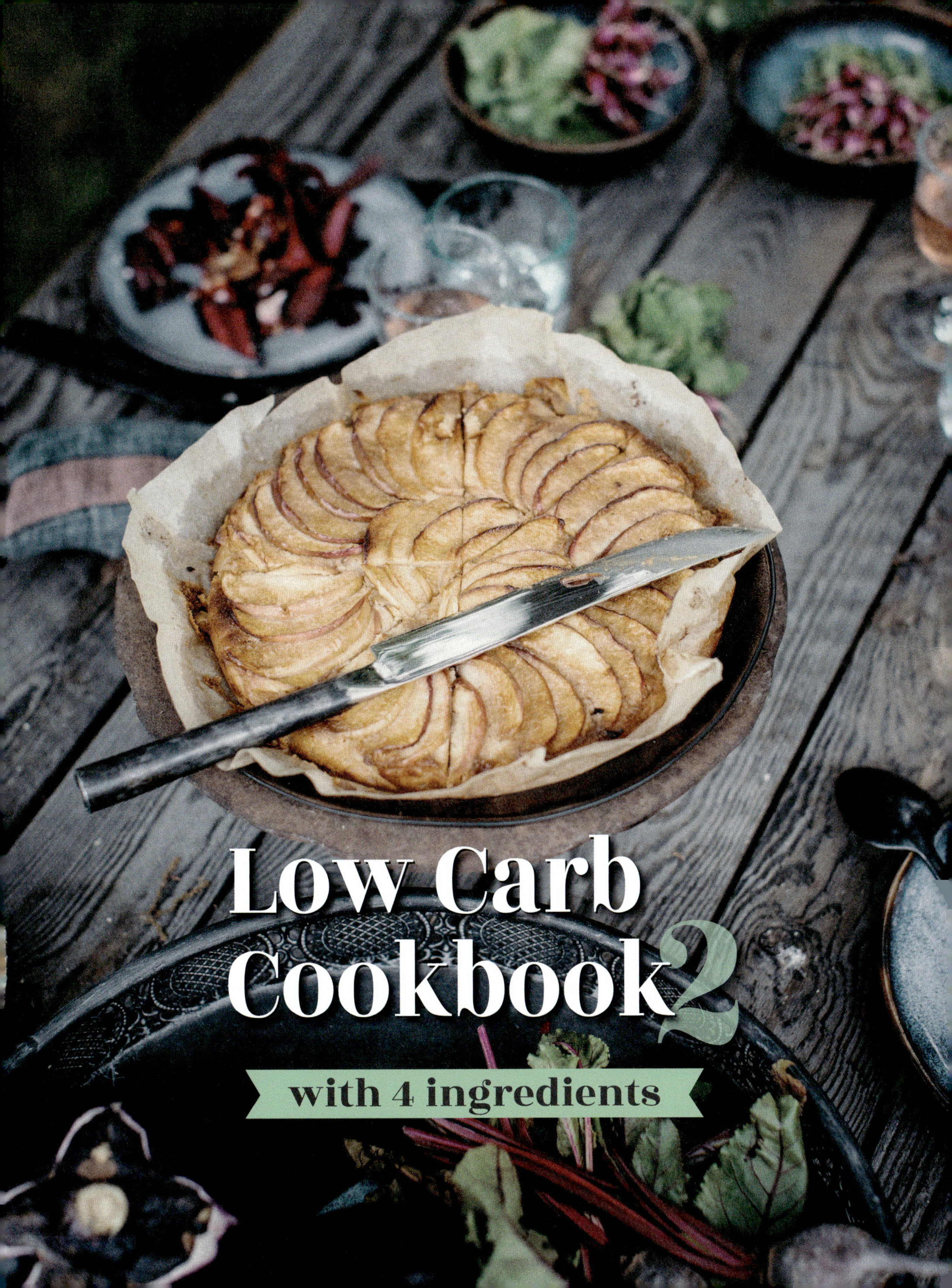

Low Carb Cookbook 2

with 4 ingredients

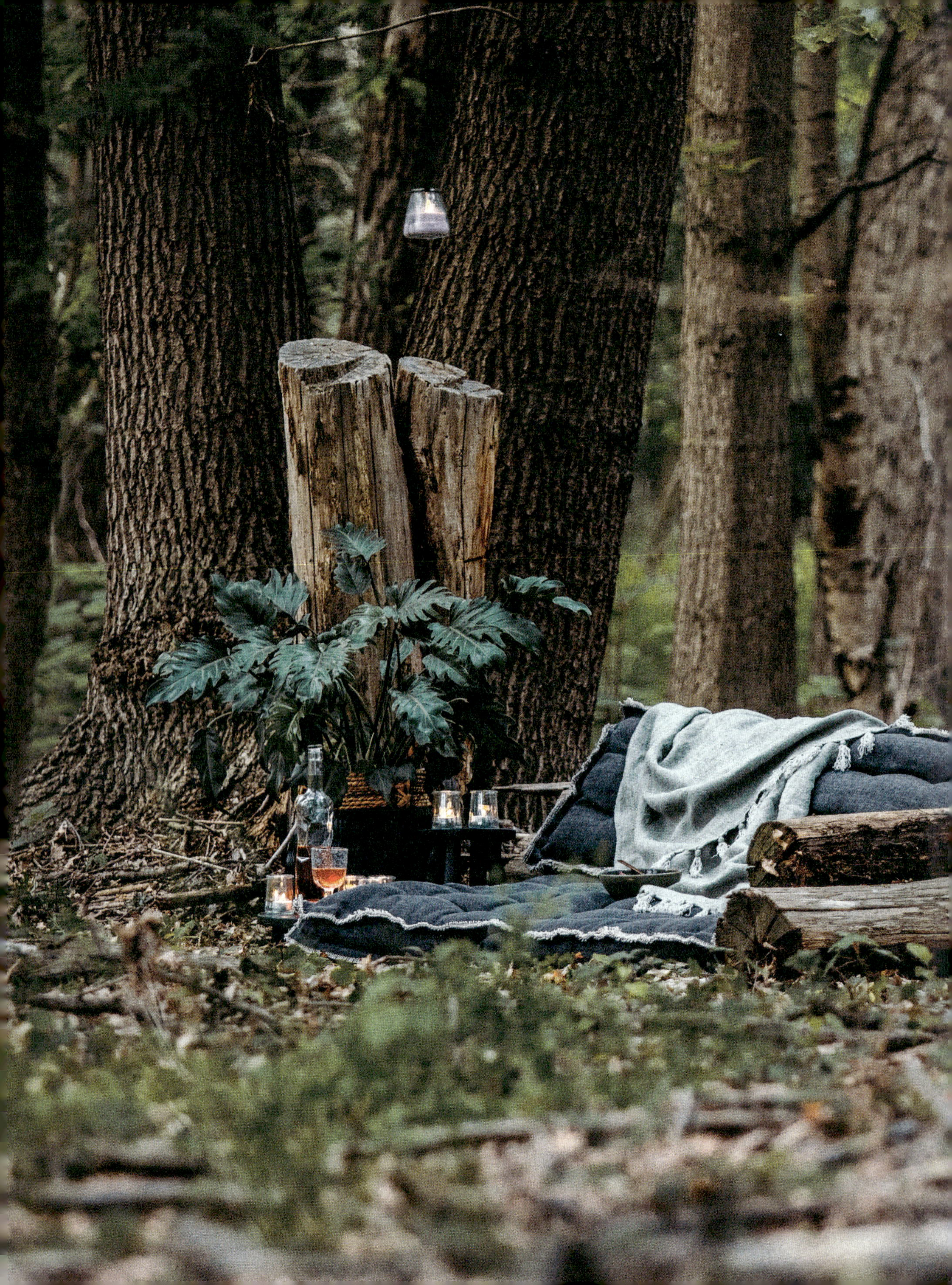

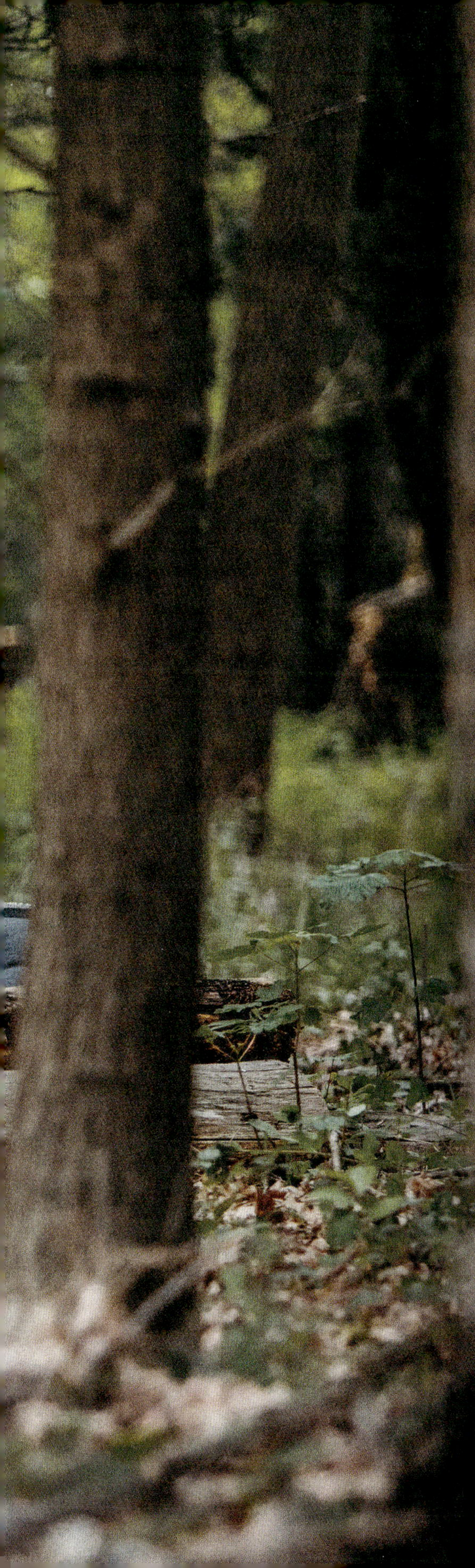

The recipes in this book are for two people.

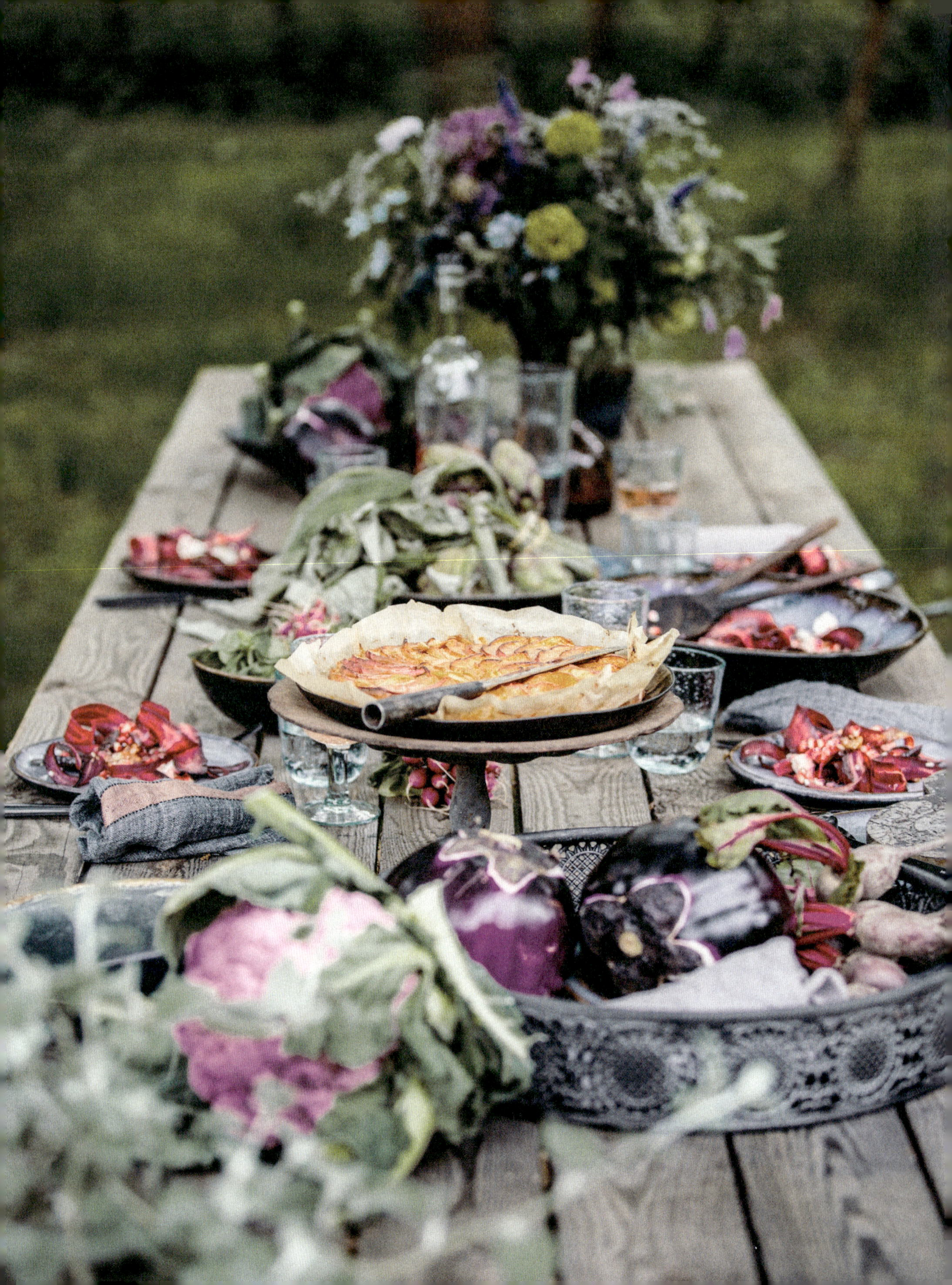

Pure enjoyment

If this book could be summed up in two words, those are the right ones. I've just invited a few friends over and prepared all sorts of recipes from this book. It shows that my approach works on all fronts. As a hostess, preparing this meal didn't take much work and not much shopping either. Each recipe only requires four ingredients, and each dish is a taste explosion in its own right. It never ceases to amaze me how you can enhance flavors by using as few ingredients as possible. The strength of each recipe lies in its pure flavors, and that's something worth appreciating.

No bells and whistles, no pretentiousness, just recipes that come straight from the heart. The guests were very enthusiastic, and the atmosphere was amazing. I enjoy such experiences to the fullest, especially when I can create the atmosphere myself. To me, cooking will always be one of the most wonderful ways to communicate with your loved ones. Which explains why I have a hard time cooking for people I don't like. Thankfully, that's not a problem for me. ☺ But when I cook for my husband, my friends and my family, I enjoy myself to the fullest and everything falls effortlessly into place. I do so love the gesture of "giving food". Perhaps that's why I love making baked dishes so much. Not only are they beautiful to look at, but they also let you share the food at the table. It's a way of dining that immediately has a casual, convivial feel to it. Everyone feels welcome, everyone feels at home.

I also really enjoy the everyday dinners with just the two of us. This book shows you how you can bring an exceptionally delicious, fresh dish to the table in practically no time, so you can relax and unwind after a busy day. It also gives you a moment to catch up with each other, which is easier to do when the food is delicious and the time in the kitchen is kept to a minimum.

Cooking will always be a magical experience for me. I hope that you will experience many wonderful and welcoming moments with the recipes from this book.

Love, Pascale

XXX

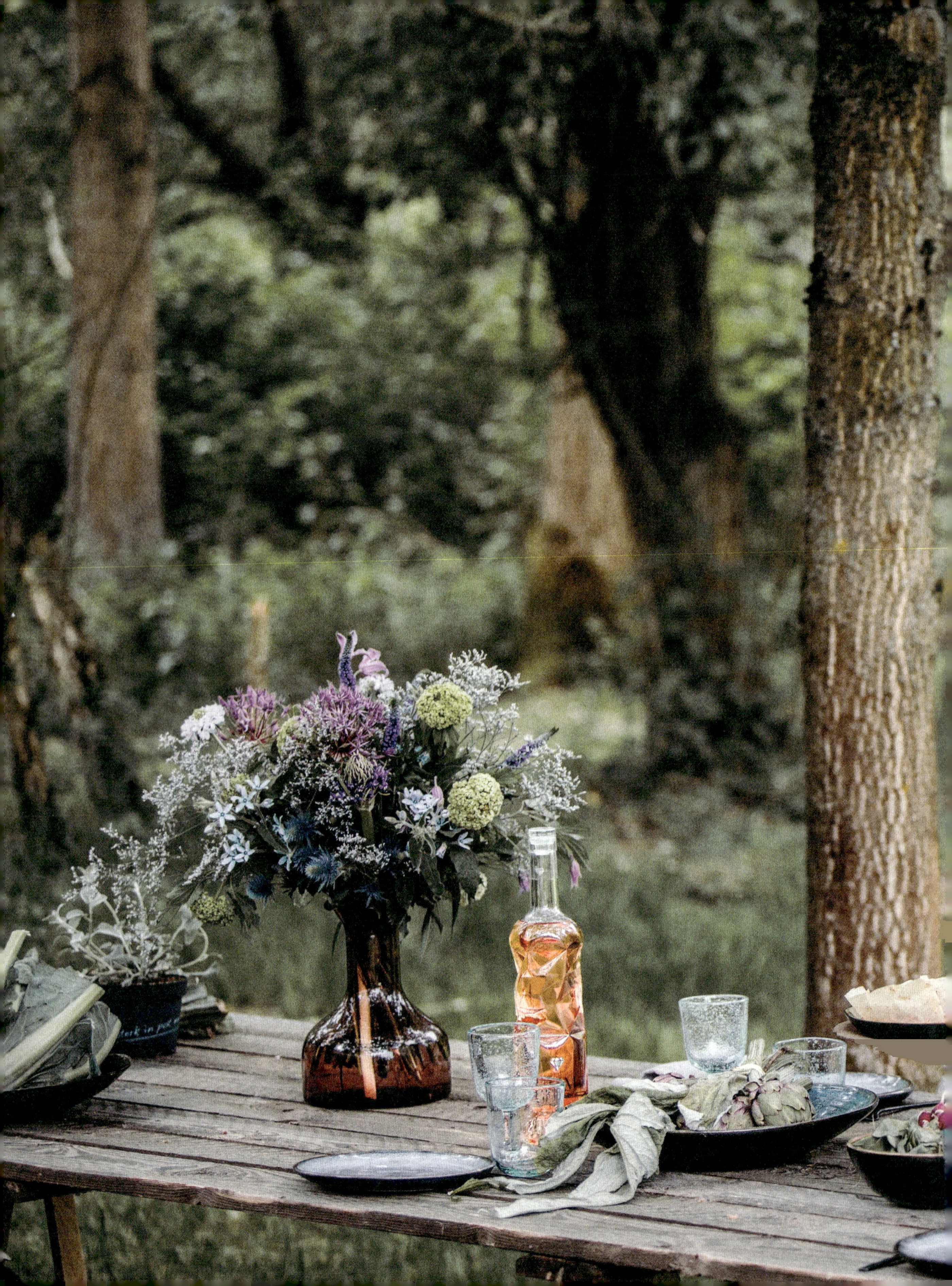

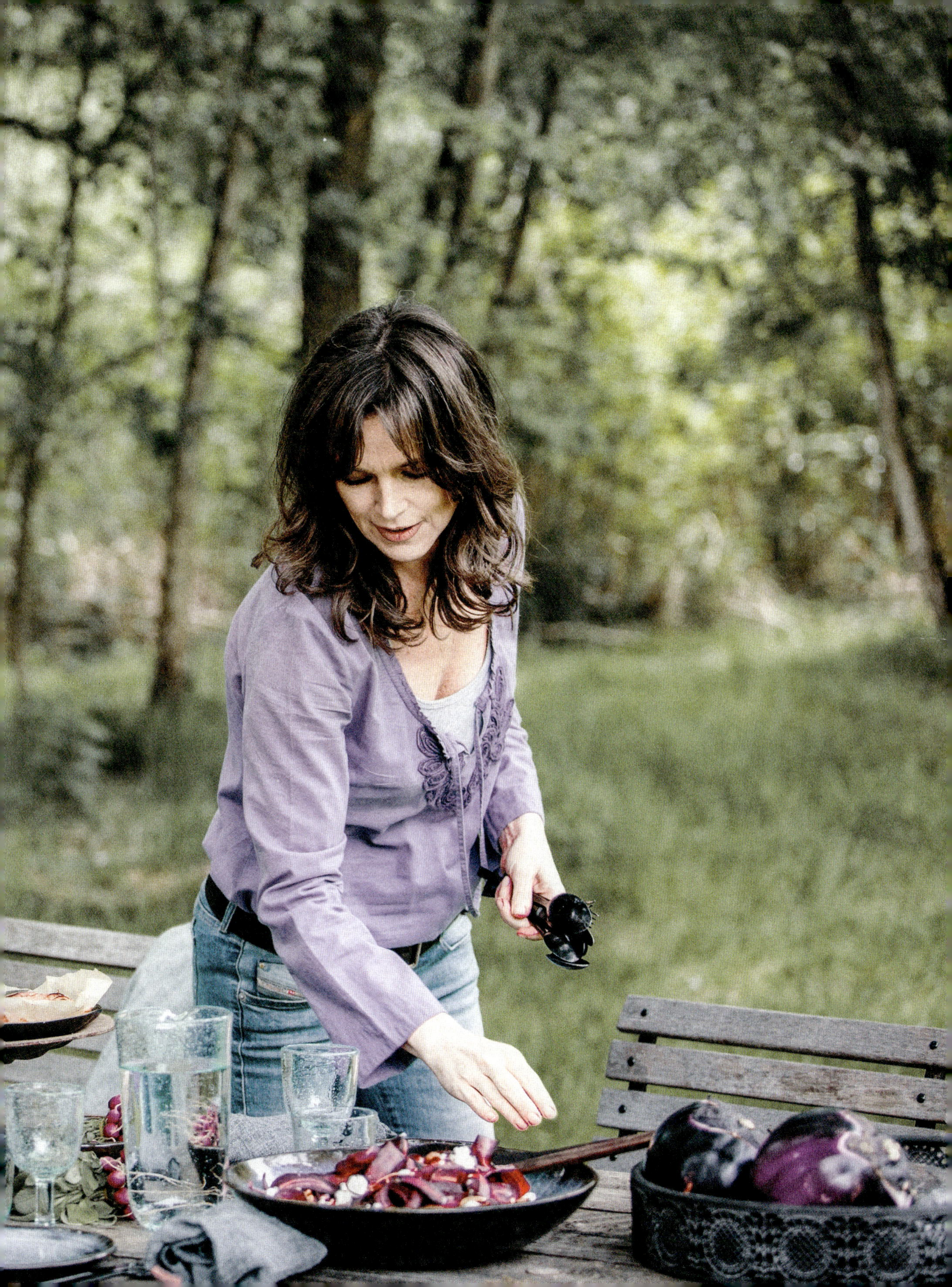

Eating well is more important than the theory behind it

Eating delicious and healthy food; in my kitchen, that's what it's all about. What's on your plate is far more important than all the theories and food fads. If you just get started and cook according to my recipes, you'll always be eating delicious, healthy food – and then you can forget about all the rest. Each recipe fits into my approach to food and will contribute to a better and healthier life. Enough said. Bon appétit!

I know some readers won't want to stop there. They want more details, to know more about the science behind healthy nutrition. They want to understand better terms such as "low carb", "keto", "resistant starch" and "intermittent fasting". For those readers, I have included additional information towards the end of the book about these terms and how they fit into my cooking style.

The way of eating I have been following for years and that you will find in all my books can best be described as a moderately low-carbohydrate Mediterranean diet. It's still my favorite cuisine, but it's also the most scientifically-researched and proven healthy way of eating.

Below you'll find an overview of my tried-and-tested approach, the same approach that's in all my books. When you use this approach, you'll automatically choose authentic, natural food and start eating "low carb", the healthiest, most delicious, and simplest cuisine out there.

all vegetables

combine well with
proteins or carbohydrates

concentrated proteins

fish
cheese
meat
soy products

not a good combination

concentrated carbohydrates

white bread
potatoes
white rice
pasta
brown rice
sweet potatoes
whole-wheat bread
wholegrain pasta
beans
chickpeas
oatmeal
quinoa
lentils

(healthier sources of carbohydrates are marked in green)

Nuts, seeds, yogurt, eggs and fats (such as olive oil, coconut oil, butter, cream and other fats) can be combined with everything.

You can combine proteins, but it's not recommended; you should not be eating more proteins.

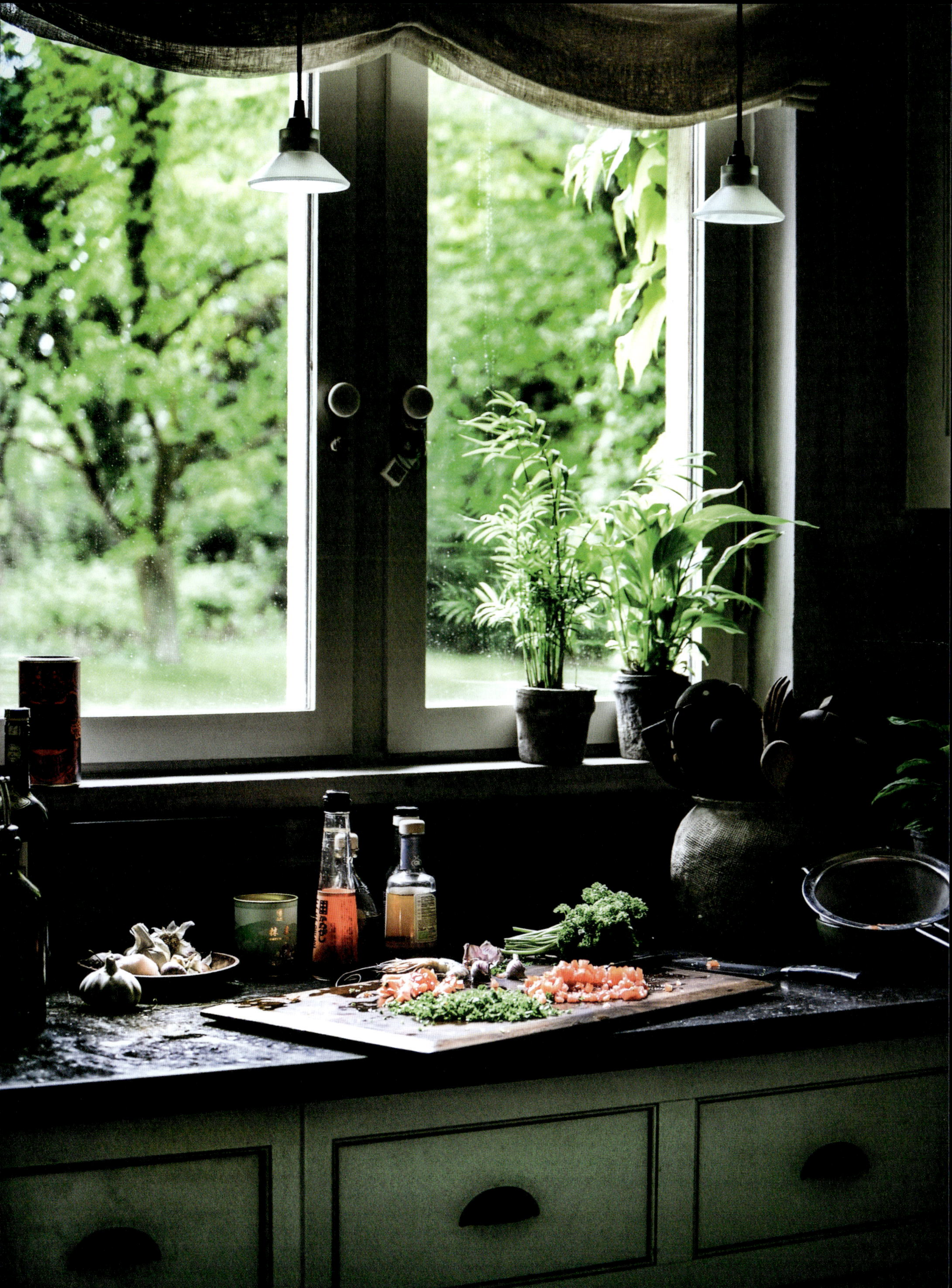

You don’t need many ingredients
to produce delicious meals.

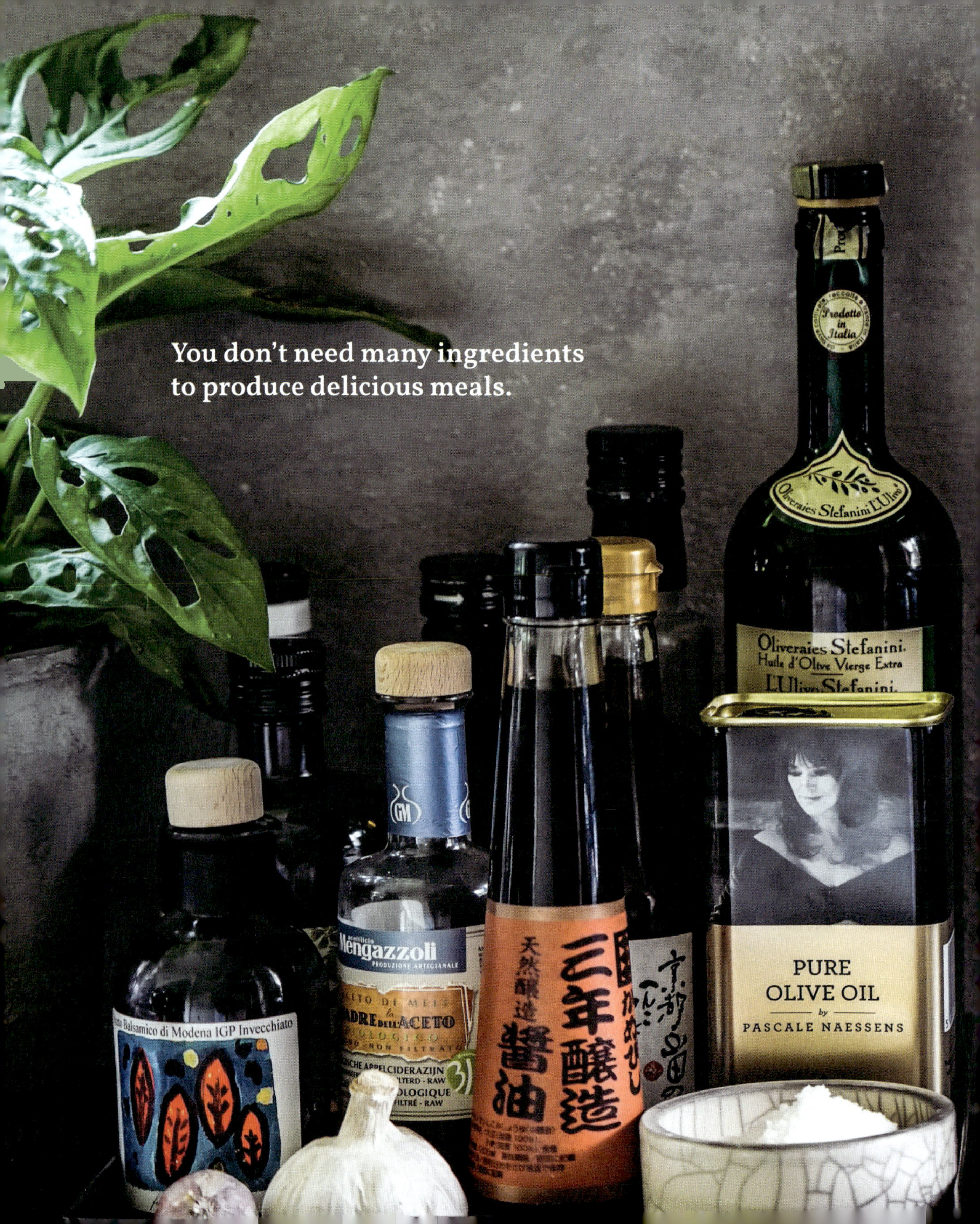

the pantry

If you have a well-stocked pantry, you only need to buy the few fresh ingredients found in these recipes to conjure up instantly the most delicious meals at the table. I have to admit, my own pantry is brimming with the wonderful flavorings, seasonings, herbs and spices; but, for this book I've stuck to the bare basics. The only difference between this and my first Low Carb Cookbook is that I have added fresh garlic to the pantry. After doing a poll on Facebook, we discovered that 94% of readers always have fresh garlic at home and have no problems with having fresh garlic in the pantry.

If you want to make the most of this book, make sure you have the following ingredients in your cupboard:

Fats	**Vinegar**	**Flavorings**	**Extra**
olive oil	balsamic vinegar	(light) soy sauce	coconut sugar
butter	apple cider vinegar	mustard	honey
coconut oil			

Herbs and spices
black pepper
fleur de sel (sea salt)
ras el hanout
dried Herbes de Provence: thyme, rosemary...
fresh garlic

The recipes in this book are delicious in their own right and don't need any extras, but I invite you to be creative and experiment with my recipes. Feel free to add additional vegetables or other ingredients. I hope that these recipes will inspire you to do so.

Amounts
The recipes in this book are for two people, but feel free to adjust the amounts to suit your own needs. Age, work, exercise and gender all play a role in how much food a person needs. My rule is: no one should leave the table hungry ☺. Try to keep to three meals a day and only eat snacks when you're hungry (unless you are doing intermittent fasting – read more about this on page 218).

Cooking times and temperatures
Every oven is different. I work with a convection oven and I have the impression that it's a lot more powerful than many other ovens. You may have to raise the temperature on your oven a little and bake the dishes in the oven for a little longer.

Why all this discussion about nutrition?

If we look around us, we see that no two people have the same body shape. We see family members in the same family who are both slim and stocky, while they all eat the same food. We are all different, so why should we all have to eat the same way?

There are people who are just fine with the classic way of eating, with plenty of fast carbs. We all probably know someone who can eat plenty of fast carbs and yet remain slim. During my lectures, I often ask the question: "Who in this room can eat bread, chips and French fries without gaining weight?" Usually only a couple of people will raise their hand. Unfortunately, most people do gain weight when they rely too much on convenience foods. The diversity within that large group of people is endless. Some of us have no trouble following the advice "everything in moderation", a classic, frequently used phrase. I believe that for that group of people, the food pyramid works well as a guideline. They don't have much trouble following the guidelines set by the Health Department. They are people whose bodies react well to carbs. They can follow the traditional nutrition guidelines and still feel energetic and healthy.

But does that advice work for everyone? When I ask, "Who regularly eats too much?" more than half the audience clearly raise their hands. I am also one of those people for whom carbs cause me to gain weight very quickly. Unfortunately, I can't get enough of them, especially those typical Western fast carbs such as bread, potatoes, pasta and French fries. They make me fat and miserable, and moreover, they're highly addictive.

That means that I have trouble with traditional guidelines like "eat plenty of carbohydrates" or "everything in moderation". They don't work for me, no matter how hard I try. And believe me, like so many others, I've tried really hard.

"We should let go of the idea that we should all eat in the same way."

I understand that this is difficult to explain to someone who has never had problems with carbs, somebody who has never felt that irresistible urge to eat carbs. If you talk about it with people, the conversation usually leads to: you don't have enough willpower, you just need to find the right motivation, get someone to coach you, you're just an emotional eater... All issues which have to do with our way of thinking, as if eating is all in the mind. If you eat too much, people tend to say that it's your own choice, or worse, your own fault.

Do we really believe that all those people who have trouble with overeating are spineless weaklings? I am afraid that sadly, most people and even a few experts would say "yes". Do they not know about other factors which may play a role? What about our genes, our hormones, our gut bacteria and other physical processes?

For those of you who think I'm in the minority, let me open your eyes.
According to doctor and scientific researcher Vera Tarman, who works with addicts and specializes in eating disorders, 50% of obese people, 20 to 30% of people who are overweight and 10% of people with a normal weight are addicted to food, especially foods containing high levels of starch and sugar, such as bread, cookies and pasta.

A study (1) dating from 2018 shows that carbohydrates with a high glycemic index can activate the neurochemical substances associated with addiction. Or as Vera Tarman says: some people, possibly due to genetic variations in the dopamine receptors in the brain, react particularly strongly to certain foods, which leads to an increased craving for that type of food. Drugs and foods trigger the systems in our brain associated with desire and rewards, causing the reaction to become increasingly stronger, despite the negative effects.

I belong to the 10% of people with a normal weight whose bodies are hypersensitive to certain types of food. At first, I thought that food in general was the problem and that I'd never be rid of my food addiction, because you simply can't survive without food. Moreover, I believed the experts who told me that it was all in my head. I was branded as having an "eating disorder". But, after a lot of research and reading, I discovered that, like most food addicts, I was only addicted to foods with high levels of starch and/or sugars, such as bread, pasta, cake, cookies and potatoes... and that I would react normally to whole natural foods such as vegetables, fruit, nuts, seeds, fish, meat and eggs.
My findings were in line with the latest scientific insights that place the blame regarding overweight primarily on processed foods.
It has also further convinced me that, in most cases, eating disorders should be treated as a (physical) addiction rather than a psychological disorder, or that the two should at least be considered separately.

What is the best solution for someone who is addicted? Reduce the intake of the foods to which they are hypersensitive to a bare minimum. That means that it's almost impossible to follow the traditional advice of "everything in moderation".

You don't go up to an alcoholic and say: drink just one glass of wine a day and one glass of whisky on the weekend. You can eat and drink anything, as long as you don't overdo it!
Why would you then recommend (fast) carbs, such as three slices of bread, three potatoes and one slice of cake per weekend? Why would you even consider recommending plenty of carbs, even the healthier ones, to someone who reacts strongly to those foods? That's just encouraging their addiction even more!

Now you understand why "everything in moderation" doesn't work for me, and probably for many others as well. So, what does work for me?

- I eat a lot of whole, natural products
  (vegetables, fruits, nuts, seeds, fish, eggs, meat ...)
- I eat carbs sparingly, even the "healthy" carbs
  (chickpeas, brown rice, lentils, quinoa ...)
- I never or very rarely eat bread, pasta, rice, cake, potatoes ...

We think too little about how our bodies physically react to food. It's not in our heads, it's in our bodies, our genes, and in our gut (bacteria). Give them the right nutrition and the problems disappear. But that's where it goes wrong. We're not getting the right nutritional advice because the current guidelines only work for part of the population.

The whole discussion around food stems from the fact that many experts are looking for one way of eating, one that is ideal for everyone. The fact that everyone thinks they're right doesn't help. But, with current developments in science and the large number of people for whom those traditional guidelines don't work, we have to let go of this one-size-fits-all mentality.

There's also no way of ignoring the success achieved by the low-carb movement, especially the many health benefits people experience when they eat fewer (fast) carbohydrates and more natural foods.

For those of you who still think that this problem concerns a small group of people, I'd like to refer to David Ludwig, a professor at Harvard University. "Recommending a carbohydrate-rich diet to a (US) population, two-thirds of which are insulin-resistant, has never made much sense. It is a disease that can be defined as glucose intolerance. It's time to introduce the low-carb diet to the broader public."

I can only agree with Professor Ludwig. It's high time that the general guidelines are expanded upon and that we take the diversity of the population into consideration. How simplistic and naïve is it to strive for a one-size-fits-all nutritional model, knowing that we couldn't be more different from one another? I'm thinking about our genes, our microbiomes, our surroundings, our digestion and our hormones, because we are all unique.

However, I have hope for the future. Many new, high-quality studies are being conducted that will provide new insights into the information I've presented above. One important thing we can already agree on is that processed food is one of the major culprits for everyone. In other words, we should all be eating more natural, whole foods. It's funny how I keep coming back to my own motto: buy fresh, cook your own meals and eat together.

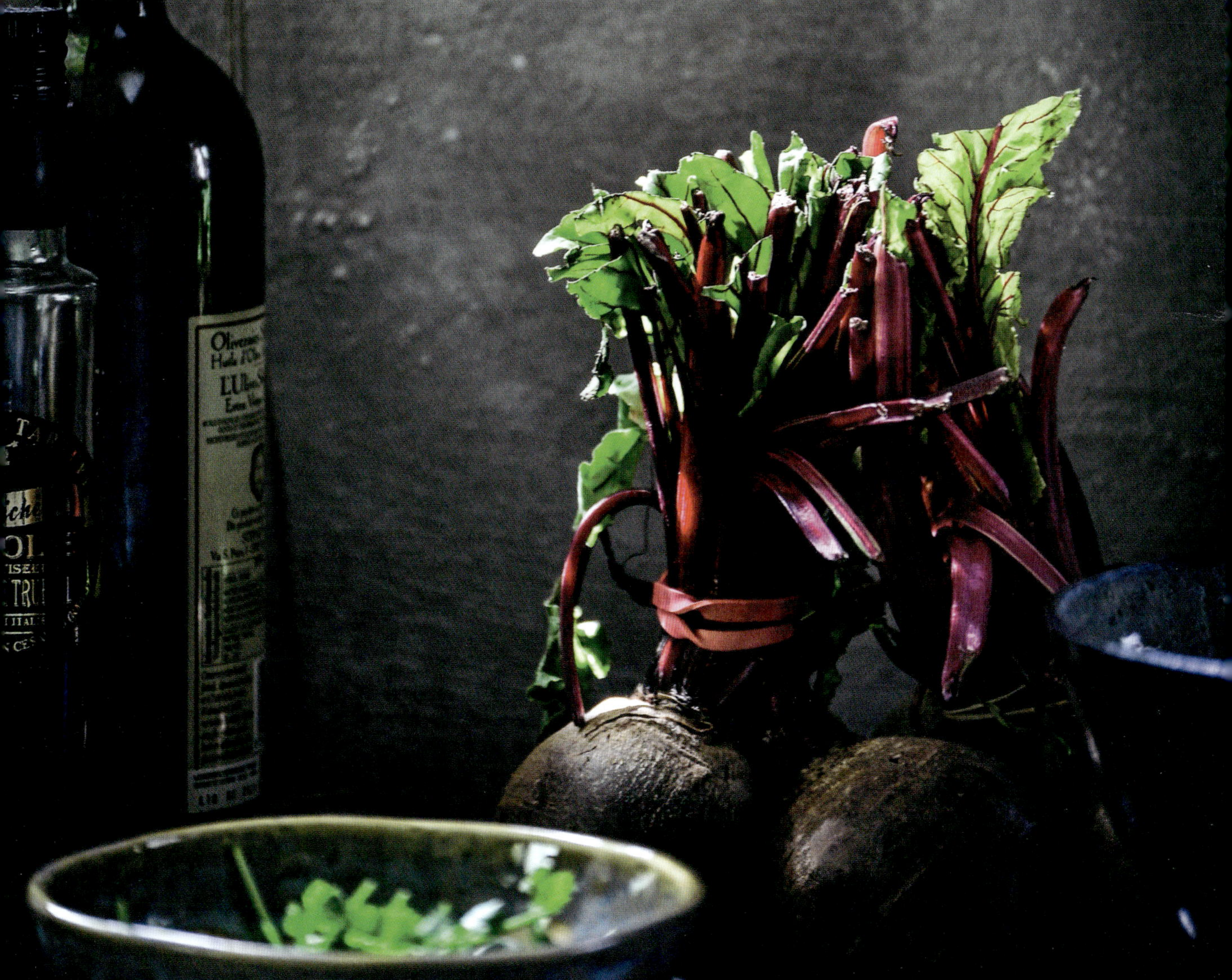

(1) Clin Chem. 2018 Jan;64(1):64-71. doi: 10.1373/clinchem.2017.273532.
Epub 2017 Nov 20. Food Addiction, High-Glycemic-Index Carbohydrates, and Obesity.
Lennerz B1, Lennerz JK2.

https://www.eurekalert.org/pub_releases/2019-06/mcg-lsn060719.php

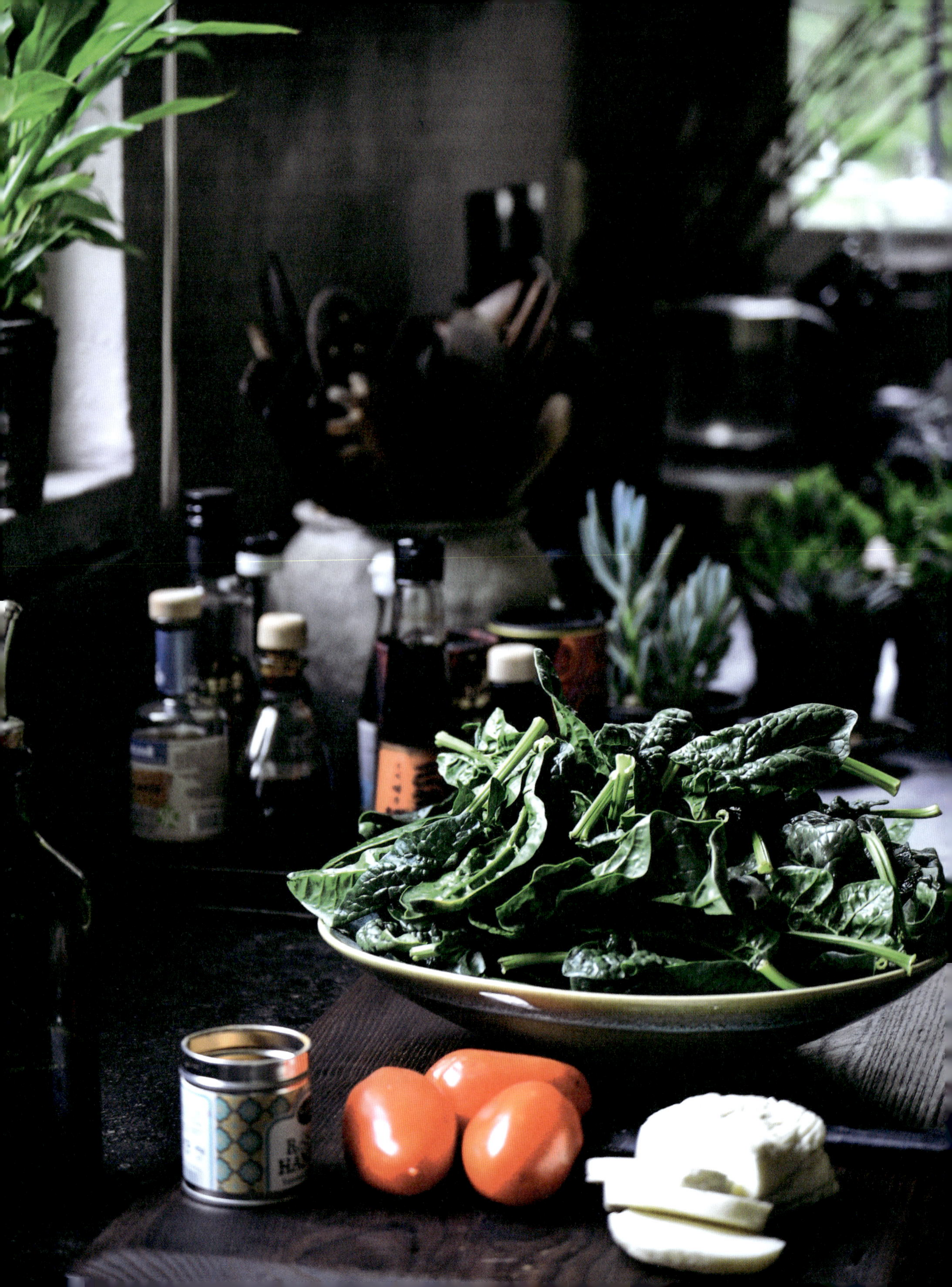

ready in 10 minutes

The chapters in this book are divided according to the time you need to make a dish. The time starts from the moment that all the ingredients are out on your kitchen counter until the dish is ready to be served. It may be that you won't be able to prepare the dish in the given time the first time round, but chances are you'll succeed the second time round, and you may even have some time left over on the third try. Cooking is not a race against the clock, but it helps if you only need to spend ten minutes getting a meal ready after a long day at work or during a short lunchbreak. Afterwards, you can take all the time you need to savor a delicious and healthy meal. This will give you peace and energy and make you happy.

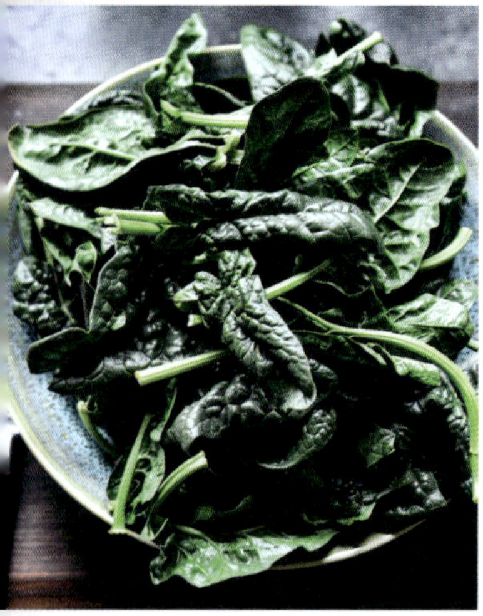

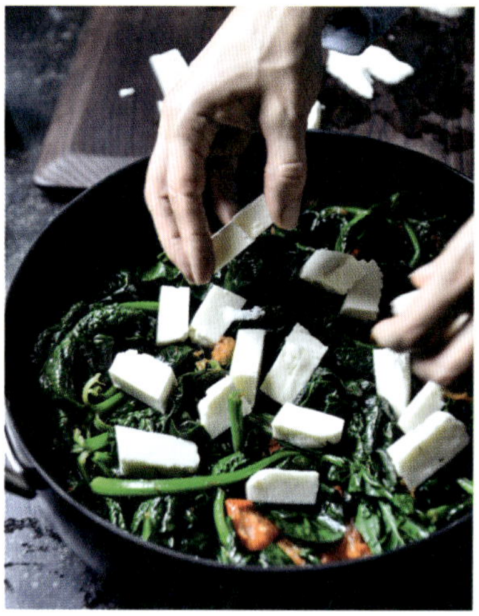

spinach ✓ keto

with tomato and halloumi

- 10½ oz (300 g) organic spinach (see tip)
- 3 plum tomatoes
- 1 package halloumi cheese

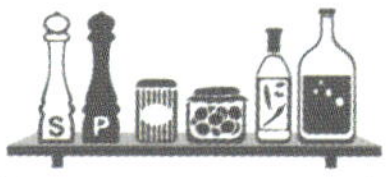

- 2 tablespoons ras el hanout -

Slice the tomatoes and sauté them in a dash of olive oil, then cover with a lid.
After 3 minutes, sprinkle 2 tablespoons of ras el hanout over the tomatoes and season with salt and pepper.
Add the spinach and another splash of olive oil, then cover the pan once more.
Sauté the vegetables for another 3 minutes.
Dice the halloumi into cubes and cook with the vegetables for an additional 2 minutes.
Serve in bowls.

TIP: SPINACH
Organic spinach has thicker leaves and contains less water, making it much tastier.
If you use regular spinach you'll find it gives off too much moisture, which will make this dish watery.

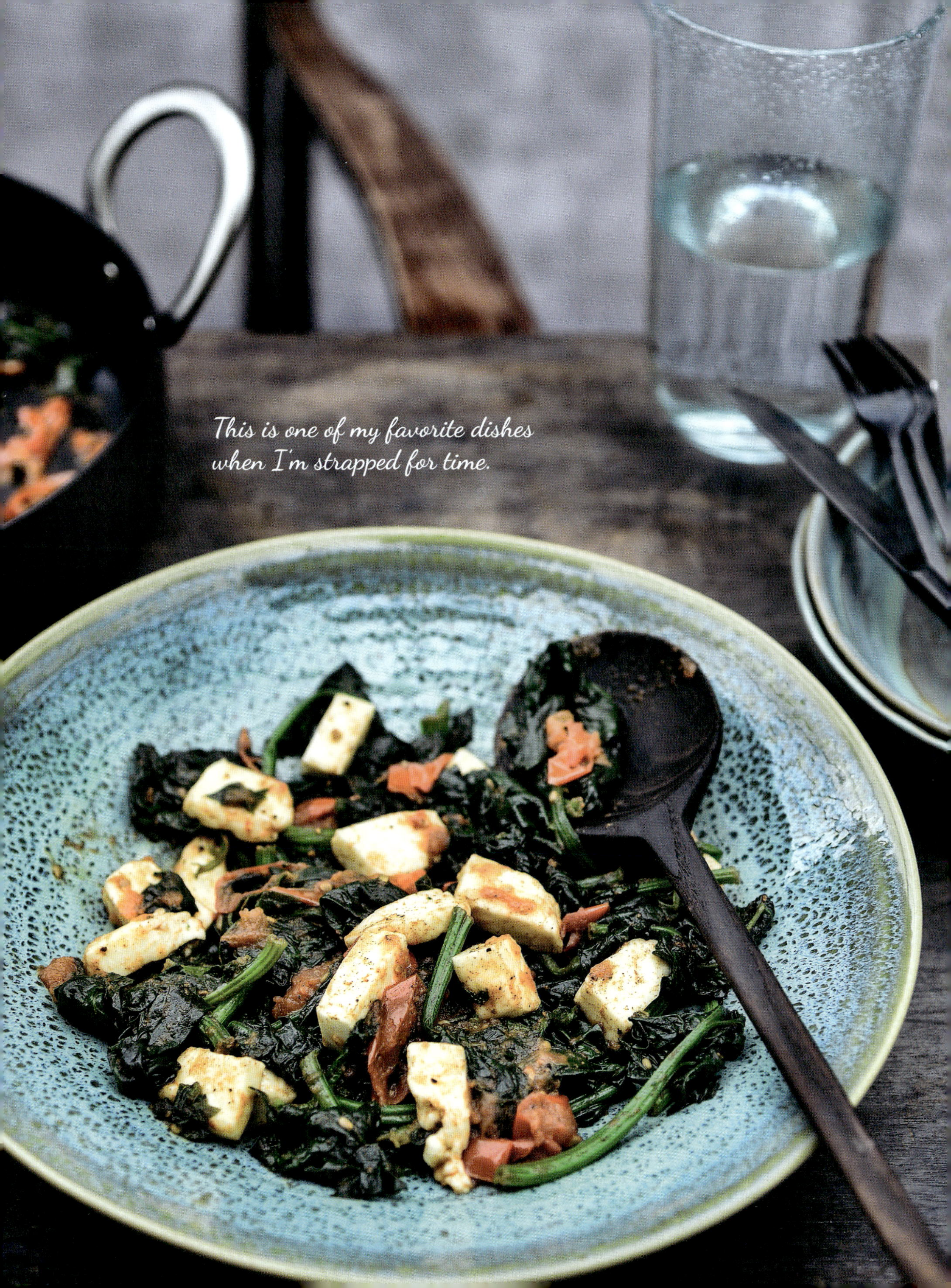

This is one of my favorite dishes when I'm strapped for time.

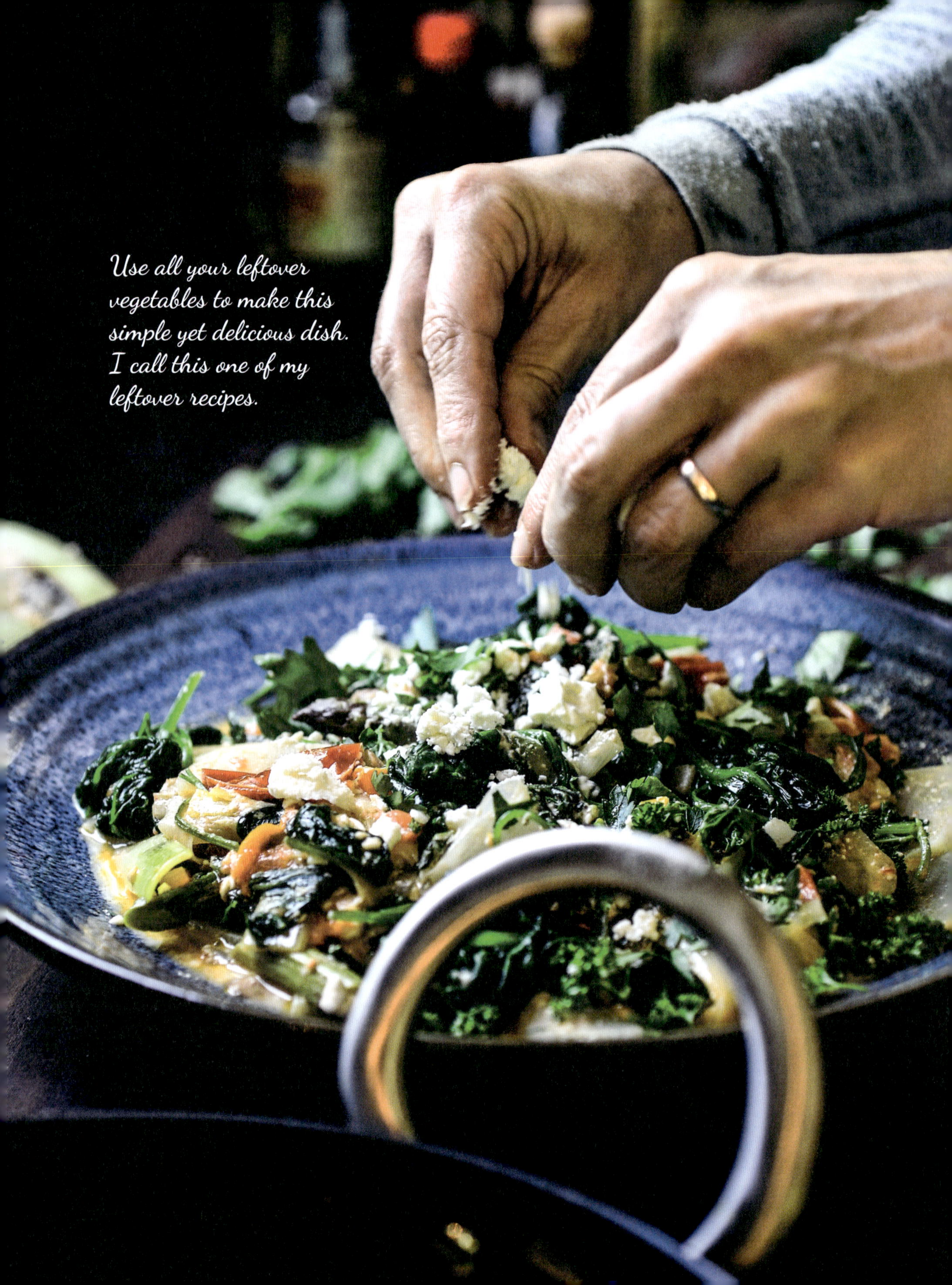

Use all your leftover vegetables to make this simple yet delicious dish. I call this one of my leftover recipes.

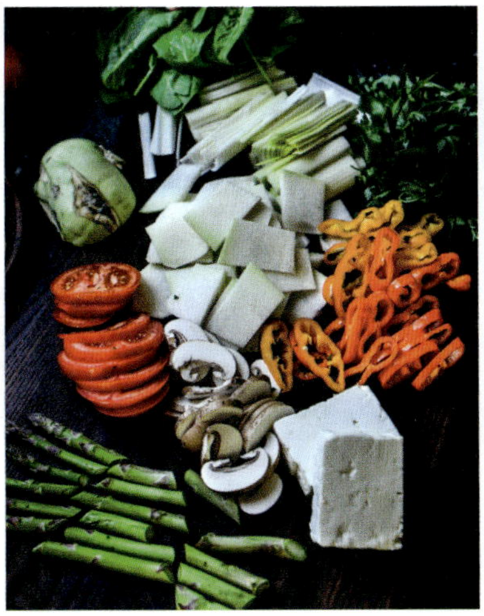
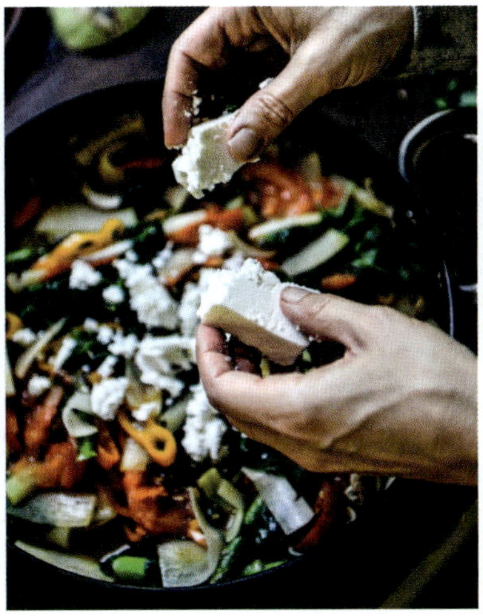
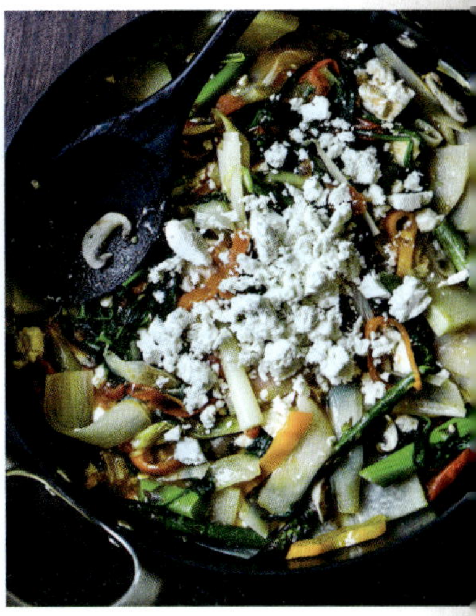

no-waste recipe

vegetables

keto

with feta and nuts

- **1 to 1½ lbs (500 to 700 g) leftover vegetables**
- **leftover fresh herbs such as parsley, chives ...**
- **1 package of feta**
- **a handful of nuts, e.g. pecans**

Dice all the hard vegetables (see tip) into small pieces and cook them, covered, in plenty of olive oil and a small amount of water. Meanwhile, cut the softer vegetables into various different shapes: slices, cubes, strips ... and add them to the hard vegetables. Season with salt and pepper and cover the pan again. Stir occasionally and add a little olive oil if necessary. Let the vegetables sauté for about 7 minutes. Crumble three quarters of the feta over the vegetables and cover once more. After a minute, remove the pan from the heat. Add the nuts and the finely chopped herbs. Serve in an attractive bowl and garnish with the remaining feta.

TIP: VEGETABLES

Hard vegetables are root vegetables such as carrots, cabbages ... Soft vegetables include tomatoes, zucchini, spinach, asparagus ...

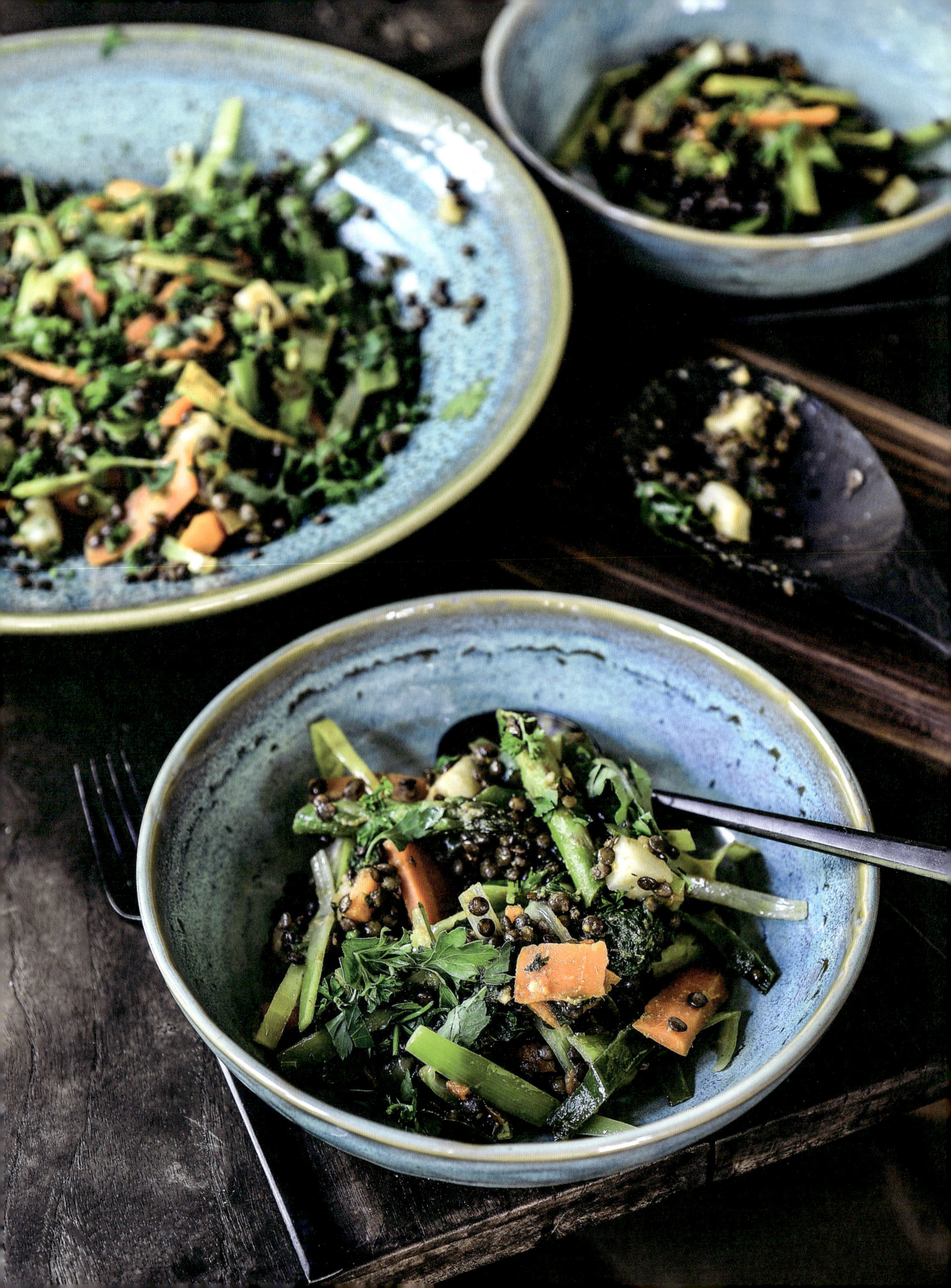

This is one of my ideal no-waste recipes. No two dishes are the same, and you get to clean out your fridge without having to throw anything away.

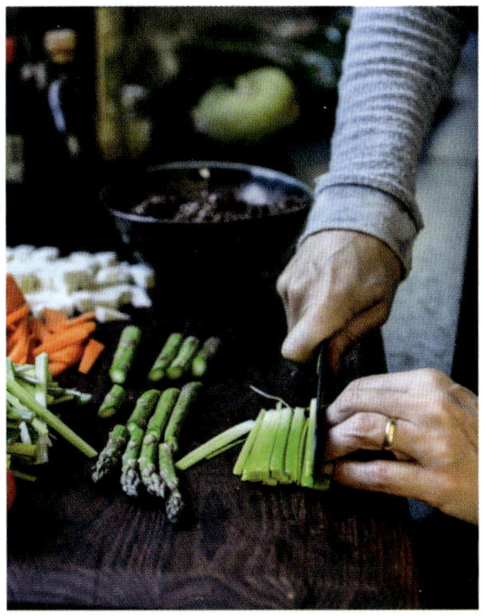

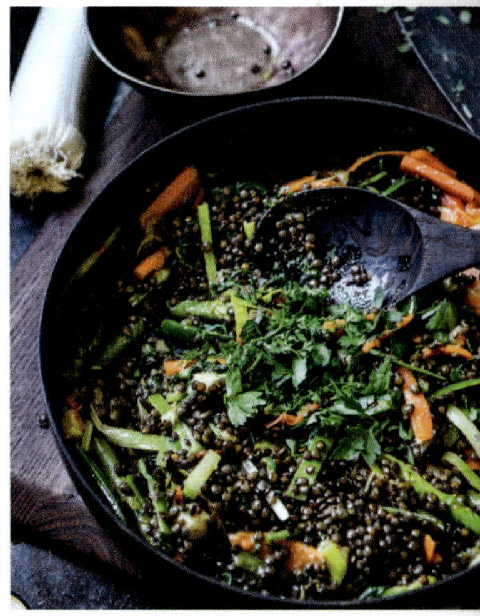

vegan no-waste recipe

curried vegetables

with lentils

- **1 to 1½ lbs (500 to 700 g) leftover vegetables**
- **leftover fresh herbs such as parsley, chives ...**
- **7 oz (200 g) precooked lentils (see tip)**
- **2 to 4 tablespoons red curry paste**

Dice all the hard vegetables (see tip) into small pieces and cook them, covered, in plenty of olive oil and a small amount of water. Meanwhile, slice the softer vegetables into various different shapes. Different shapes make the dish more fun! Add them to the pan, season with salt and pepper, then cover. Sauté the vegetables for about 7 minutes. Stir the red curry paste and the lentils into the vegetables. Stir in some finely chopped fresh herbs just before serving. I like to serve recipes like this in an attractive dish.

TIP: PRECOOKED LENTILS

I always have a can of precooked lentils in my cupboard in case I'm short on time. But you can, of course, cook your own lentils.

TIP: HARD AND SOFT VEGETABLES

Hard vegetables are root vegetables such as carrots, cabbages ... Soft vegetables include tomatoes, zucchini, spinach, asparagus, mushrooms ...

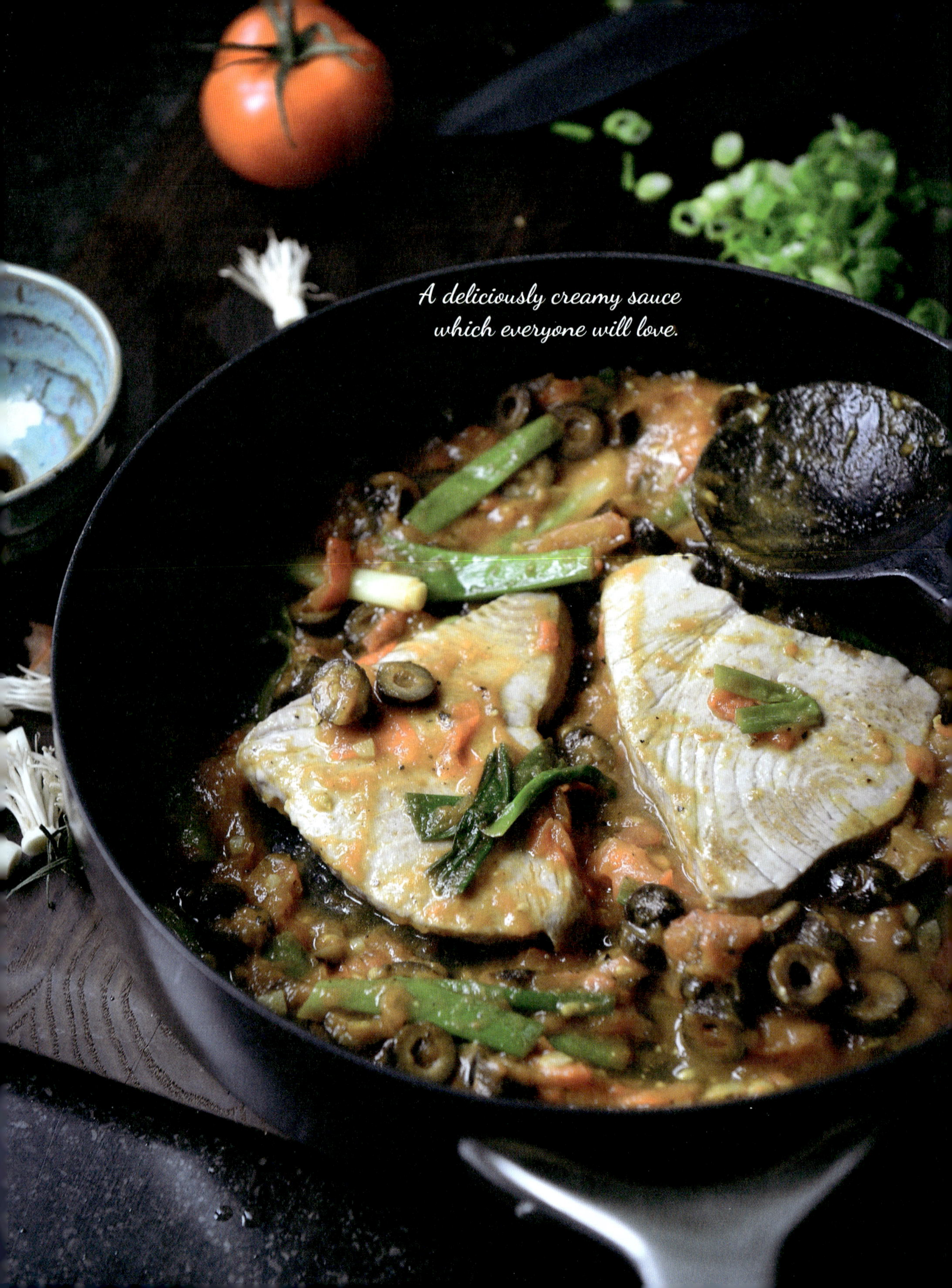
A deliciously creamy sauce
which everyone will love.

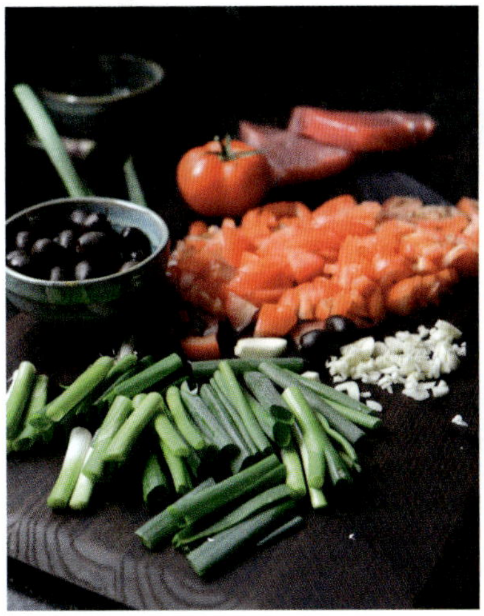

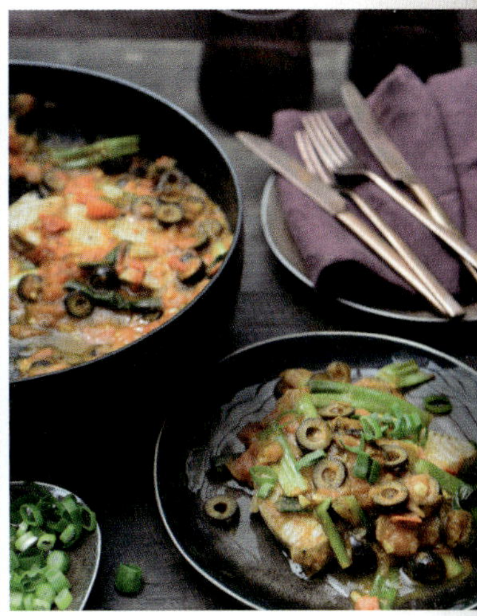

tuna

keto

with herbed tomato sauce

- **2 pieces of tuna (see tip)**
- **a handful of pitted black olives**
- **4 tomatoes**
- **8 spring onions**

- fresh garlic -

- ras el hanout -

Slice seven of the spring onions into 2-inch (5 cm) pieces.

Briefly sauté the spring onions in a pan with some olive oil. Finely chop 2 cloves of garlic and add to the spring onions.

Dice the tomatoes, remove the hard, white core and add them to the pan.

Cover the pan with a lid each time as this speeds up the cooking process.

Slice the olives into rings and add to the pan. Stir the tomatoes until you have a thick sauce.

Add 2 teaspoons of ras el hanout and season with salt and pepper. Stir everything together well.

Place the tuna in the sauce and cook for another 3 minutes or so.

Serve and garnish the tuna with the remaining finely chopped spring onion.

TIP: TUNA

Buy tuna with the MSC label. This label guarantees that the fish comes from a sustainable fishing source. Tuna with the MSC label is usually caught using the pole-and-line fishing method.

You can also use another type of firm-fleshed fish for this recipe.

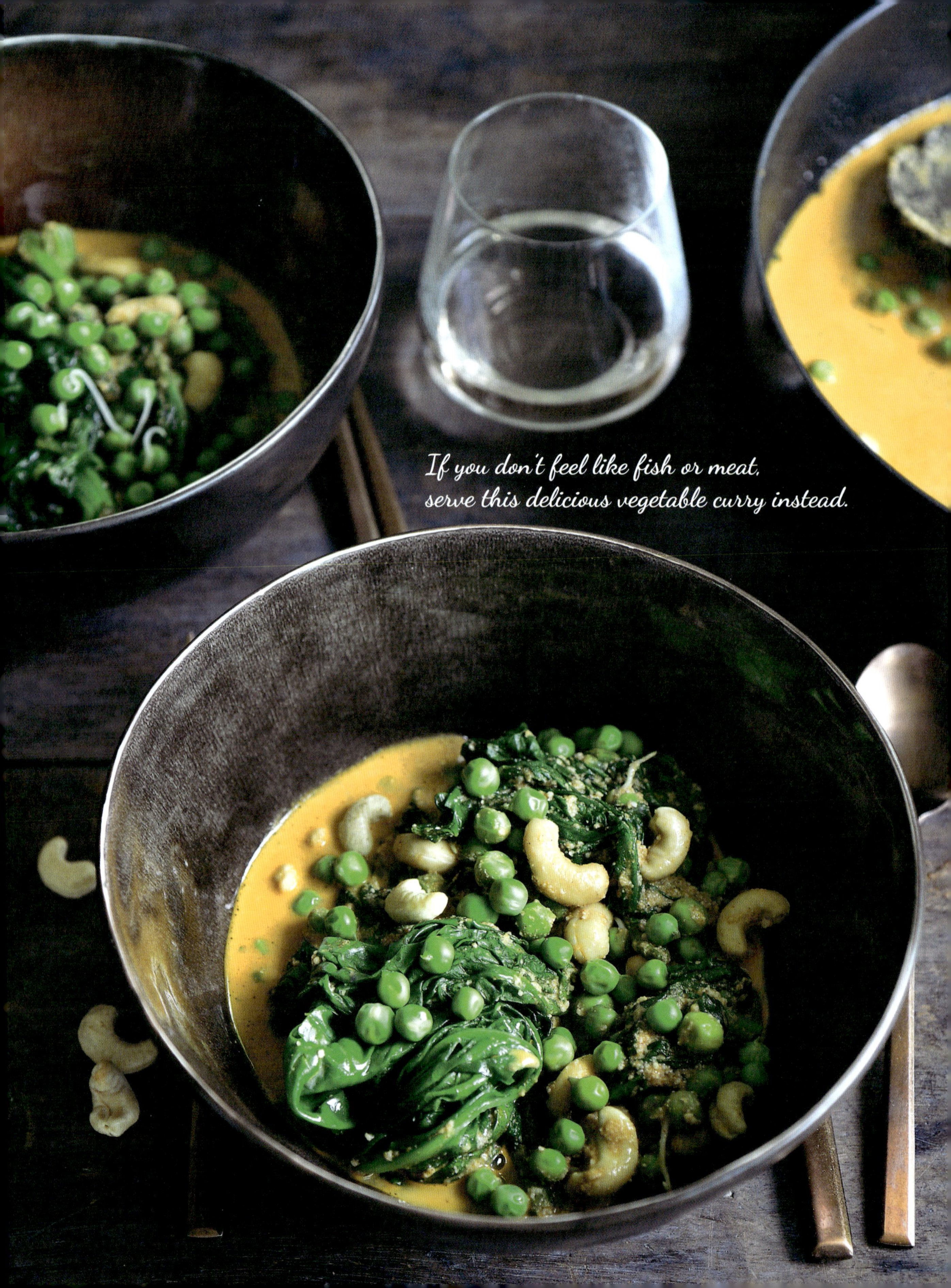
*If you don't feel like fish or meat,
serve this delicious vegetable curry instead.*

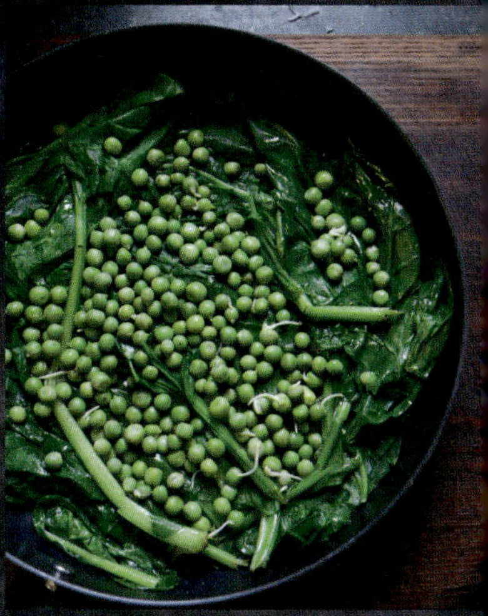

vegan

spinach

and cashews with red curry paste

- 10½ oz (300 g) organic spinach (see tip)
- 5 oz (150 g) cashews
- 3 to 4 tablespoons red curry paste
- 3½ oz (100 g) garden peas (fresh or frozen - see tip)

In a pan, sauté the spinach with some olive oil, salt and pepper until it has wilted. Put half the cashew nuts in a blender and add 10½ fl oz (300 ml) of water. Blend to create a milky mixture (there will always be some lumps, but that's fine). Add 3 to 4 tablespoons of curry paste to taste. Add the curried cashew milk to the spinach and add the peas and the remaining nuts to the pan. Cook for a few minutes and serve.

TIP: SPINACH
Organic or wild spinach is thicker and contains less moisture, and it tastes better too.

TIP: FROZEN VEGETABLES
Frozen vegetables are healthy, but because of the risk of infection from the listeria bacteria, it is crucial to cook all frozen vegetables for at least 2 minutes above 160 °F (70 °C). This kills any remaining bacteria in the vegetables.

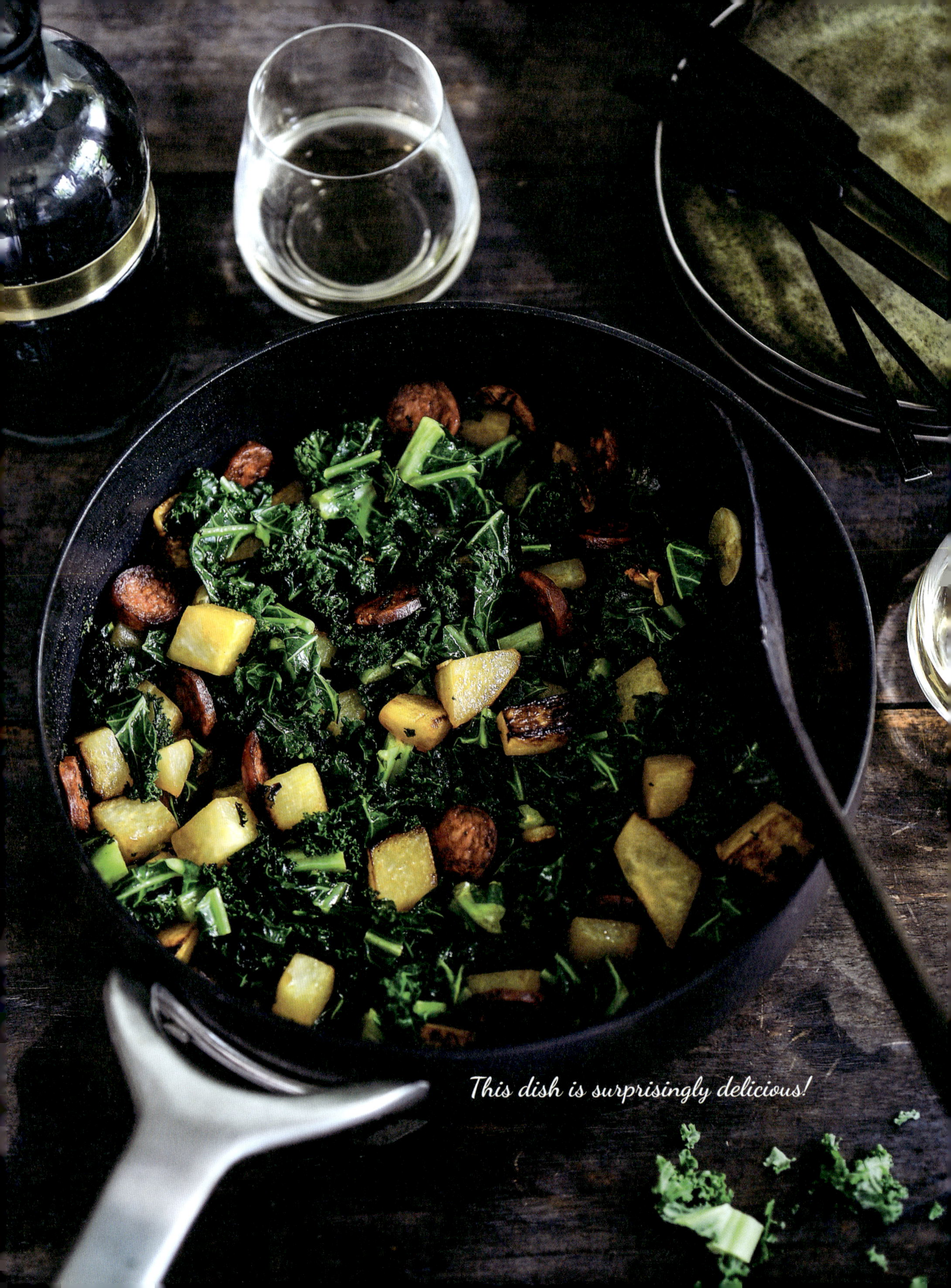
This dish is surprisingly delicious!

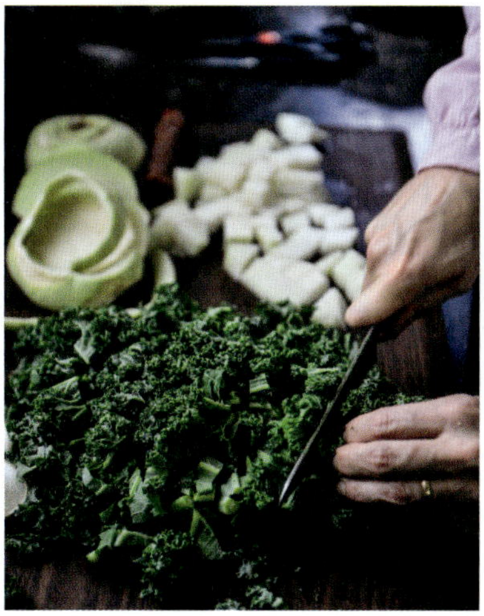
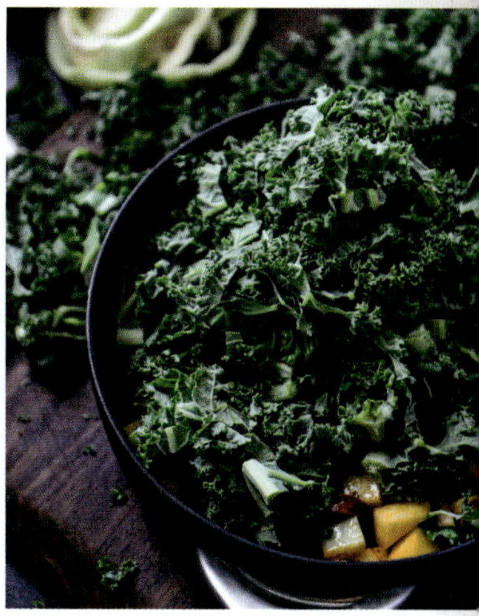

kale

keto

with kohlrabi and chorizo

- **8-inch (20 cm) piece of chorizo (see tip)**
- **1 bunch of kale (about 14 oz/400 g)**
- **1 large kohlrabi**

– fresh garlic –

Peel and dice the kohlrabi and sauté in olive oil.
Slice 2 cloves of garlic and slice the kale into thin strips.
Add the garlic and kale to the kohlrabi and cover the pan. Stir occasionally and add a little olive oil if necessary. Slice the chorizo and add to the pan. Season with salt and pepper.
The dish is ready once the kale has wilted.

TIP: CHORIZO
Chorizo is minced pork sausage seasoned with garlic, paprika (hence its red color) and other seasonings. I don't usually cook with sausage, but I have to admit, this dish is really delicious. You don't need much sausage, because it has plenty of flavor.

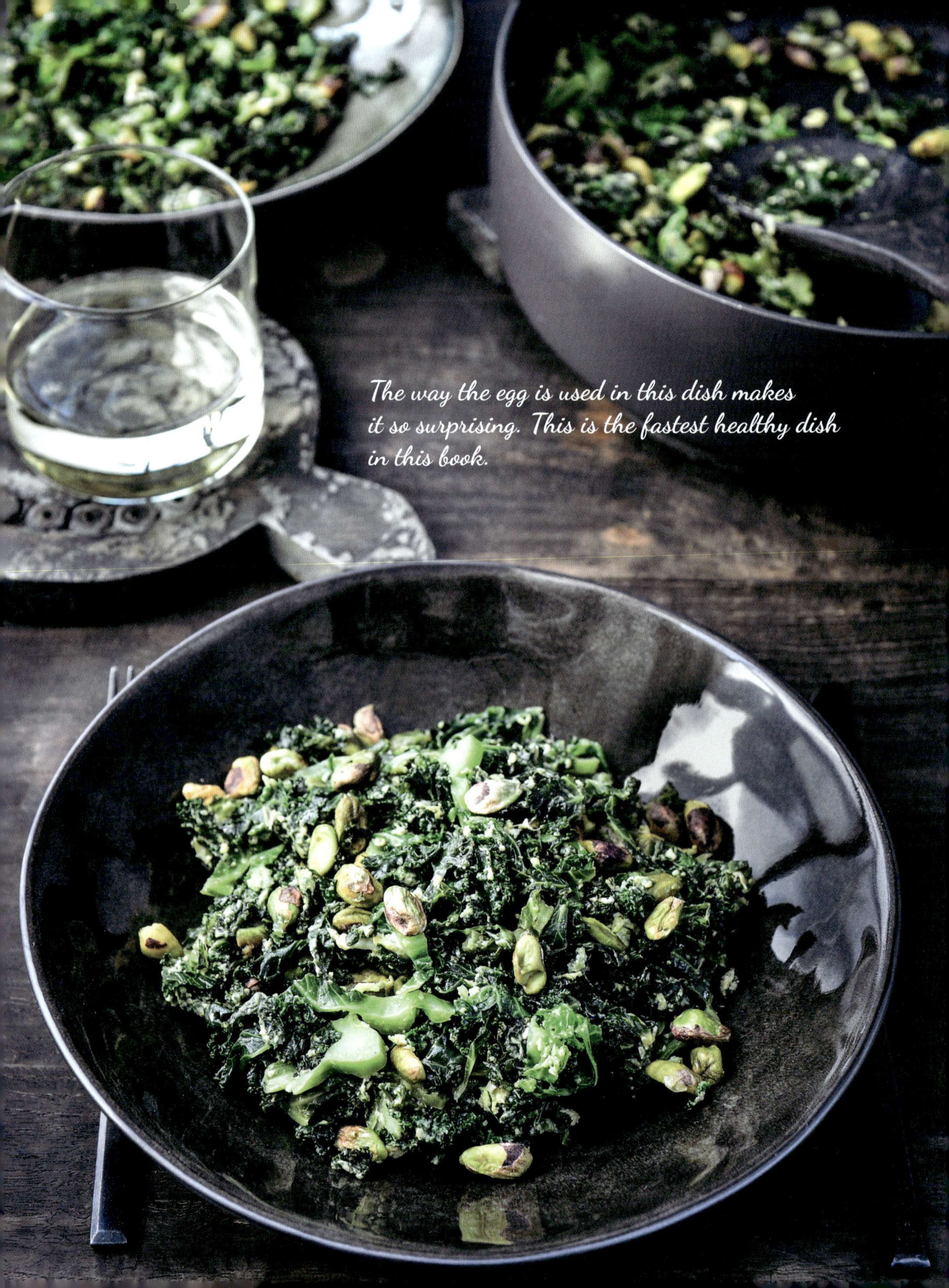

The way the egg is used in this dish makes it so surprising. This is the fastest healthy dish in this book.

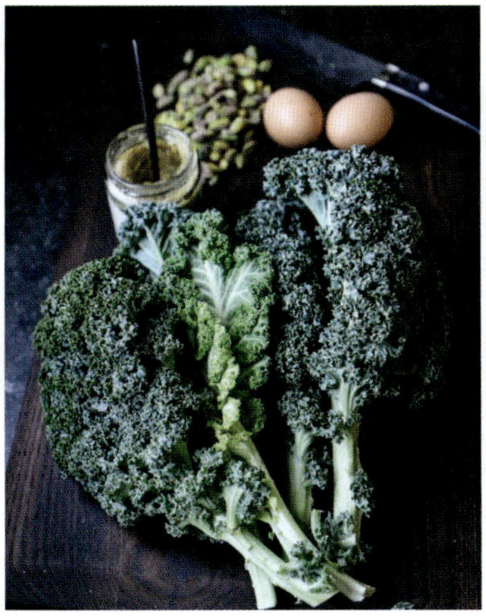

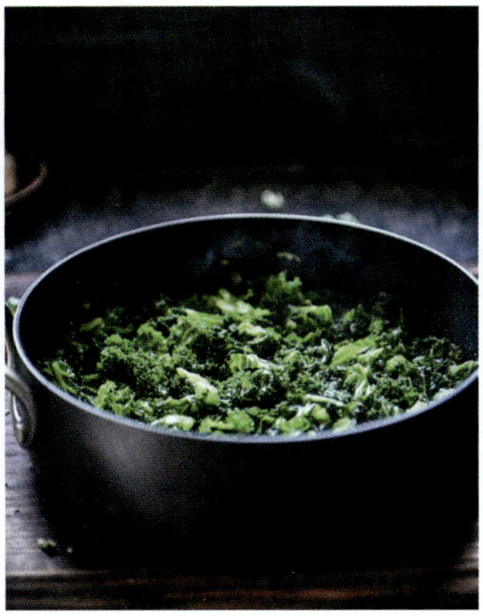

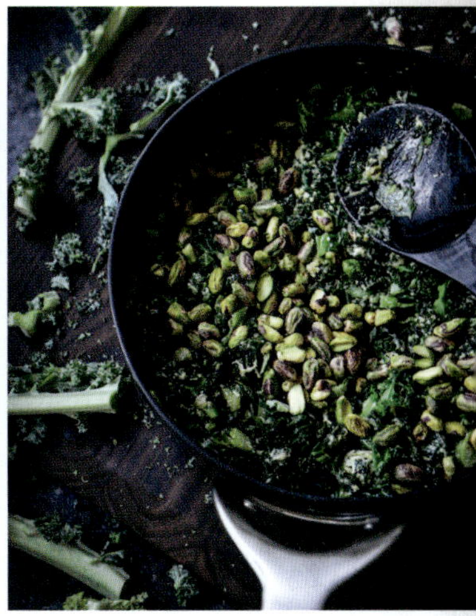

keto

curried kale

with egg and pistachios

- **a little over 1 lb (500 g) kale**
- **2 eggs**
- **2 tablespoons green curry paste (see tip)**
- **a handful of pistachios**

Finely shred the kale and put in a pan with a generous splash of olive oil and half a glass of water. Season with salt and pepper and cover the pan with a lid, so the kale cooks quicker. Cook the kale, stirring regularly. After about six minutes, the kale should be tender and the water evaporated.
If necessary, add a little more olive oil.
Stir the green curry paste into the kale.
Break an egg over the kale and stir it in quickly until the egg has set. Do the same with the second egg.
Stir the pistachios into the kale and serve.

TIP: GREEN CURRY PASTE
Be careful with green curry paste! Taste the curry first to see how spicy it is, then add more to taste.

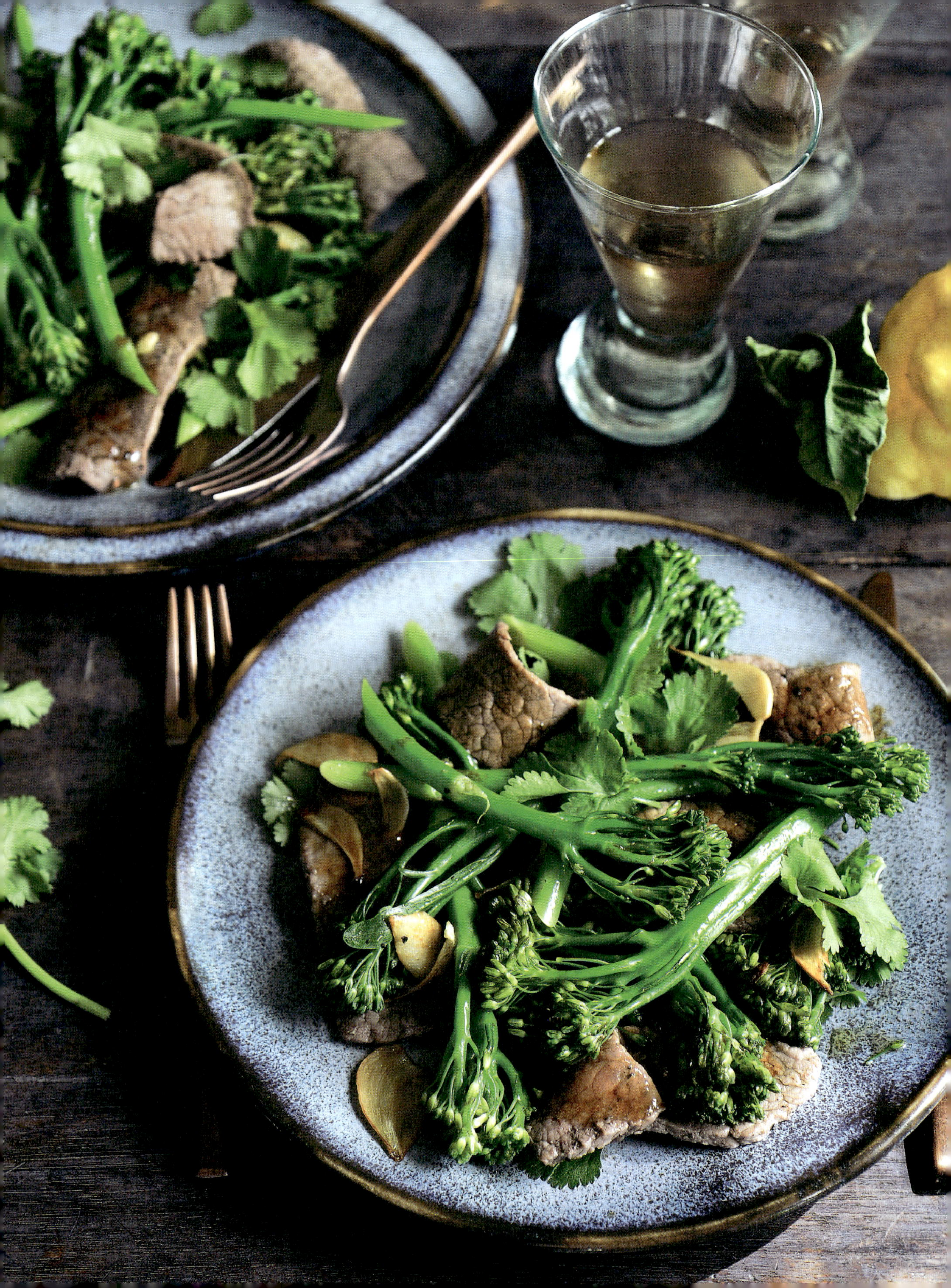

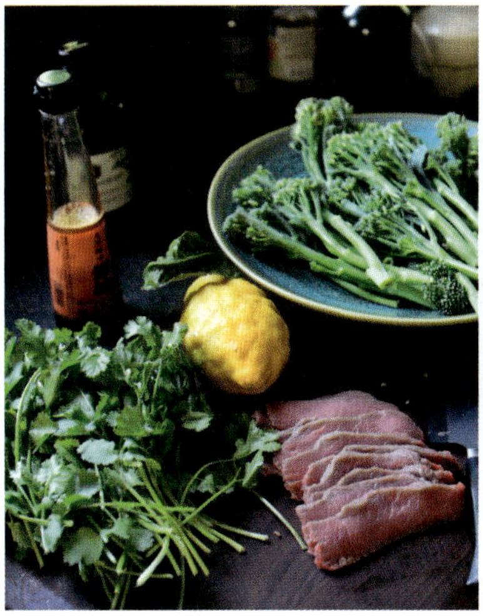

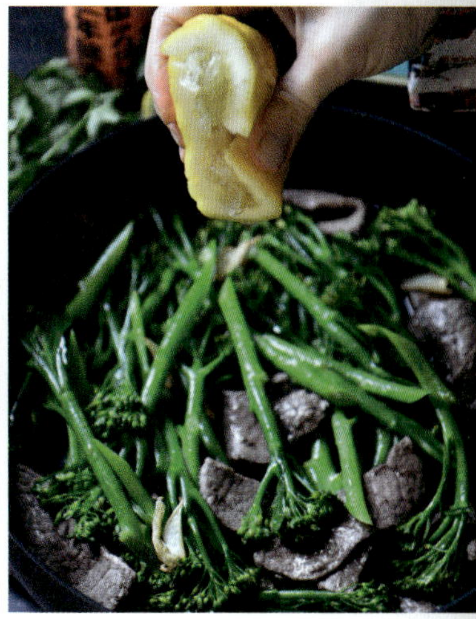

stir-fried beef ✓ keto

and broccoli

- **about 1 lb (400 to 500 g) broccoli or broccolini**
- **9 oz (250 g) steak (see tip)**
- **1 lemon**
- **1 bunch of cilantro**

– soy sauce –
– fresh garlic –

In a pan, combine the broccoli or broccolini with plenty of olive oil and a splash of water (see tip). Cover the pan. Slice 2 cloves of garlic and add to the broccoli. Stir occasionally. Slice the steak into strips and add to the pan. Stir-fry for about 2 to 3 minutes. Squeeze the juice of ½ lemon over the ingredients in the pan, add a generous splash of soy sauce and season with black pepper. Remove the pan from the heat. Roughly chop the fresh cilantro and mix it in with the beef and broccoli. Serve.

TIP: MEAT PORTIONS
I usually use one serving of meat for the two of us, especially in dishes that have plenty of vegetables. That way I still get to enjoy meat but without overindulging.
Feel free to change the serving size to suit your needs.

TIP: BROCCOLI
Broccoli should be cooked al dente. If you prefer your broccoli a little softer, steam it a little longer.

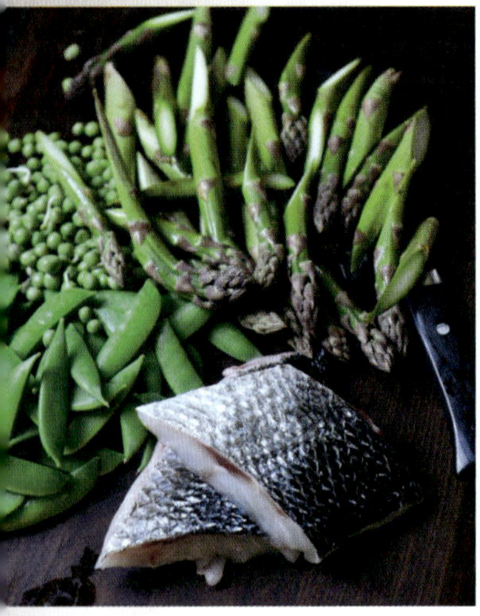

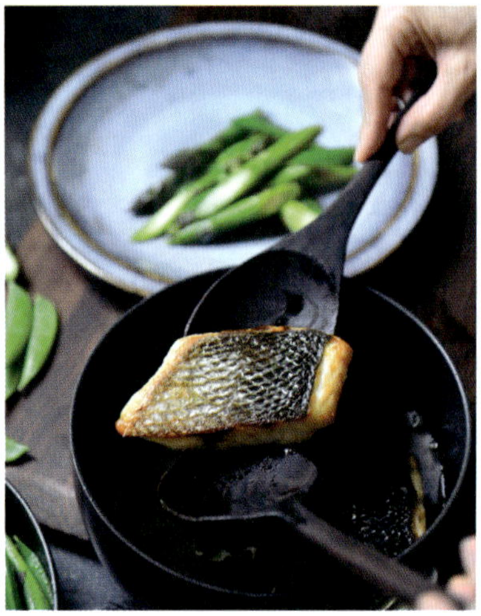

This dish always makes me happy for some reason. Is it the colors, the gorgeous sea bass, or the simplicity of the dish?

pan-seared sea bass
with green vegetables

- **2 sea bass fillets, with skin**
- **3½ oz (100 g) sugar snap peas**
- **1 bunch of green asparagus**
- **3½ oz (100 g) peas (fresh or frozen - see tip)**

– soy sauce –

Chop the green asparagus into pieces and throw away the tough ends. In a pan, combine the asparagus with plenty of olive oil and a splash of water. Add the sugar snap peas and green peas. Cover the pan. Stir occasionally and add a little olive oil if necessary. I like to cook my vegetables al dente, so 4 to 5 minutes is more than enough. Towards the end of the cooking time, add a generous splash of soy sauce and season with black pepper. In another pan, fry the sea bass for 2 minutes with the skin side down, and then for another 2 minutes on the other side. Arrange the vegetables on a plate and place the sea bass next to it.

TIP: FROZEN VEGETABLES
Frozen vegetables are healthy, but because of potential infection from the listeria bacteria, it is crucial to cook all frozen vegetables for at least 2 minutes above 160 °F (70 °C). This prevents any potential infection.

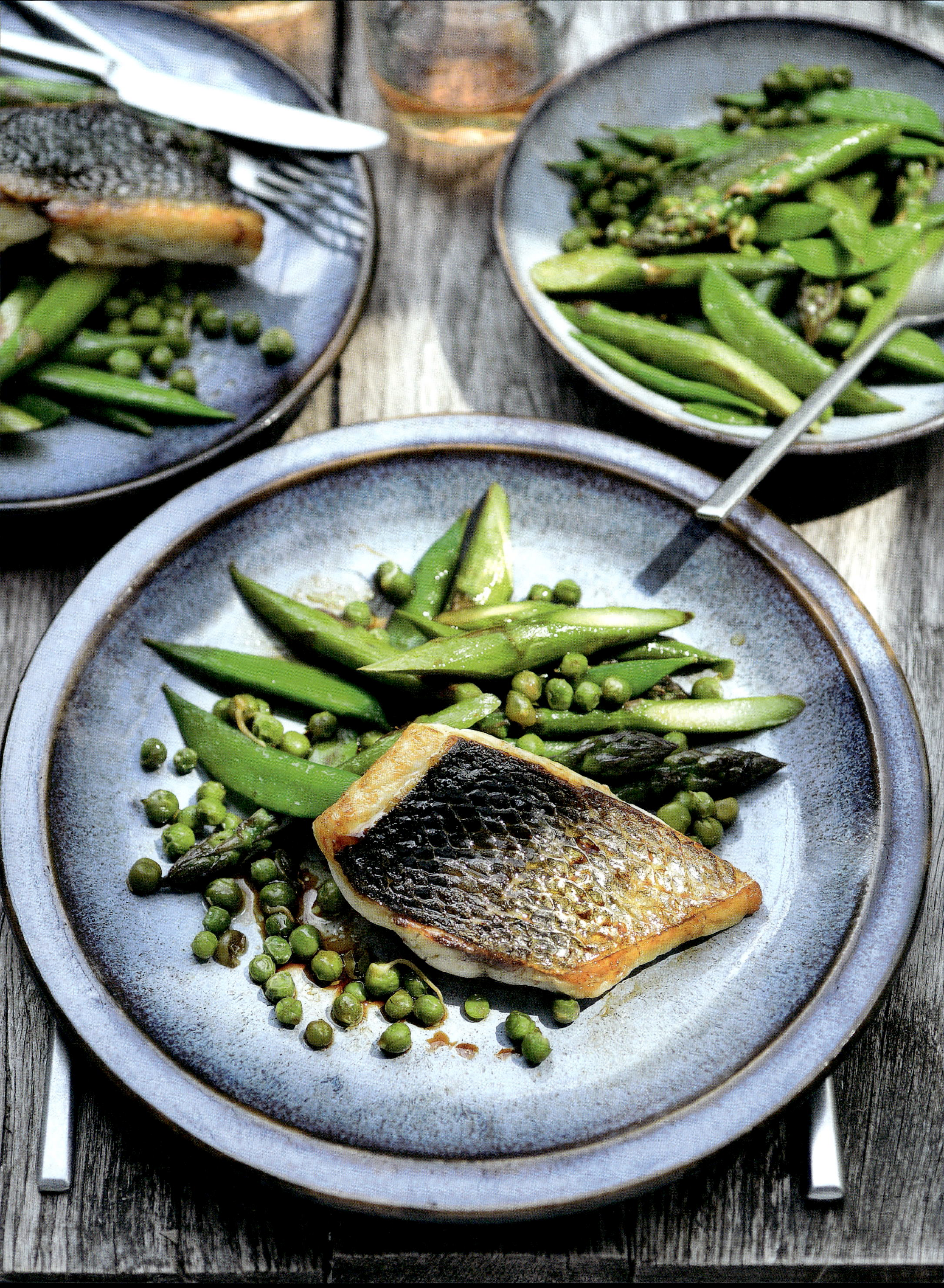

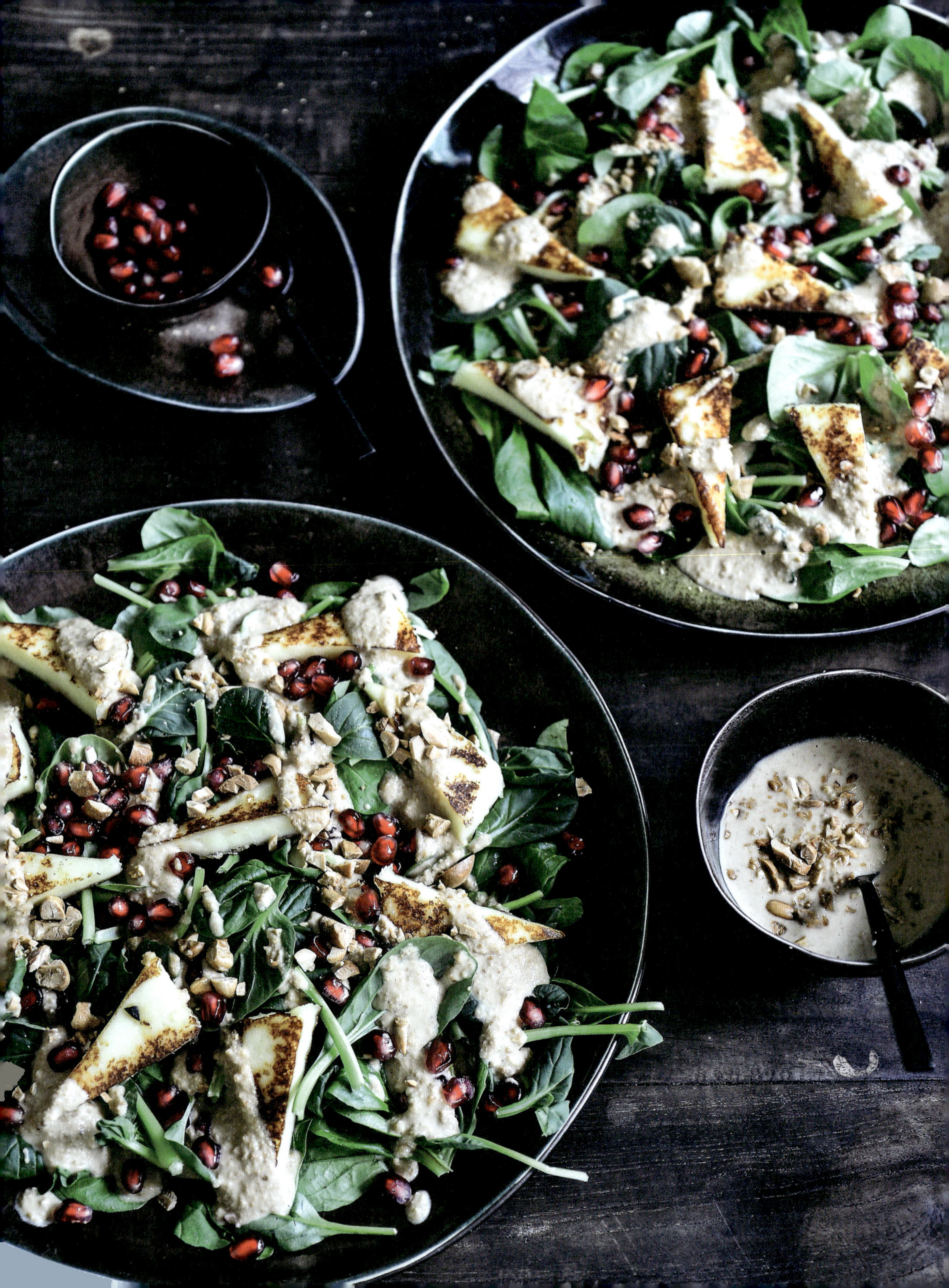

ready in
15 minutes

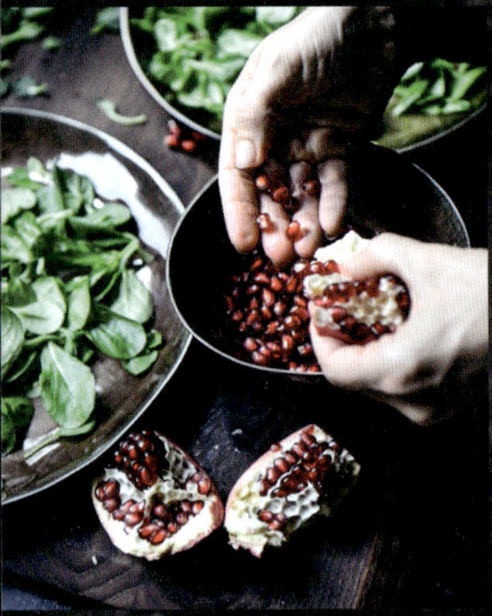

A delicious combination of cheese and nuts with a sweet hint of pomegranate.

salad

with paneer and peanut sauce

- **7 oz (200 g) paneer (see tip on page 57)**
- **3½ oz (100 g) lamb's lettuce**
- **a handful of peanuts**
- **½ pomegranate**

- fresh garlic -

First, make the peanut sauce. Sauté 4 finely chopped cloves of garlic until browned. Put them in a food processor together with a handful of peanuts, a splash of olive oil and a small amount of water. Blend until you have a thick sauce. Add a little water if the sauce is too thick. Cut the paneer into slices and then into triangles. Take the pan which you used to sauté the garlic and fry the paneer for 2 minutes on each side until nice and golden brown. Remove the seeds from the pomegranate (see tip).
Place some lamb's lettuce on the plates and arrange the paneer on the lettuce. Sprinkle some pomegranate seeds over the top and finish with the peanut sauce.

TIP: REMOVING POMEGRANATE SEEDS
Slice away the top of the pomegranate and make four vertical cuts into the skin, as if you're slicing the fruit into quarters. Make sure to slice only into the skin, not the pulp. Break the pomegranate open and remove the seeds.

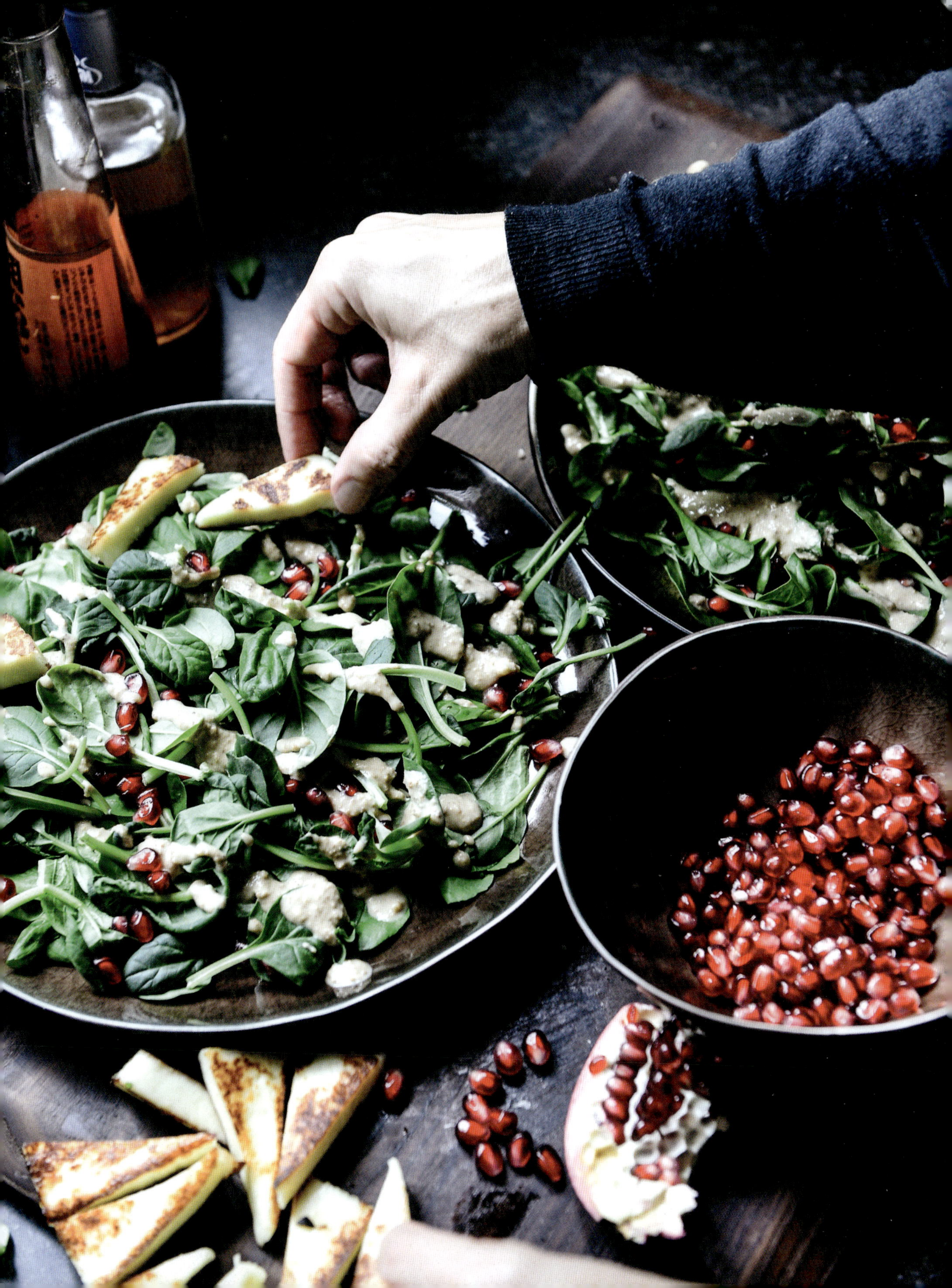

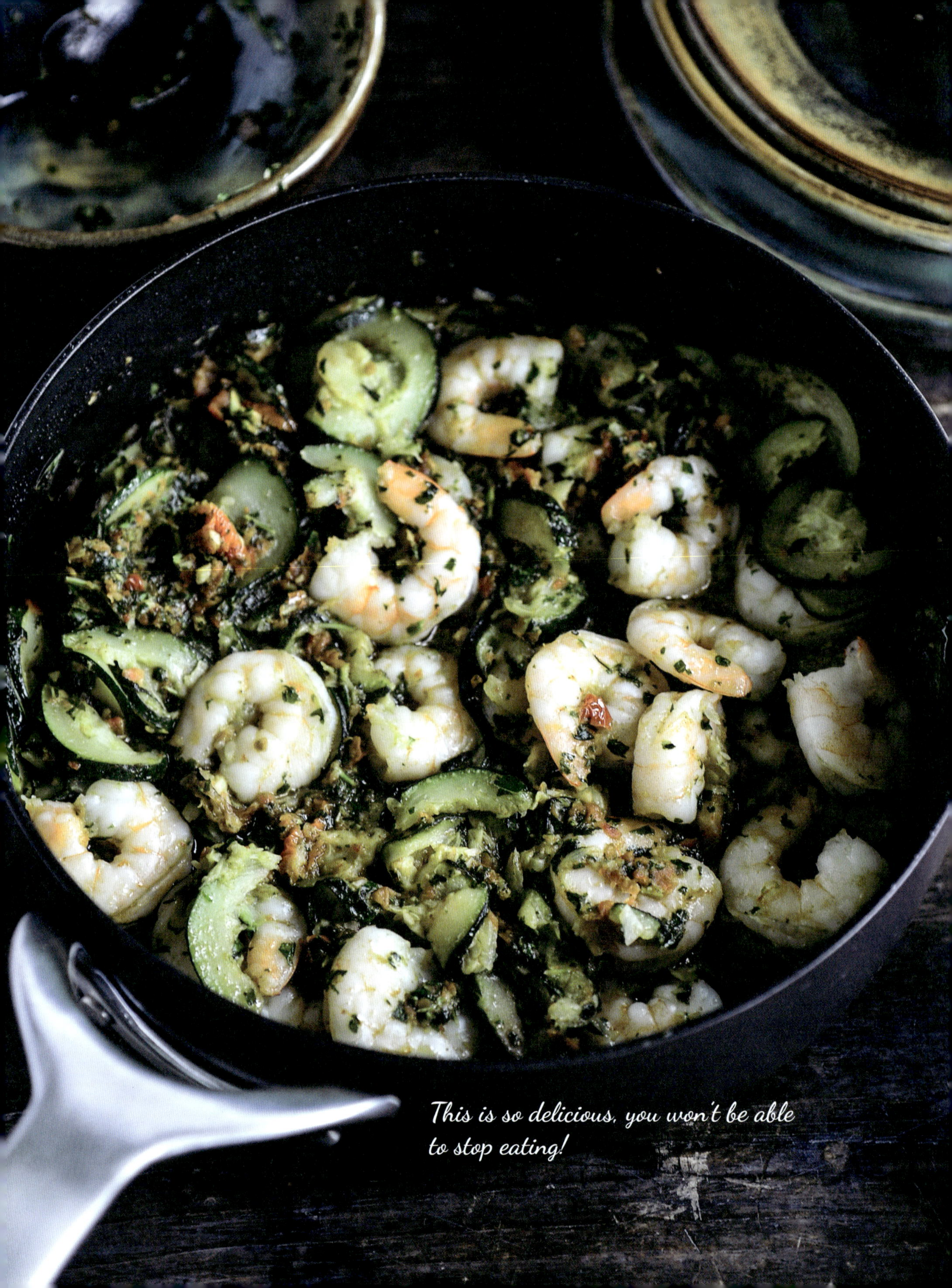
This is so delicious, you won't be able to stop eating!

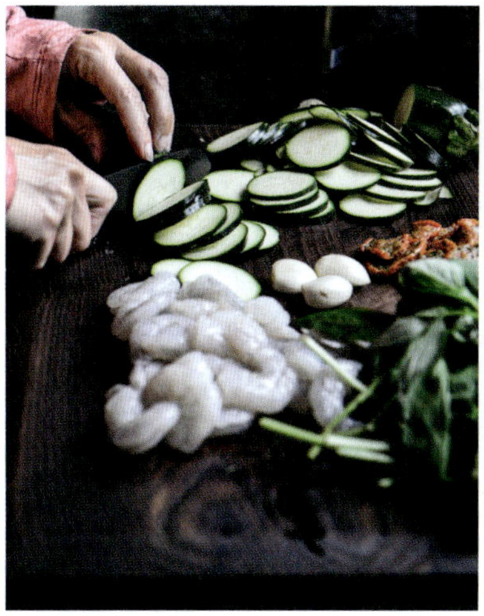

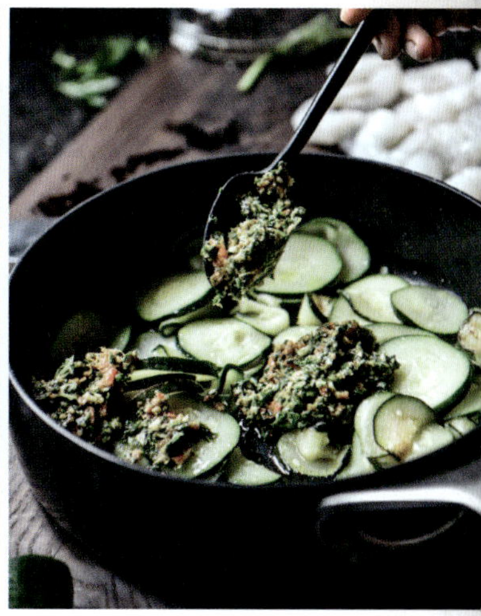

large shrimp

keto

with zucchini in herb sauce

- **14 oz (400 g) large shrimp, peeled**
- **3½ oz (100 g) sundried tomatoes (about 10 pieces - see tip)**
- **3 bunches of basil (2 oz/60 g)**
- **2 zucchini**

- fresh garlic -

Slice the zucchini and sauté in olive oil.
Combine 2 cloves of garlic, the tomatoes and basil in a blender and blend together with a generous splash of olive oil to make a thick mixture.
After about 7 minutes, when the zucchini is cooked, add the herb and tomato mixture and stir it in gently. Season with salt and pepper and add the raw shrimp. Let them cook with the vegetables for another 3 minutes.
Serve in deep dishes.

TIP: SUNDRIED TOMATOES
Use sundried tomatoes that have been soaked in oil, as these are soft. Other sundried tomatoes may be quite tough.

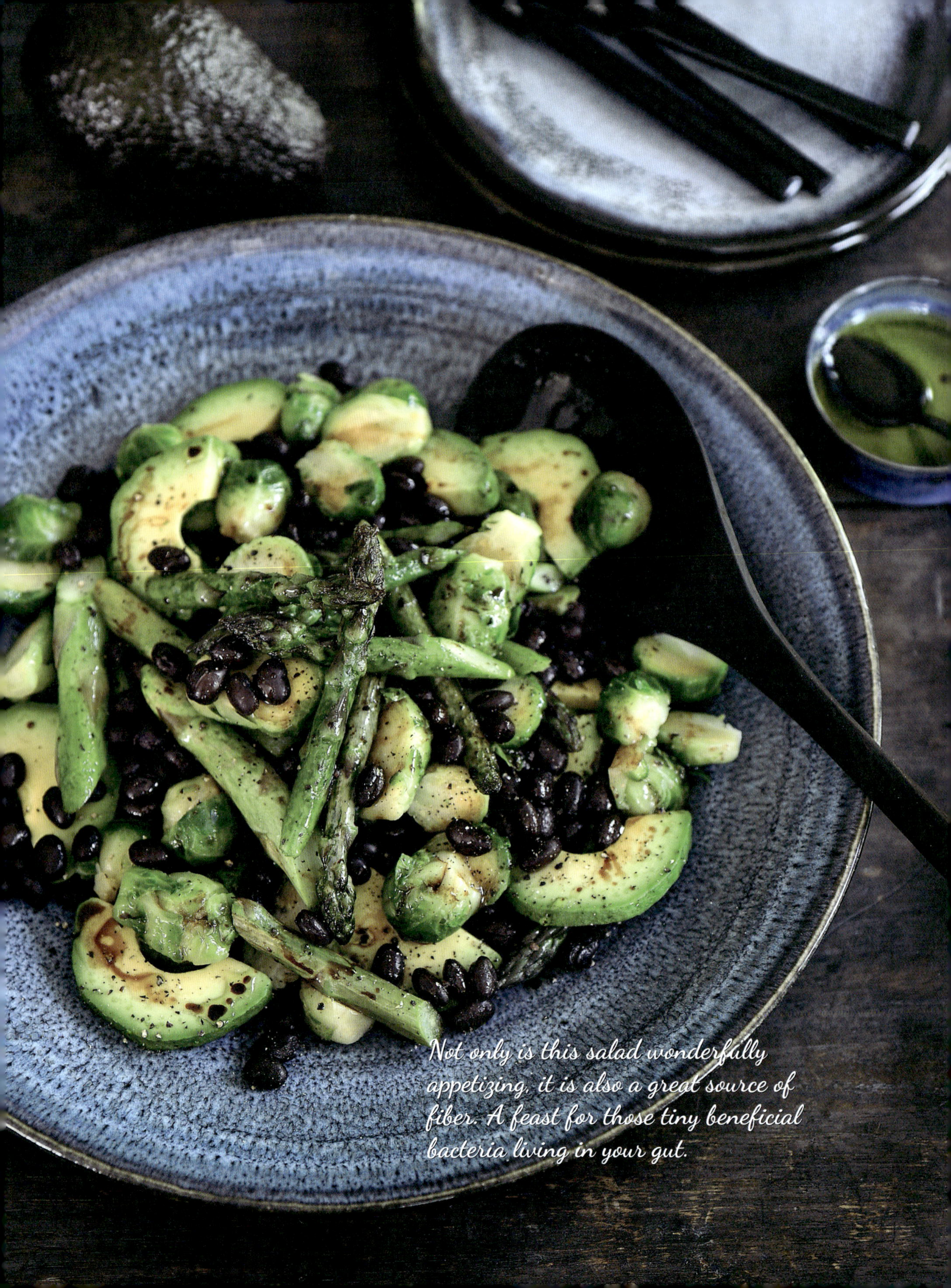

Not only is this salad wonderfully appetizing, it is also a great source of fiber. A feast for those tiny beneficial bacteria living in your gut.

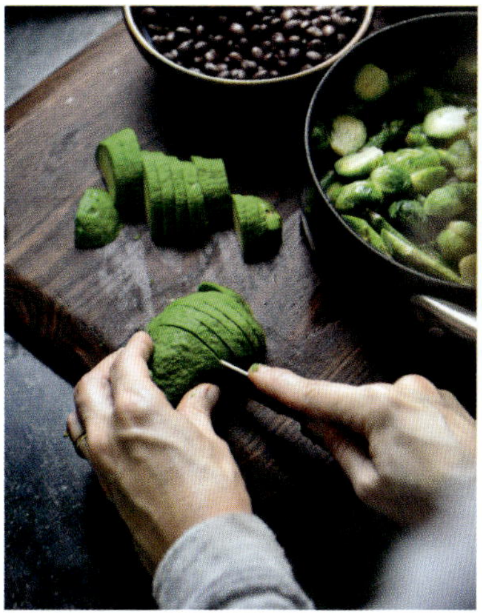

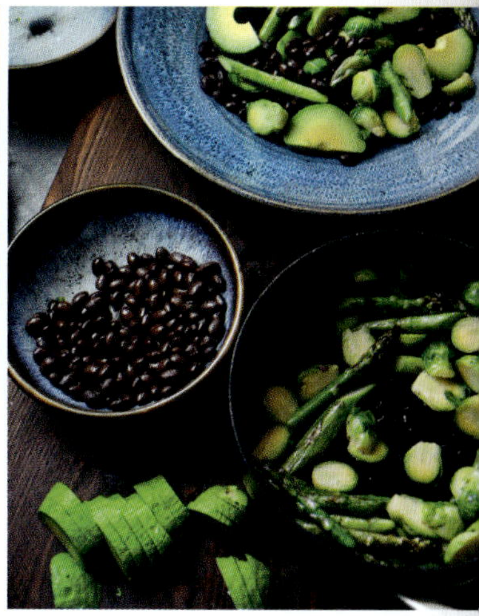

vegan & extra fiber

black bean salad

- **9 oz (250 g) cooked black beans (drained)**
- **1 avocado**
- **10½ oz (300 g) Brussels sprouts**
- **1 bunch of green asparagus**

– balsamic vinegar –

Cut the Brussels sprouts in half and cook them for 2 to 3 minutes in water seasoned with salt, pepper and a splash of olive oil.
Halve the avocado, remove the seed and skin and cut the flesh into strips.
Cut the asparagus into pieces and throw away the tough ends. Drain the Brussels sprouts and stir-fry them together with the asparagus in plenty of olive oil for 3 to 4 minutes. Season with salt and pepper. Combine the vegetables with the avocado and the drained black beans and spoon into an attractive dish. Make a vinaigrette with 4 tablespoons of olive oil and 2 tablespoons of balsamic vinegar. Pour some of the vinaigrette over the vegetables and serve the rest separately.

TIP: FIBER
All the ingredients in this recipe are excellent sources of fiber. Black beans are also one of the best sources of resistant starch. Brussels sprouts, asparagus and avocados contain both soluble and insoluble fiber (read more about fiber on page 210). This makes those little beneficial bacteria that live in your gut happy.

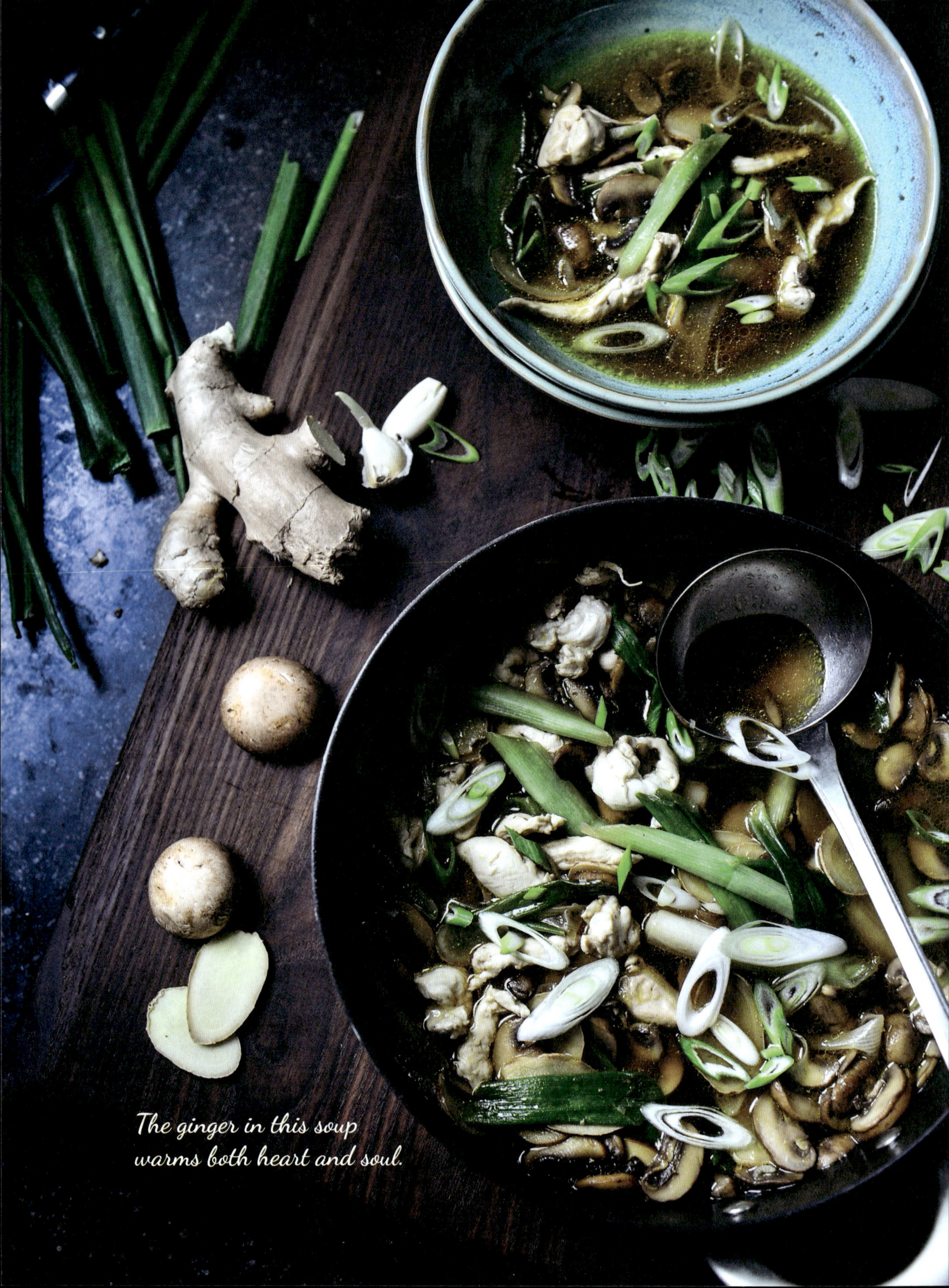
The ginger in this soup
warms both heart and soul.

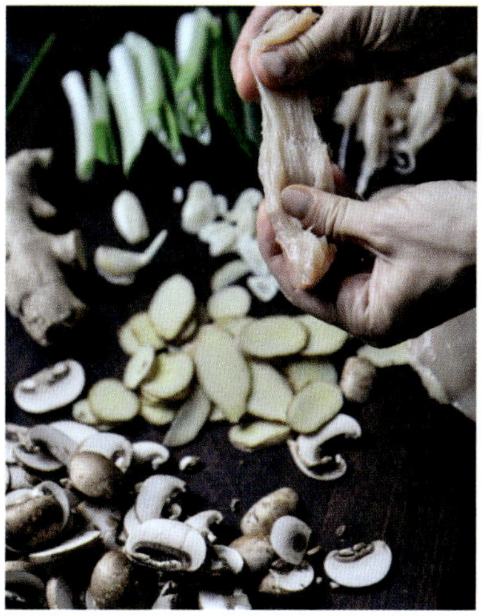

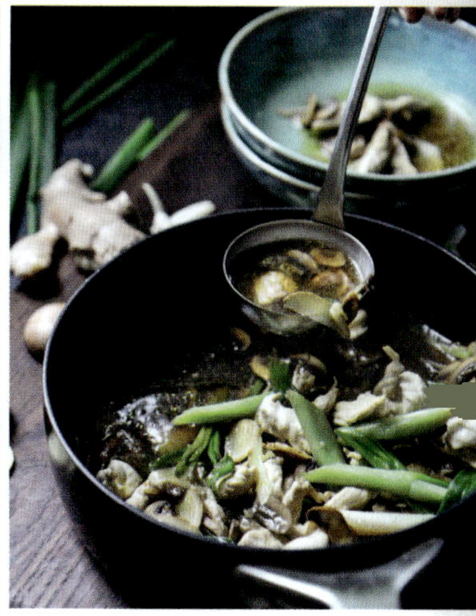

chicken soup

keto

with vegetables

- **10½ oz (300 g) pre-cooked chicken breasts**
- **14 oz (400 g) brown mushrooms**
- **8 spring onions**
- **2-inch (5 cm) ginger root**

- soy sauce -
- fresh garlic -

Slice the mushrooms and sauté them in plenty of olive oil. Slice seven of the spring onions into 3-inch (8 cm) pieces and add them to the mushrooms. Slice 2 cloves of garlic and the ginger and add those as well. Stir regularly. Pull or cut the pre-cooked chicken into pieces (see tip) and add to the mushroom mixture. Spoon in 3 tablespoons of soy sauce and add water until everything is just covered. Season with black pepper. Let the soup simmer for 2 minutes. Pour the soup into two bowls. Finely chop the remaining spring onion and sprinkle over the soup.

TIP: CHICKEN

I like to pull my chicken into different-sized pieces. But if that's too much work for you, just cut the chicken into bite-sized pieces with a knife.

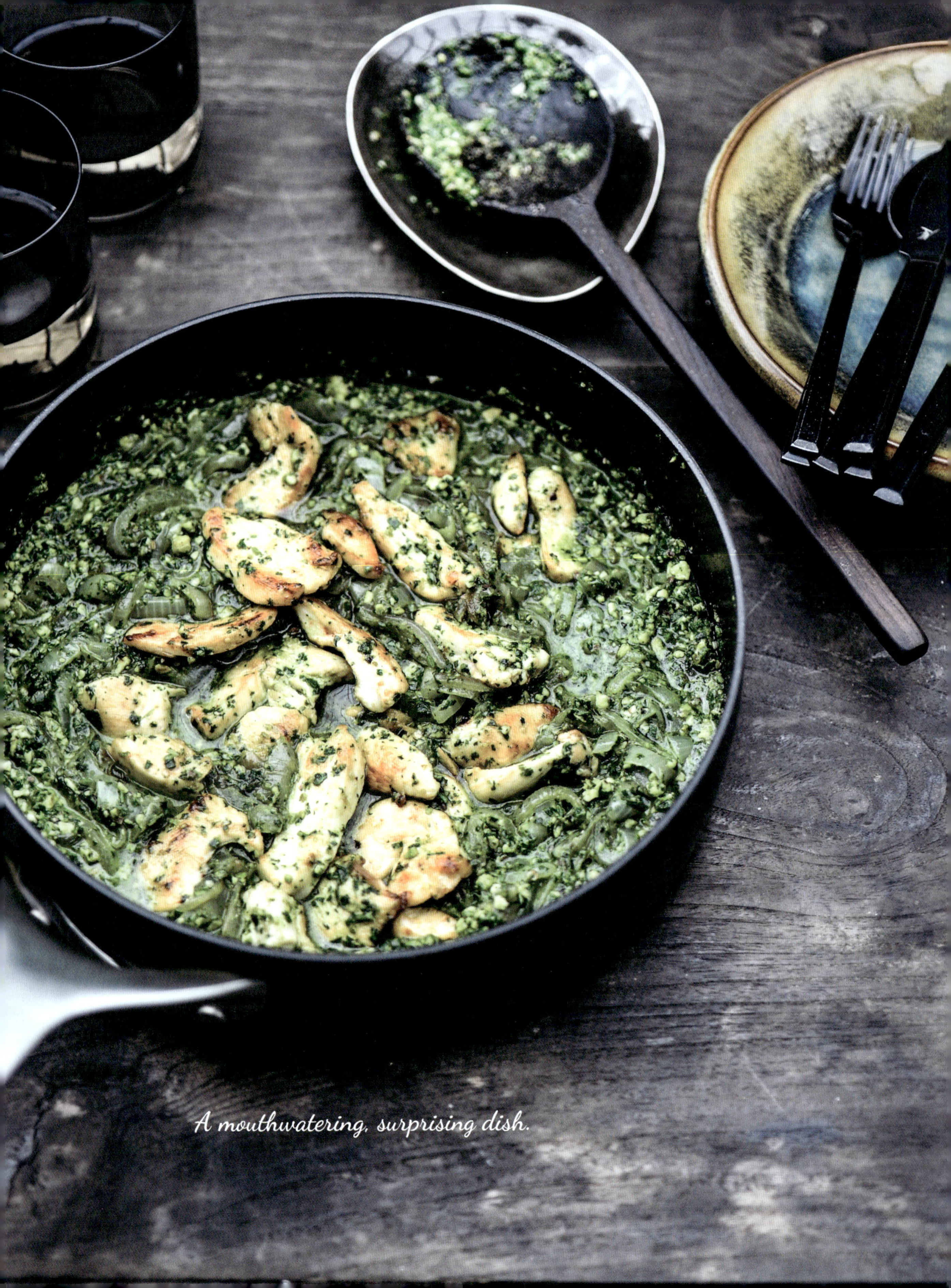
A mouthwatering, surprising dish.

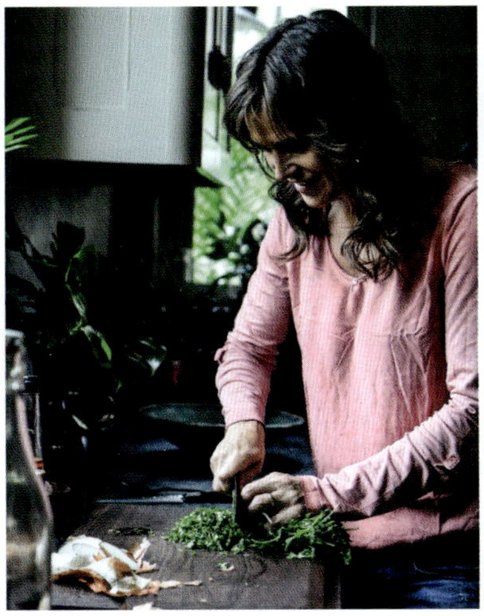 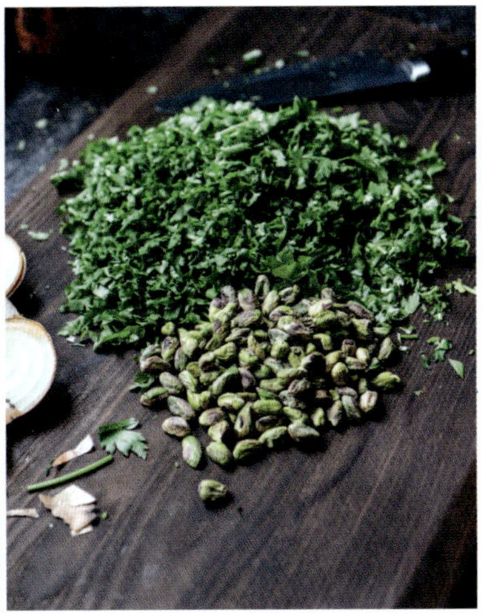 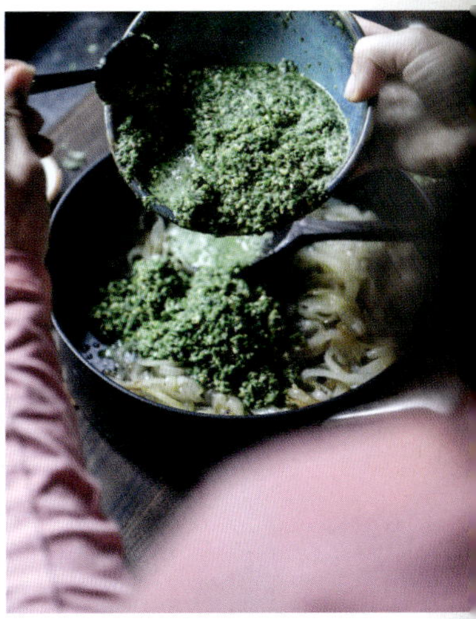

chicken with onion, pistachios and cilantro

✓ keto

- **2 large onions**
- **2 chicken breasts**
- **a handful of pistachios**
- **5 bunches of cilantro (3½ oz/100 g - see tip)**

- fresh garlic -

Slice the onions into rings and sauté them in olive oil, stirring regularly to make sure they don't burn. Cover the pan as this allows the onions to cook more quickly. Cut the chicken into pieces, brown them in a separate pan and add the chicken to the onions (see tip). Put the cilantro, pistachios and 3 cloves of garlic in a blender and blend with a splash of water and olive oil to make a thick, grainy paste. Add the paste to the chicken, season with some salt and plenty of black pepper and simmer briefly.

TIP: COOKING CHICKEN
If you don't have a lot of time and want to save on the dishwashing, add the chicken to the onions. However, it's easier to brown the chicken pieces in a separate pan.

TIP: CILANTRO
Hunt down some high-quality cilantro! I usually buy cilantro at the market or at a specialty store. That's where you'll find full bunches with that real cilantro flavor. If you're not a fan of cilantro, you can replace it with flat-leaf parsley.

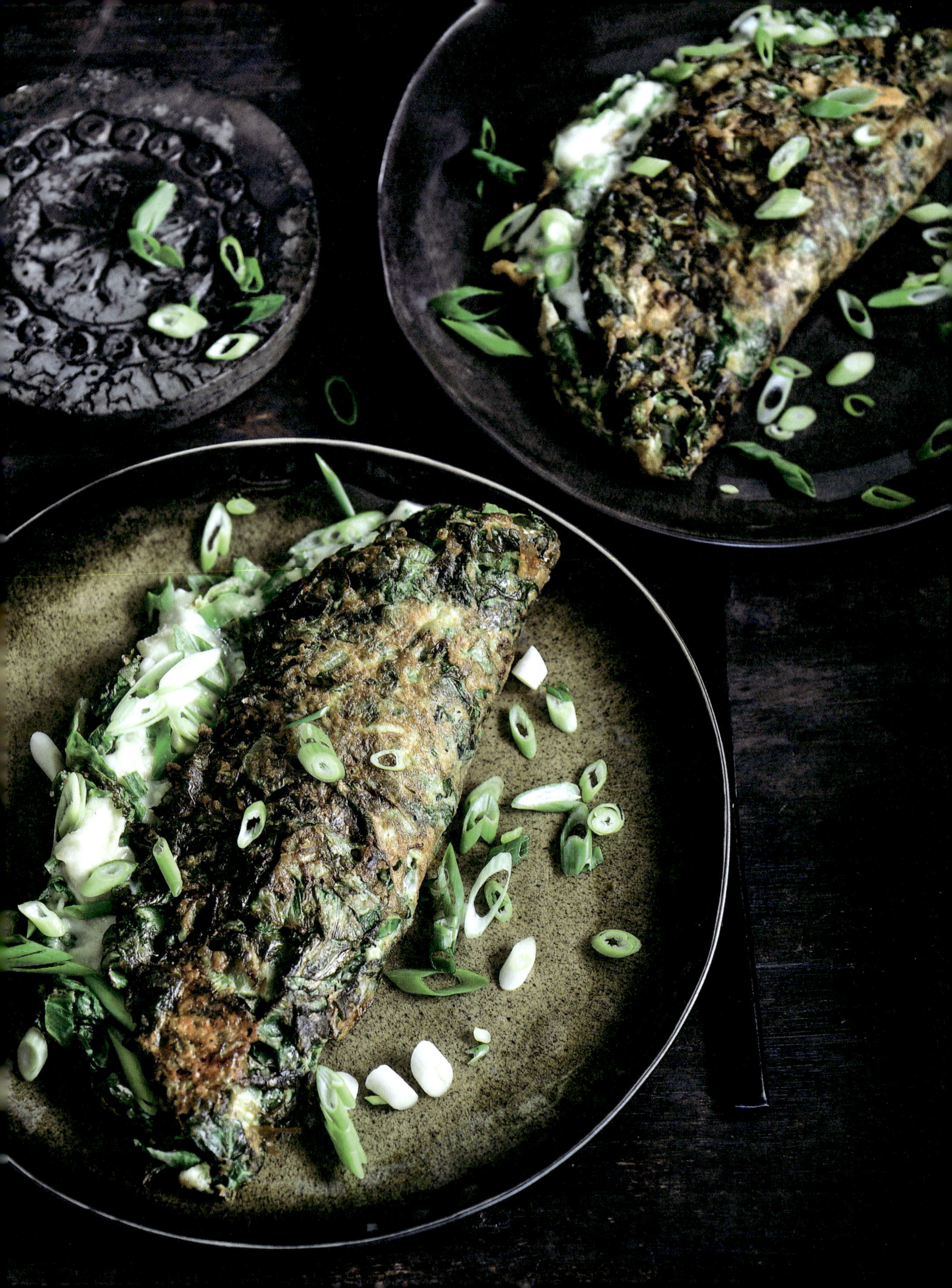

This is undoubtedly
one of the best omelets ever.
This is my favorite vegetable omelet;
the cheese makes it deliciously light and creamy.

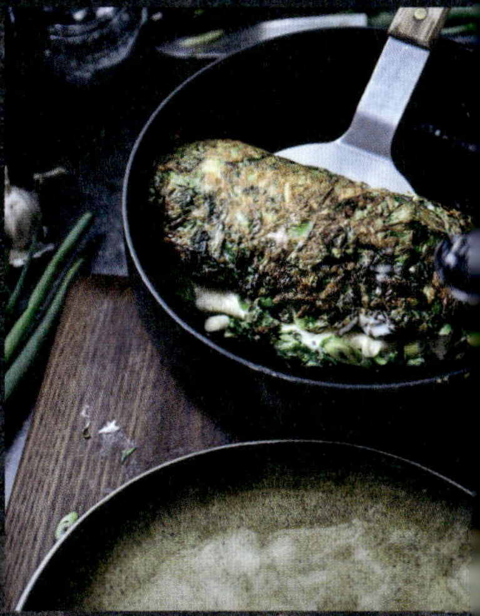

✓ keto

omelet

with Swiss chard and goat cheese

- 10½ oz (300 g) Swiss chard (see tip)
- 4 eggs
- 7 oz (200 g) creamy goat cheese
- 6 spring onions

Preheat the oven to 400 °F (200 °C). Slice the Swiss chard into thin strips. Dice the goat cheese into small cubes. I like to slice the goat cheese and then pull it into pieces, a sticky job because of the creamy cheese. Separate the eggs, fold the egg yolks into the Swiss chard and then stir half the goat cheese into the chard. Season with salt and pepper. Beat the egg whites until stiff and fold them into the Swiss chard.

Bake two omelets. Pour one half of the egg mixture into a greased pan, distribute half of the remaining goat cheese over the top and cook, covered, for 3 minutes. Place the pan in the oven for another 2 minutes. Do the same with the second omelet. Finely chop the spring onions.

Sprinkle the spring onions over the omelets. Fold the omelets over and serve.

TIP: SWISS CHARD

Swiss chard comes in many varieties. They all have plenty of leaves and look a lot like spinach. The season for Swiss chard runs from May to October, so if you can't find any Swiss chard, use spinach instead. I like preparing dishes with Swiss chard because they have firm leaves, plenty of flavor and not much moisture.

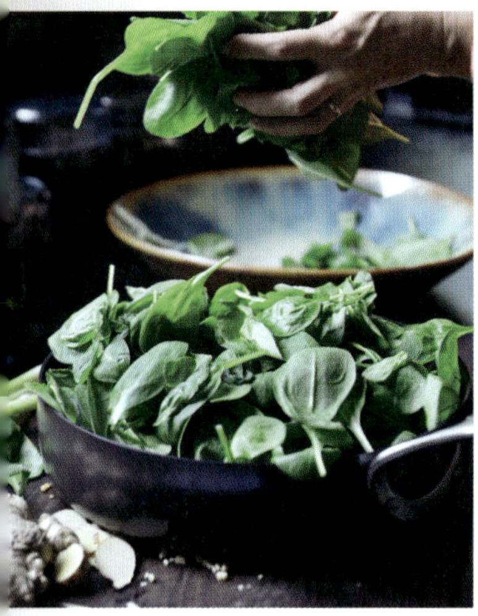 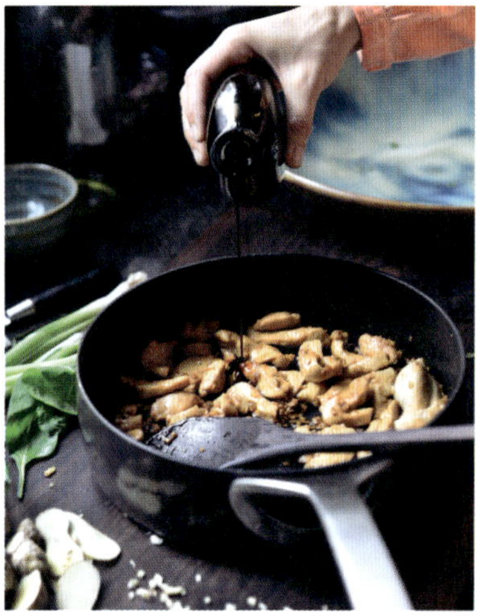

Ginger makes this chicken dish ultimate comfort food.
Sweet and spicy chicken.
Delicious!

chicken with ginger

and spinach

- **2 chicken breasts**
- **3-inch (7 cm) ginger root**
- **10½ oz (300 g) spinach**
- **2 spring onions, finely chopped**

– soy sauce –
– balsamic vinegar (see tip) –
– fresh garlic –

Cut the chicken into pieces and brown in olive oil. Meanwhile, finely chop the ginger and 3 cloves of garlic. You don't have to peel the ginger. Add 8 tablespoons of soy sauce to the chicken and immediately add the ginger and garlic. Season with plenty of pepper, but don't add salt; the soy sauce is salty enough. Sauté the spinach in a separate pan with some olive oil and season with some black pepper and a little bit of salt. Just before serving, add 5 tablespoons of balsamic vinegar to the chicken and simmer for another minute until the sauce becomes syrupy. Serve and garnish with the finely chopped spring onion.

TIP: BALSAMIC VINEGAR
Use a high-quality, thick balsamic vinegar, otherwise the sauce will be too thin. The sauce needs to be thick and syrupy.

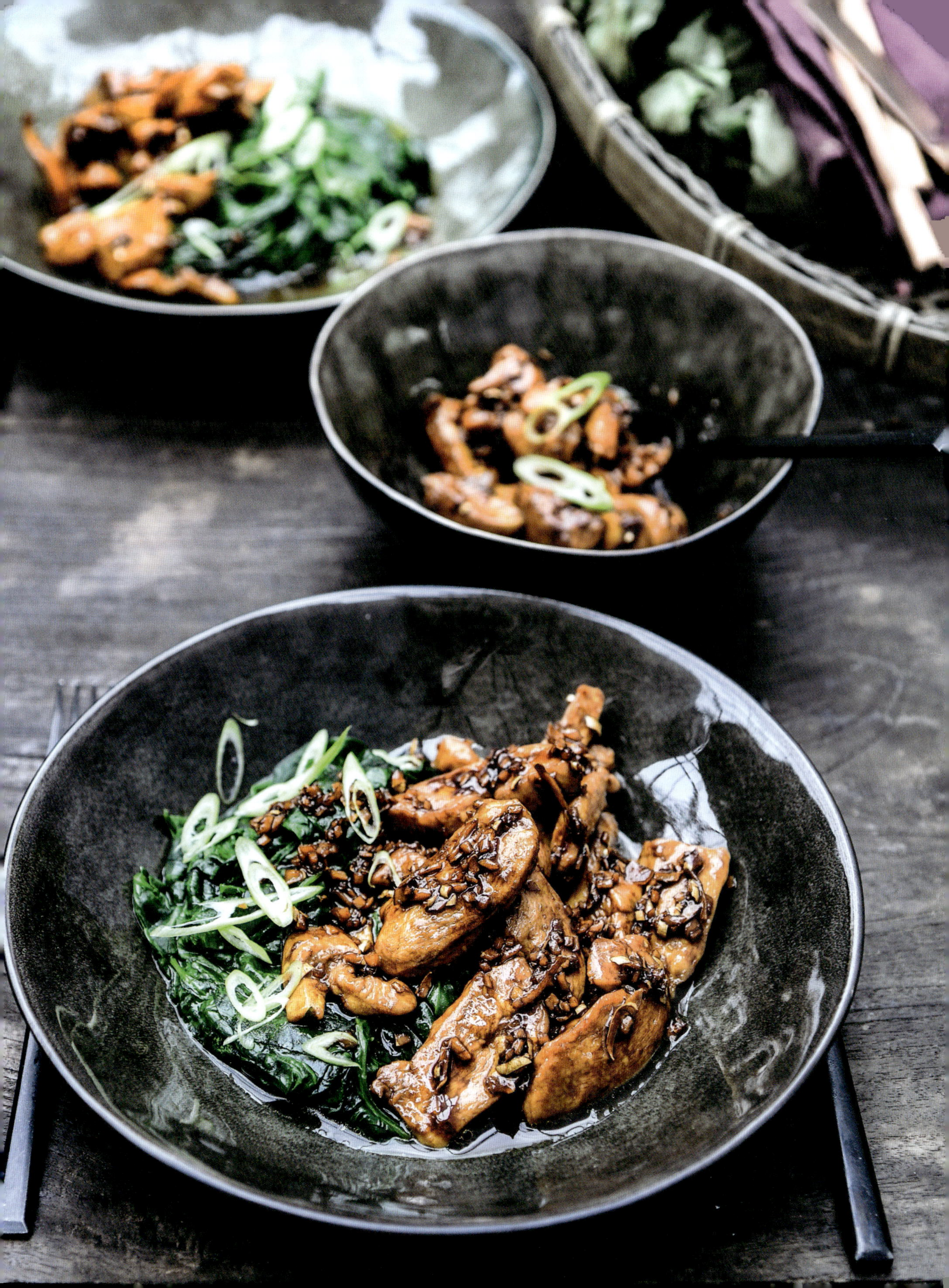

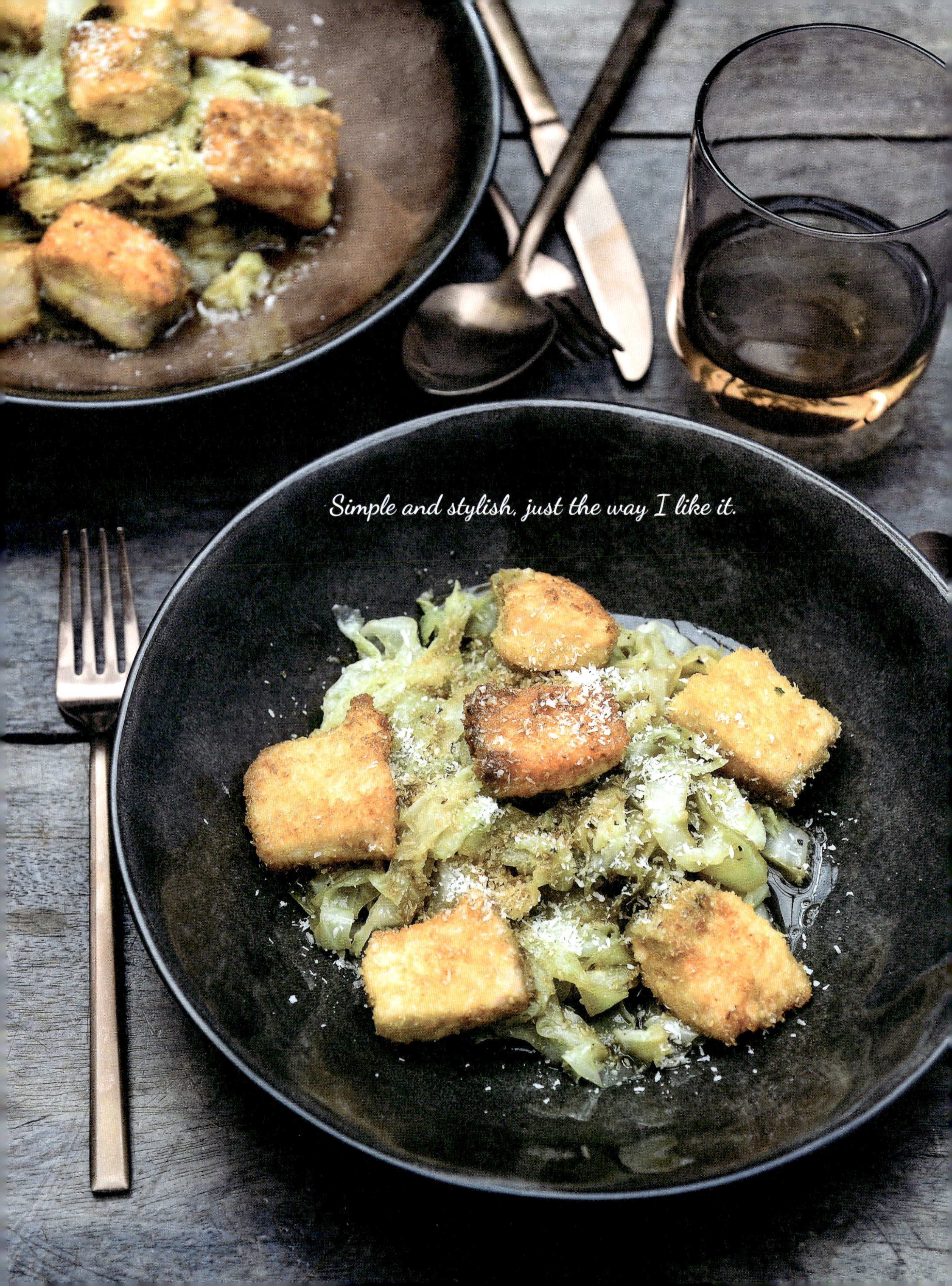
Simple and stylish, just the way I like it.

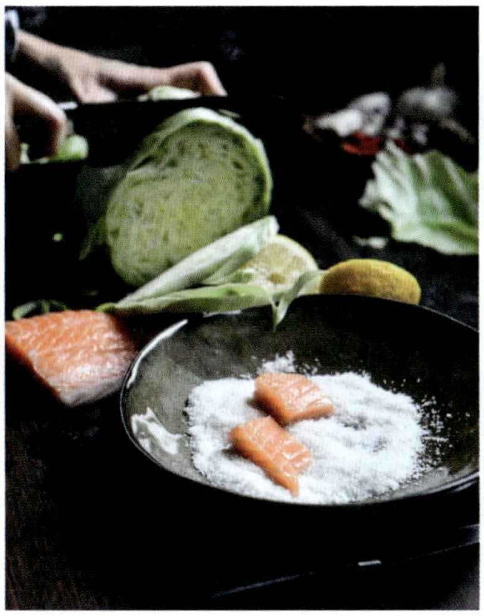

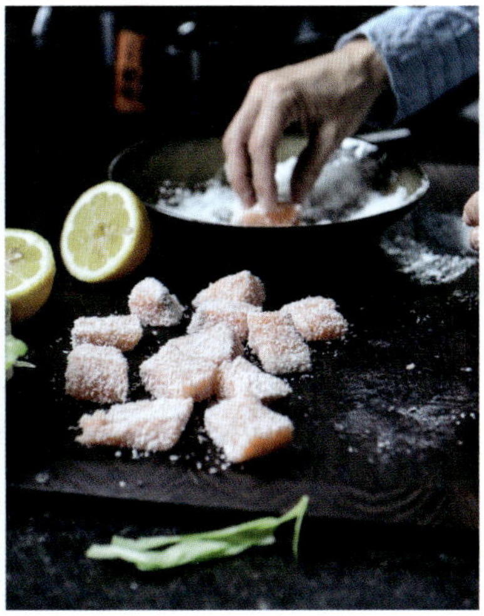

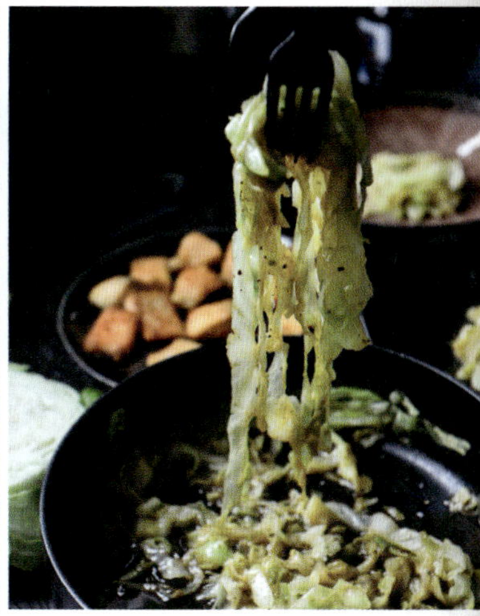

crispy salmon ✓ keto

with vegetable spaghetti

- **10½ oz (300 g) salmon fillet, without skin**
- **3½ oz (100 g) grated coconut**
- **½ lemon**
- **1 pointed (or Napa) cabbage**

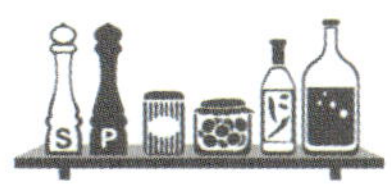

– soy sauce –

Shred the pointed or Napa cabbage and cook it, covered, in plenty of olive oil and some water. After 5 minutes, add the juice of ½ lemon and 3 tablespoons of soy sauce. Season with some black pepper. Cook for another few minutes.

Cut the salmon into cubes, coat them with the grated coconut and briefly sauté them in plenty of olive oil until lightly browned.

Spoon the cabbage onto a plate, place the crispy salmon cubes on top and garnish with some extra soy sauce and grated coconut.

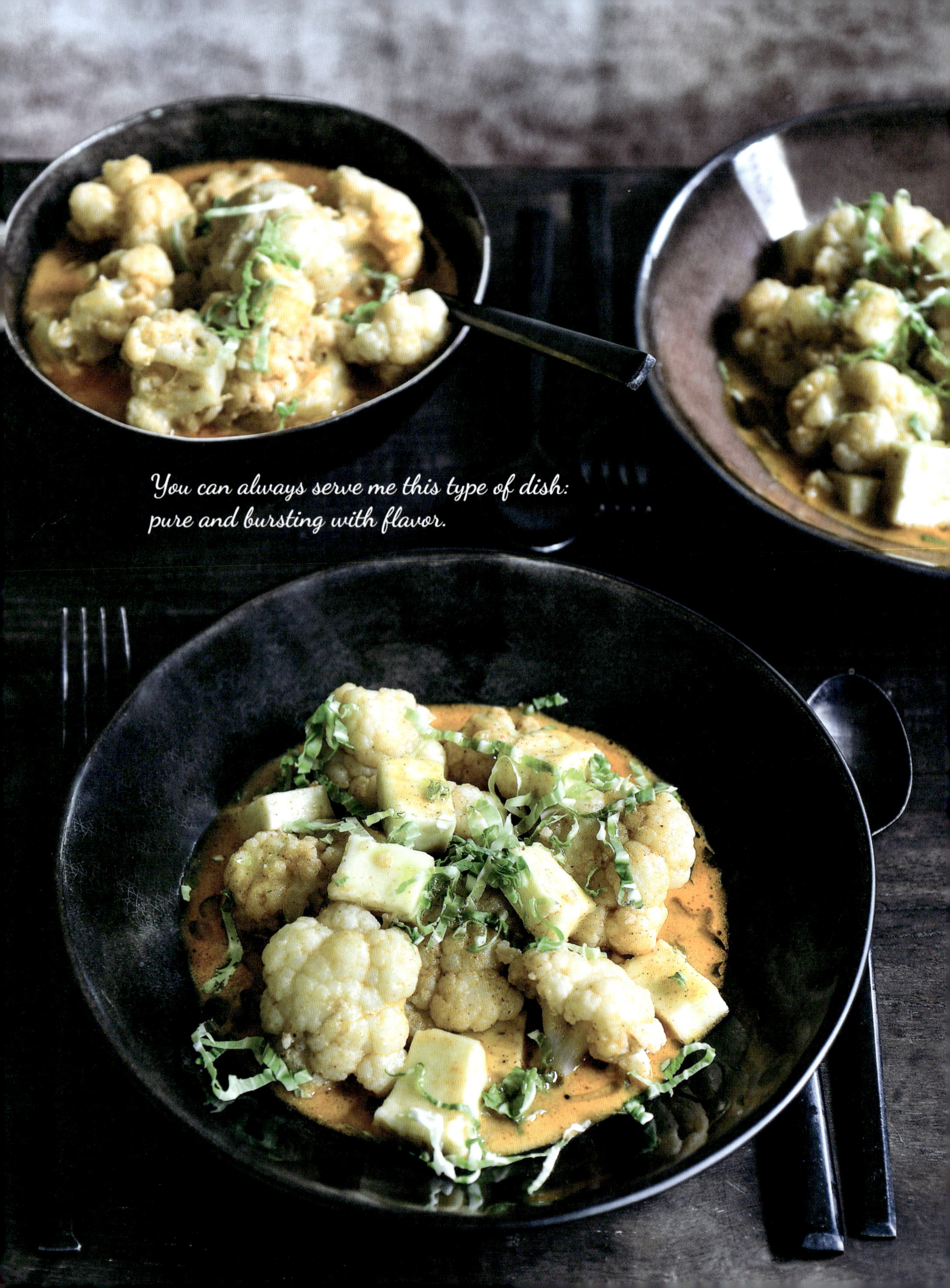

You can always serve me this type of dish: pure and bursting with flavor.

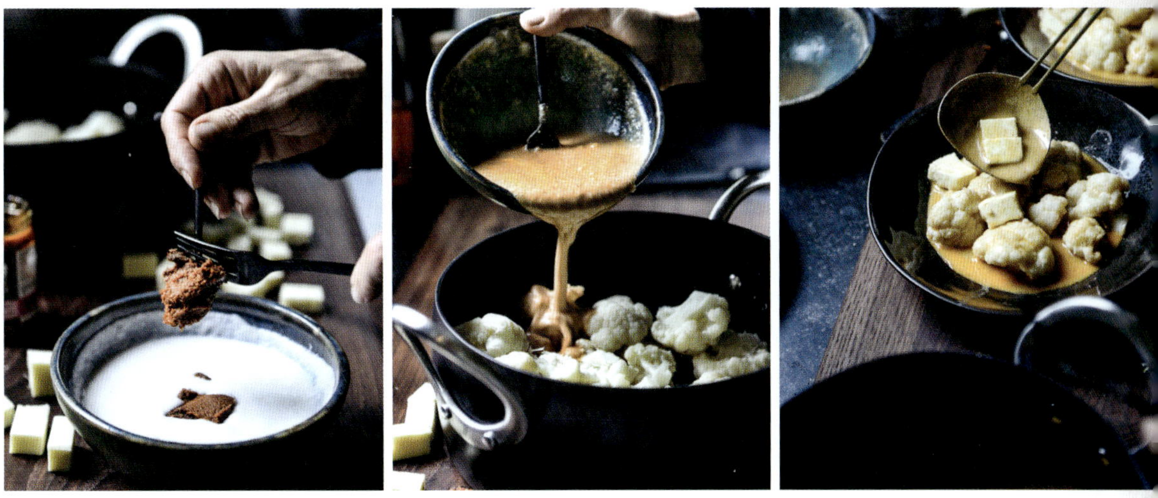

cauliflower curry ✓ keto

with paneer

- 1 cauliflower
- 14 fl oz (400 ml) coconut milk
- 2 to 3 tablespoons red curry paste
- 7 oz (200 g) paneer (see tip)

Cook the cauliflower florets until tender in water with a generous splash of olive oil and some salt. Dice the paneer into ½-inch cubes. Stir 2 to 3 tablespoons of red curry paste into the coconut milk in a bowl. Keep tasting to make sure it doesn't get too spicy. Drain the cauliflower florets and return the pan to the heat. Pour in the coconut milk and add the diced paneer. Season with salt and pepper. Simmer gently for a few moments and serve. Garnish with some of the green leaves from the cauliflower and a drizzle of olive oil.

TIP: PANEER

Paneer is a fresh, curd cheese made from cow's milk and it's a well-known ingredient in Indian cuisine. Paneer has a high protein content and doesn't contain a lot of fat and salt. This cheese is a softer and less salty version of halloumi but it's also suitable for frying. Paneer is usually diced into small cubes and used in curries. You should be able to find it in most supermarkets.

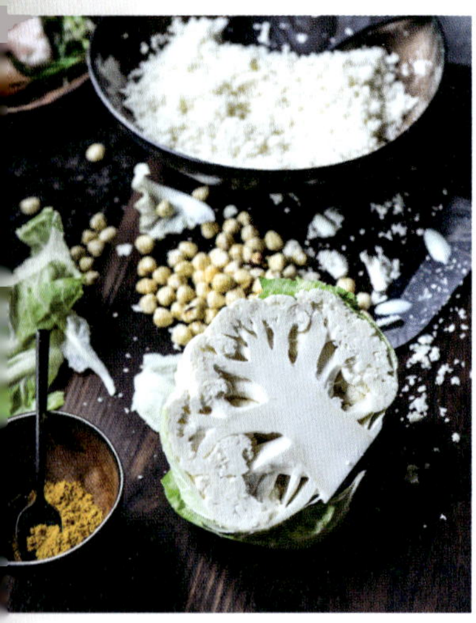

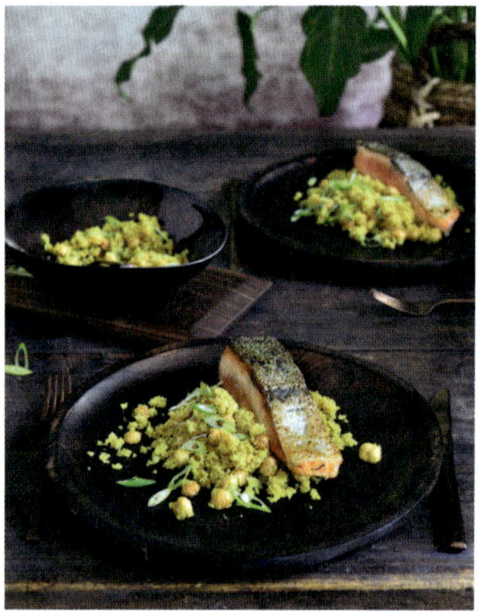

salmon

keto

with cauliflower rice and ras el hanout

- **2 salmon fillets, with skin**
- **½ cauliflower**
- **a handful of hazelnuts**
- **2 spring onions, finely chopped**

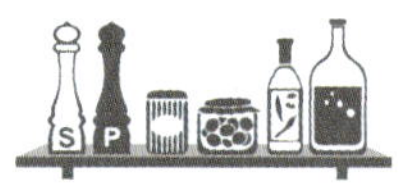

- ras el hanout -

Finely chop the cauliflower to make cauliflower rice.
Cook the cauliflower and hazelnuts in plenty of olive oil, stirring regularly.
In a separate pan, sear the salmon on both sides, making sure that the inside remains pink.
Season with salt and pepper.
When the cauliflower is almost tender, stir in 2 teaspoons of ras el hanout, plenty of black pepper and a little bit of salt. Add another splash of olive oil and keep stirring until everything is cooked through.
Spoon the cauliflower rice onto a plate and place the salmon on top.
Garnish with the finely chopped spring onions.

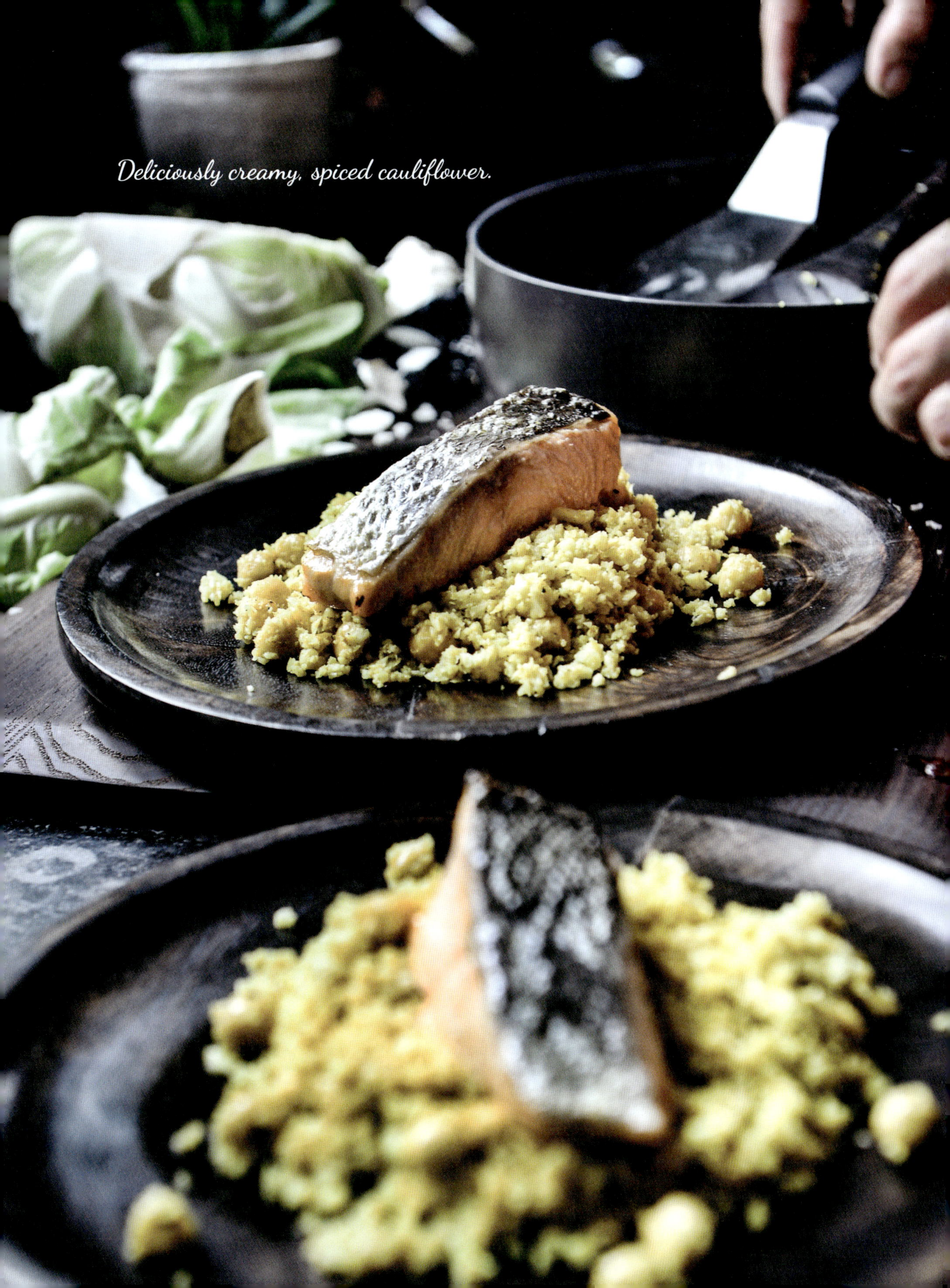

Deliciously creamy, spiced cauliflower.

You don't usually associate an omelet with crab meat or caviar; that's why this dish is so surprising.

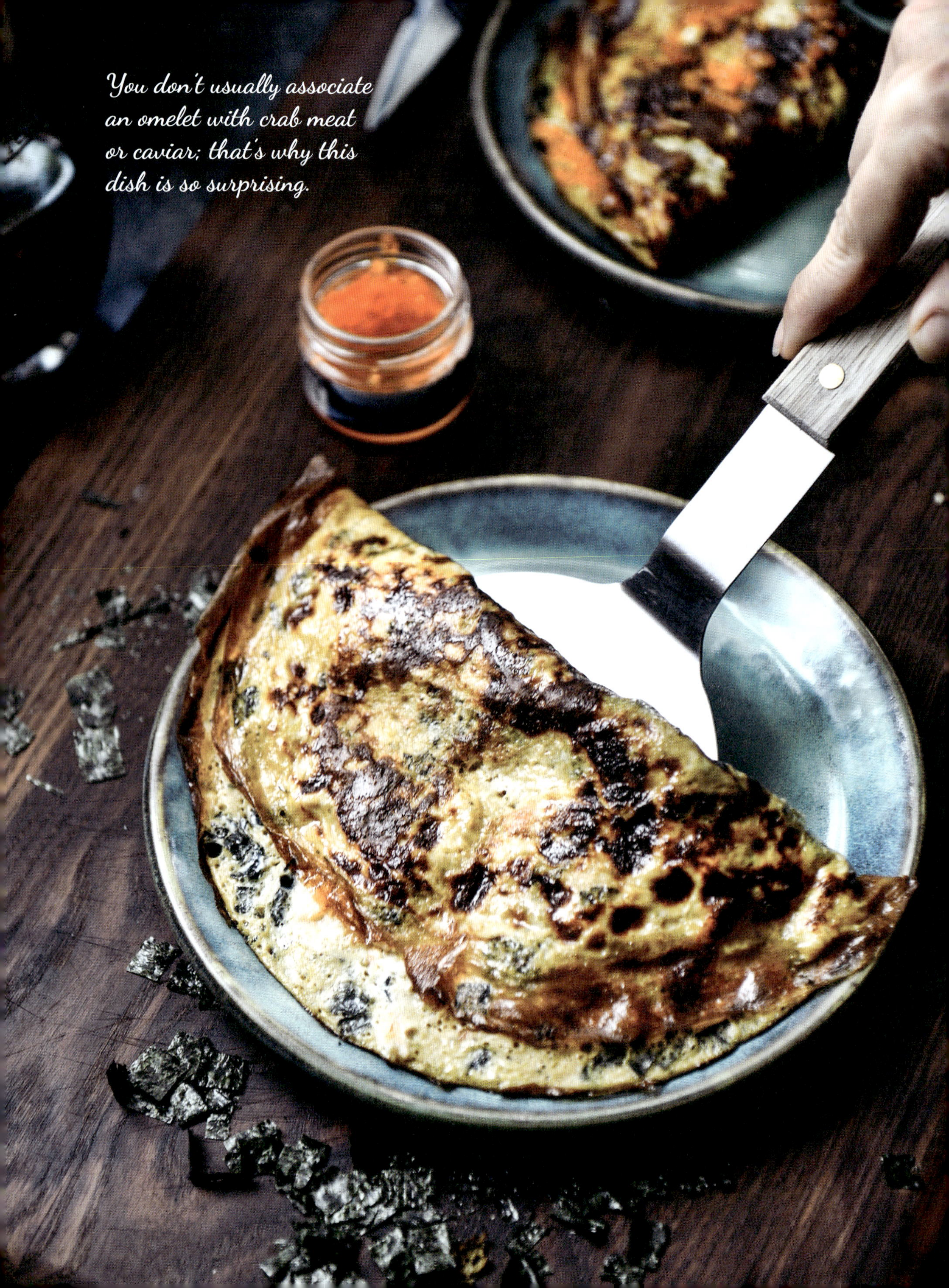

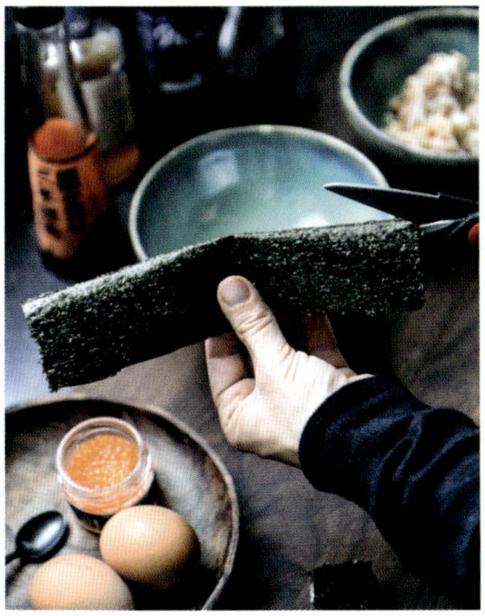
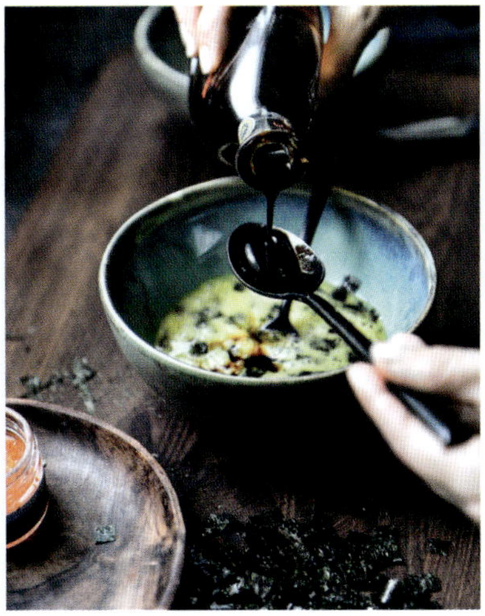
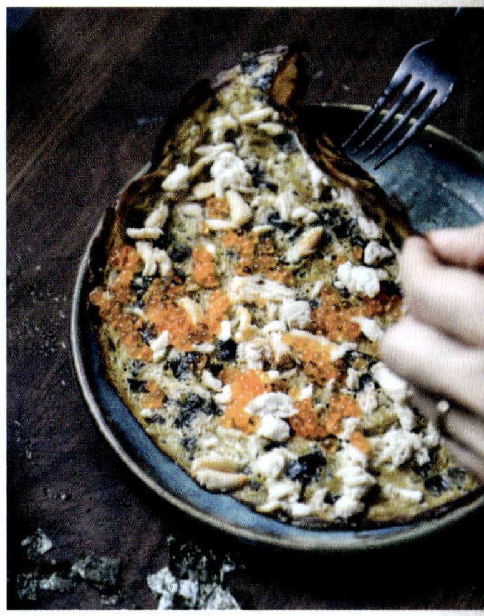

omelet ✓ keto

with nori, crab, and fish roe

- **4 eggs**
- **1 can of crab meat (4 oz/120 g - see tip)**
- **1 jar of fish roe**
- **1 sheet of nori (seaweed)**

- soy sauce -
- balsamic vinegar -

Beat the eggs with 2 tablespoons of soy sauce and 2 tablespoons of balsamic vinegar. Season with black pepper (no salt, the soy sauce is salty enough). Cut the nori sheet into small pieces with a pair of scissors and add to the eggs. Pour half the egg mixture into a pan. Distribute half the crab meat over the top and cook gently, covered, for 2 to 3 minutes. Do not turn the omelet over. Make two omelets in total.
Place the omelets on a plate, spoon some of the fish roe on top and fold over the omelets.

TIP: CRAB MEAT
You can also replace the crab meat with canned tuna.

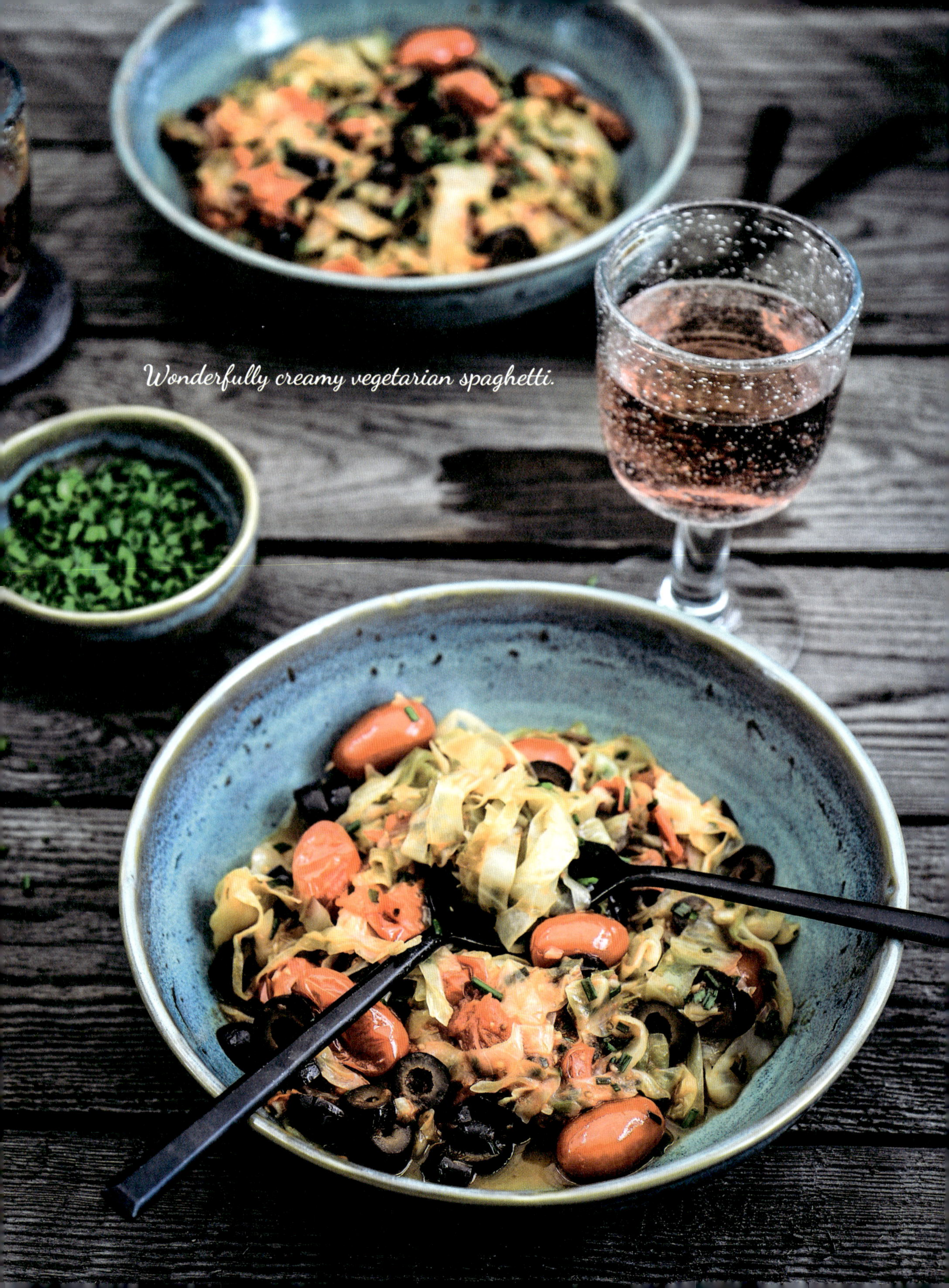
Wonderfully creamy vegetarian spaghetti.

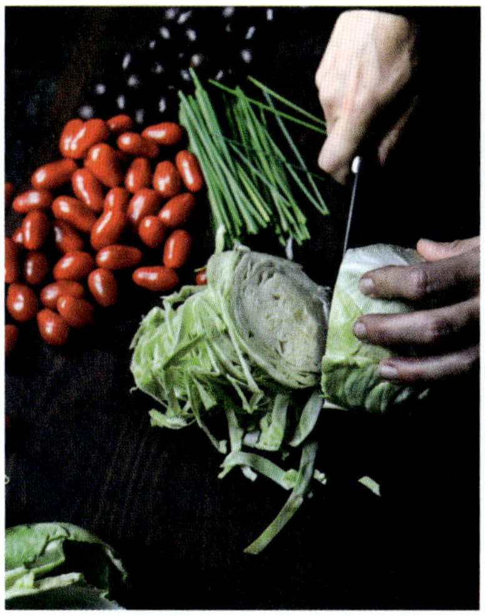

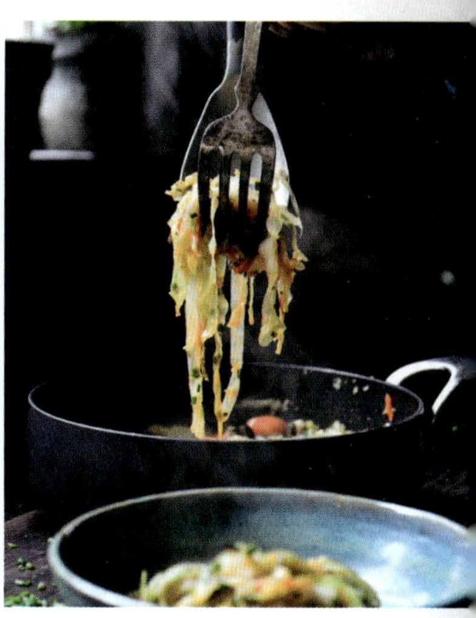

vegan

✓ keto

pointed cabbage spaghetti

with tomatoes and olives

- **1 pointed (or Napa) cabbage**
- **14 oz (400 g) cherry tomatoes**
- **a handful of pitted black olives**
- **1 bunch of chives (¾ oz/20 g)**

S P

- fresh garlic -

Slice the cabbage into long strips. Start at the top of the cabbage to get nice, long, strips.
Halve three quarters of the tomatoes and finely chop 3 cloves of garlic.
Put the tomatoes and garlic in a large pan and lay the cabbage on top.
Add a generous splash of olive oil and half a glass of water, cover the pan, and cook the cabbage for about 5 minutes. Make sure that the cabbage doesn't burn; add a little olive oil if necessary.
Meanwhile, slice the olives into rings and finely chop the chives. Add the olives, the remaining tomatoes and the chives to the cabbage, but keep some of the chives aside to garnish.
Stir everything thoroughly, season with salt and pepper and cook for another two minutes.
Serve in a deep plate or dish and garnish with some chives.

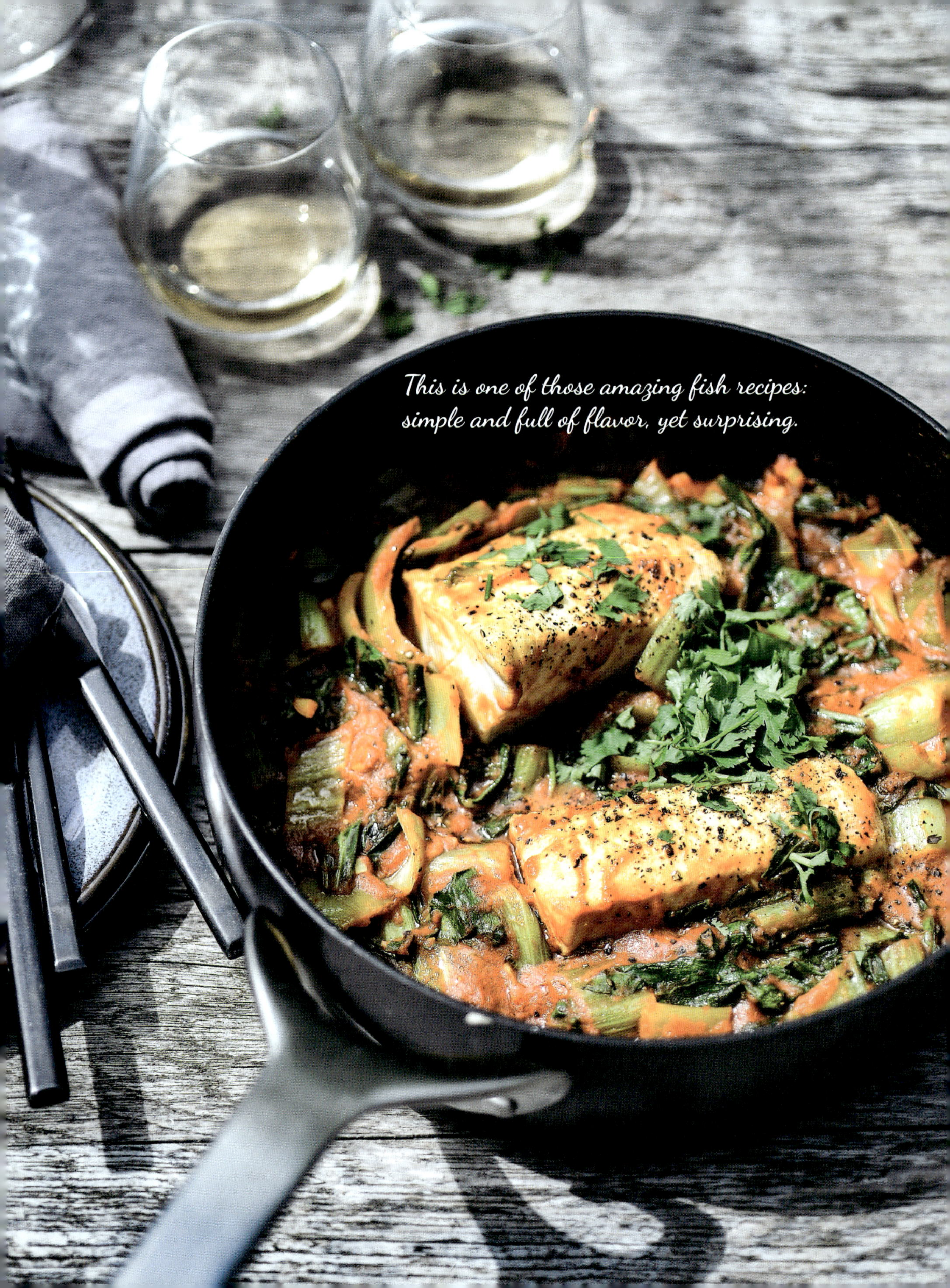
This is one of those amazing fish recipes:
simple and full of flavor, yet surprising.

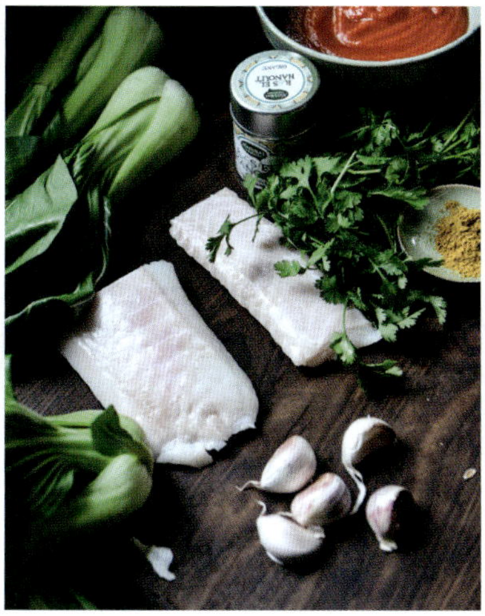

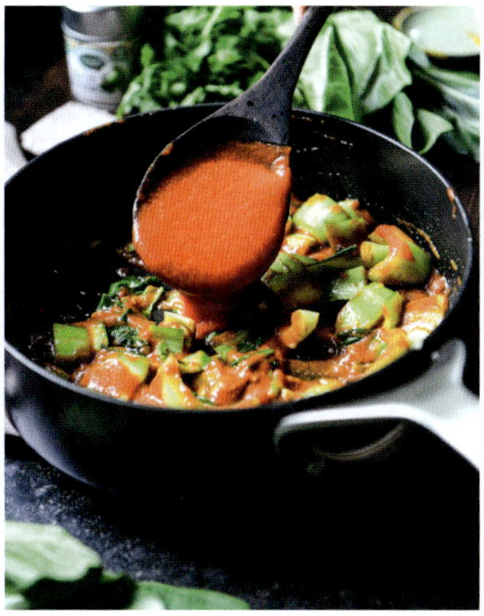

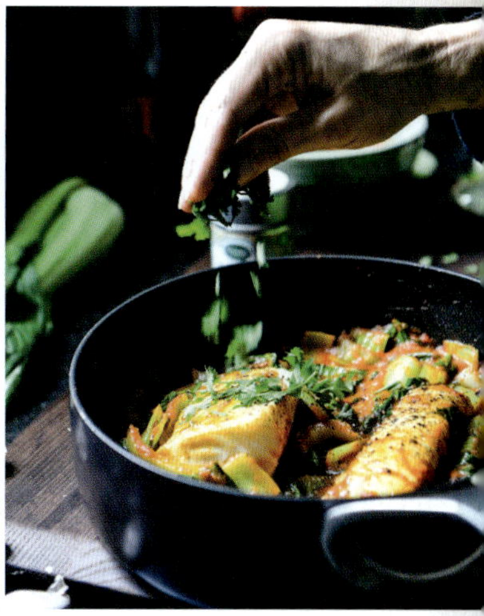

fish ✓ keto

with bok choy in tomato sauce

- **10½ oz (300 g) firm white fish (e.g. wolffish)**
- **10½ oz (300 g) strained tomatoes or tomato puree**
- **1 bunch of cilantro, finely chopped**
- **14 oz (400 g) bok choy (see tip)**

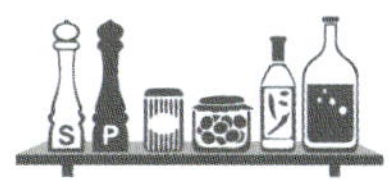

– fresh garlic –
– ras el hanout –

Slice the white part of the bok choy into thin strips and sauté in plenty of olive oil.
Finely chop 2 to 3 cloves of garlic and add to the bok choy. Season with 1 tablespoon of ras el hanout, salt and pepper, and add the strained tomatoes. Bring to a simmer over a low heat. Slice the green leaves from the bok choy into strips and add to the pan. Allow to cook for a little longer.
Put the fish fillets in the pan and cook them for 1 to 2 minutes on each side.
Add the finely chopped cilantro just before serving.

TIP: BOK CHOY
If you can't find any bok choy, use spinach.

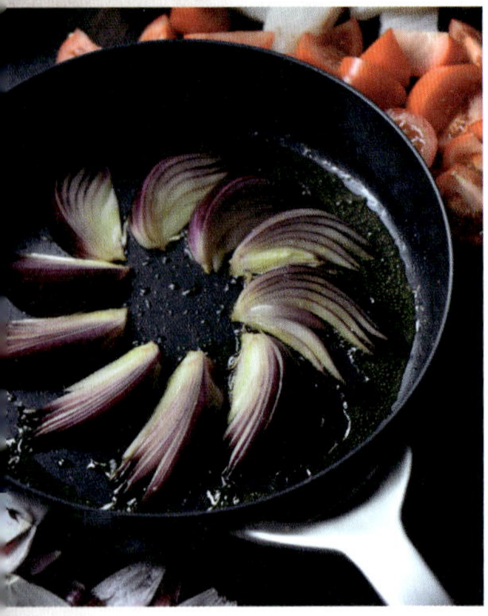

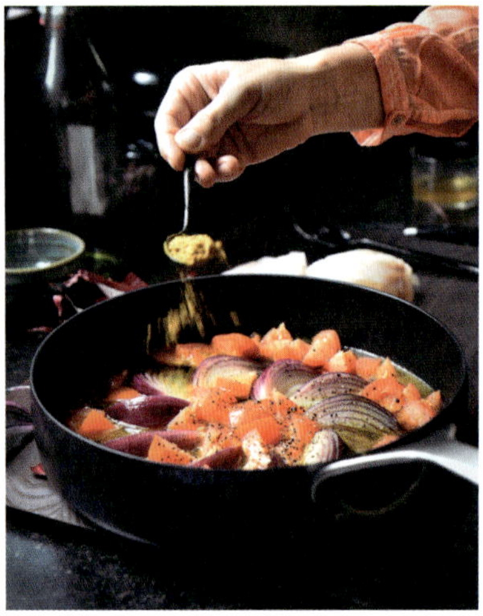

fish soup

✓ keto

- **2 firm white fish fillets (e.g. cod fillet)**
- **3 red onions**
- **3 tomatoes**
- **white wine**

- fresh garlic -
- ras el hanout -

Slice the onions into wedges (see tip) and sauté them, covered, in a large pan with some olive oil. Dice 2 tomatoes, remove the hard, white core and add them to the pan. Cover the pan. Finely chop 2 cloves of garlic and add to the pan. Cook for another 2 minutes, then add the white wine until all the vegetables are covered. Add 2 tablespoons of ras el hanout, plenty of black pepper and a little bit of salt. Carefully stir everything together and cook, uncovered, over a low heat.
Meanwhile, slice the third tomato into wedges, remove the hard, white core and add to the soup. Cut the fish into large pieces, place them in the soup and let everything cook for another 2 minutes.

TIP: SLICING ONIONS
I don't peel the onions right away, instead I slice them into wedges all the way down through the base, so everything holds together. It's much easier to remove the outer layers once the onion has already been sliced.

TIP: TOMATOES
By not adding all the tomatoes at once, you get a richer tomato sauce with both cooked and partially cooked tomatoes.

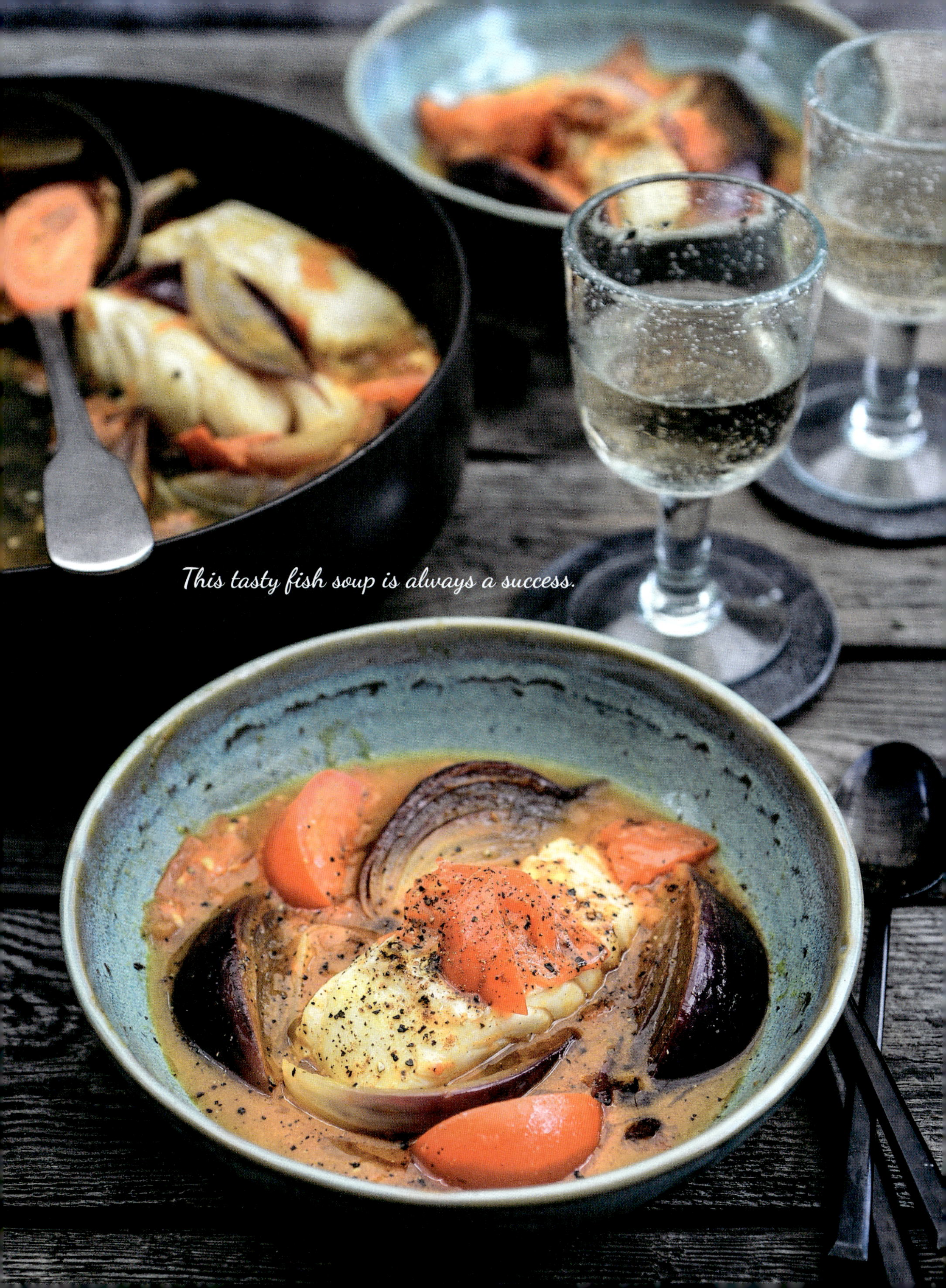
This tasty fish soup is always a success.

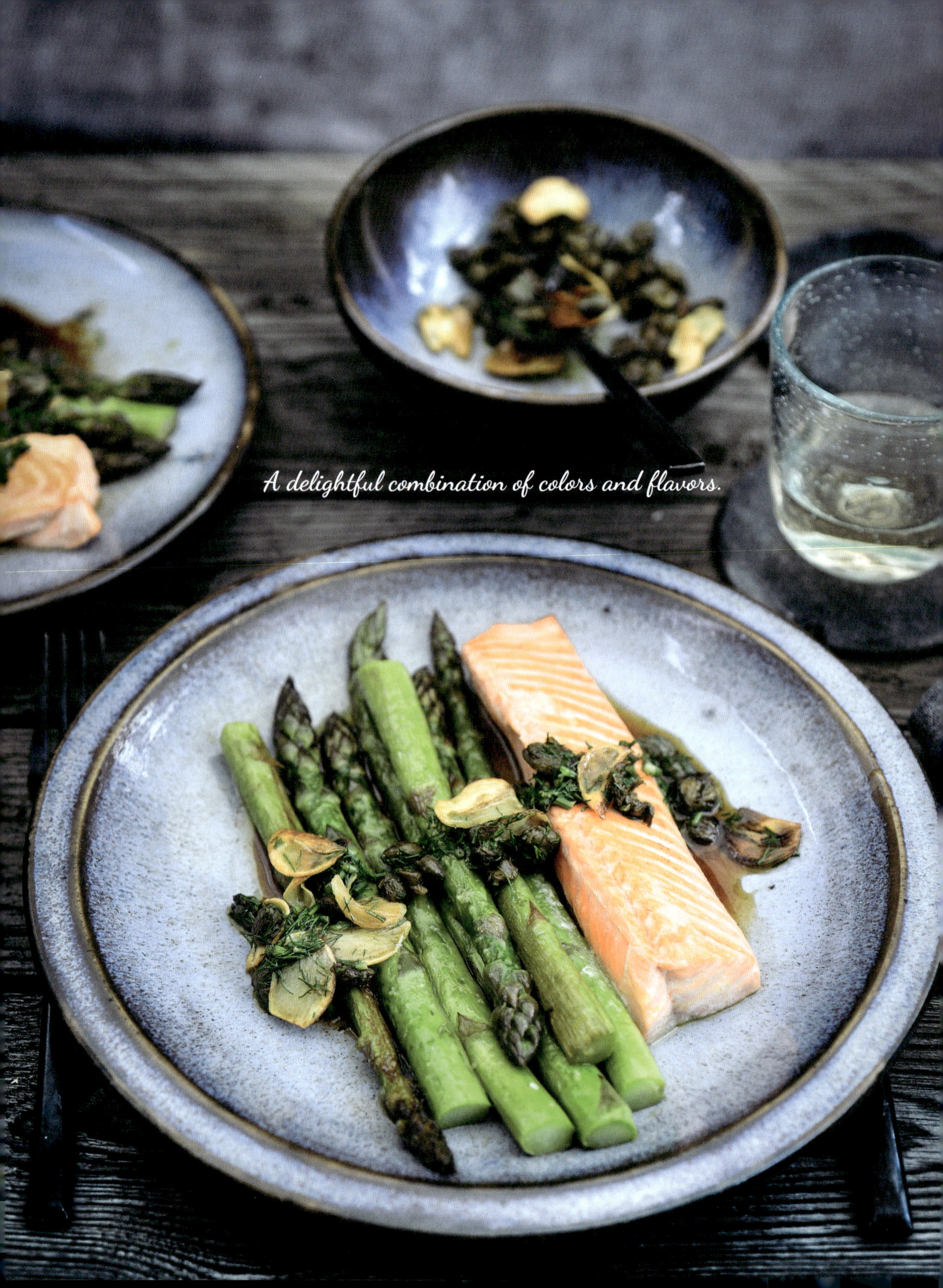
A delightful combination of colors and flavors.

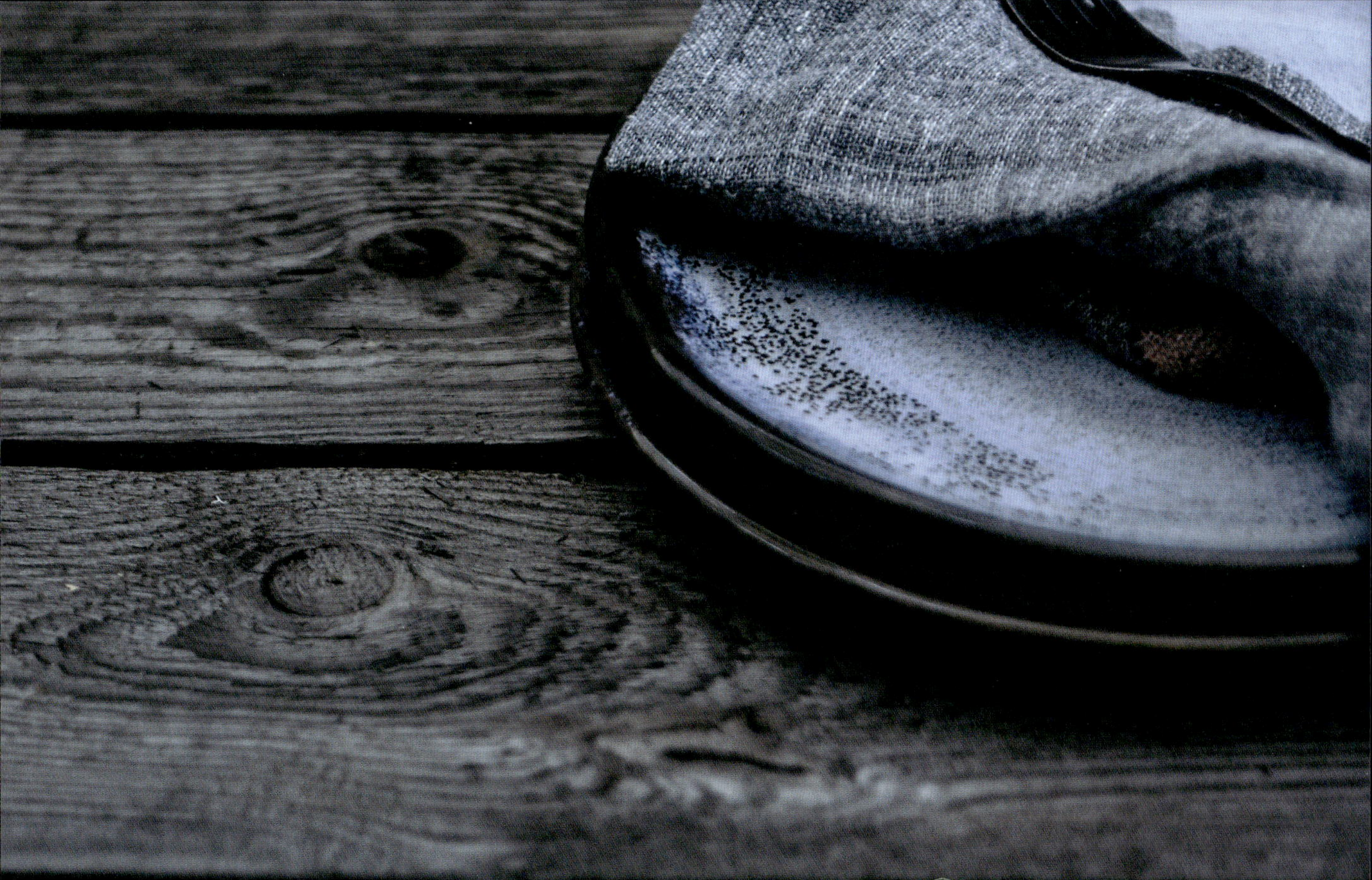

salmon trout

✓ keto

with asparagus

- 2 salmon trout fillets
- 1 bunch of green asparagus
- 1 bunch of dill
- a handful of capers

- fresh garlic -
- soy sauce -

Cut off the hard ends of the asparagus. Cook the asparagus, covered, in a pan with some olive oil and a small amount of water. Season with pepper (no salt) and cook for about 5 minutes until al dente, or a little longer if you prefer them softer. Slice 3 cloves of garlic. Place the capers between two paper towels and press out the moisture. In a separate pan, sauté the capers and garlic in plenty of olive oil until the garlic turns light brown.

Add the fish to the asparagus and cook, uncovered, until cooked through. Season with black pepper and turn the fish over only once during the cooking process. Finely chop the dill, add this to the garlic and capers and add a generous splash of soy sauce. Arrange the fish and the asparagus on a plate and spoon the sauce over the top.

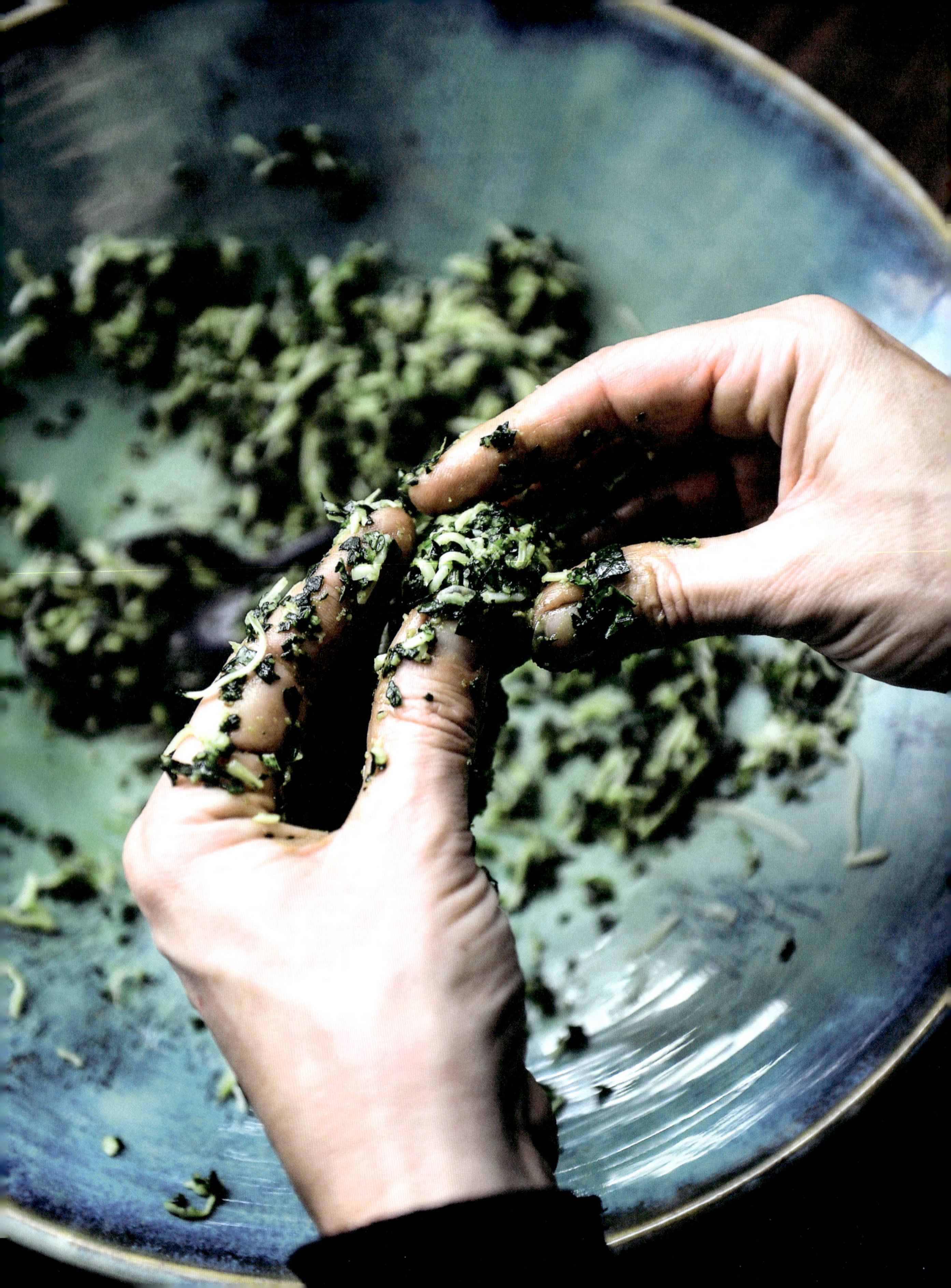

ready in
20 minutes

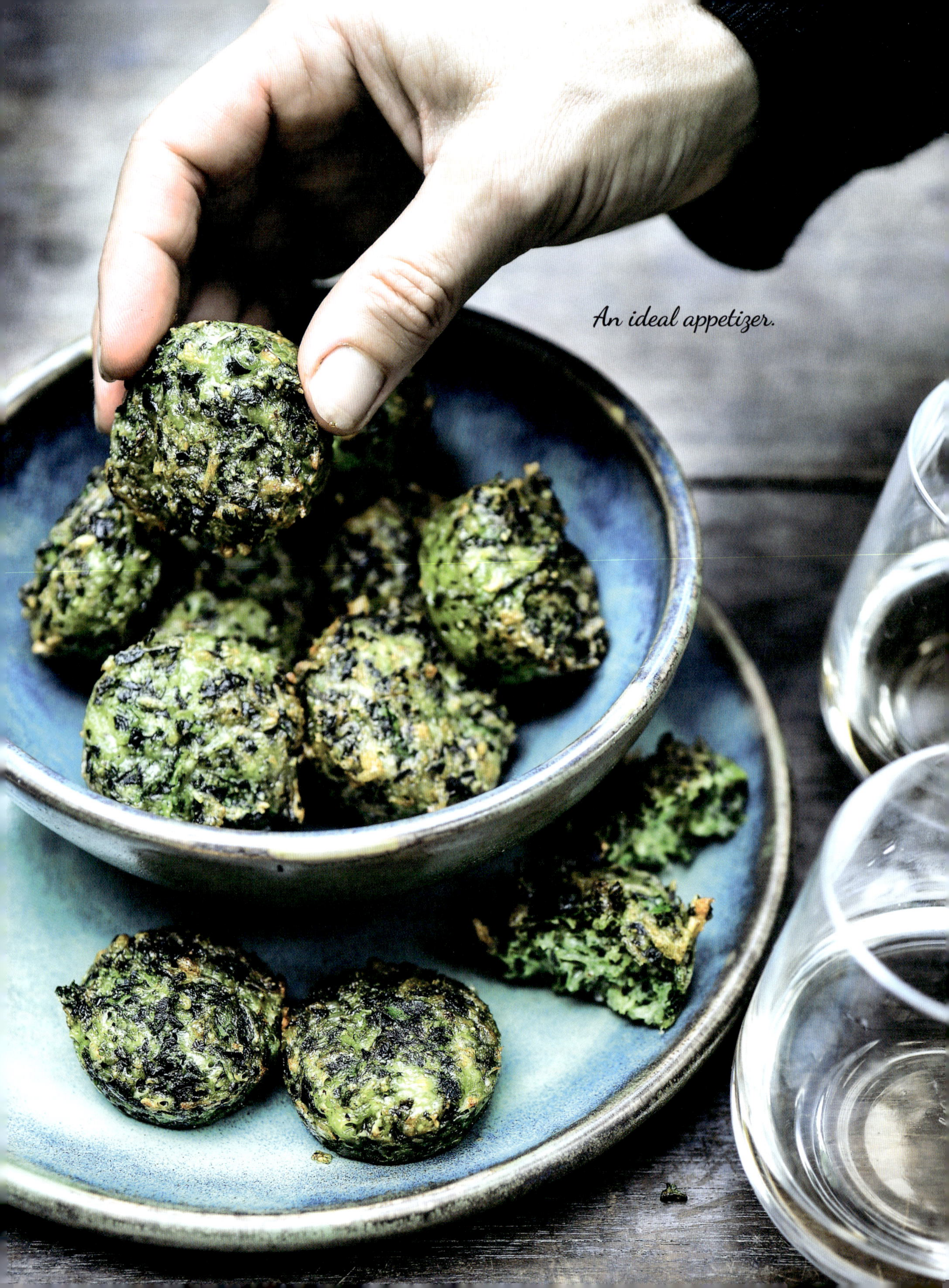

An ideal appetizer.

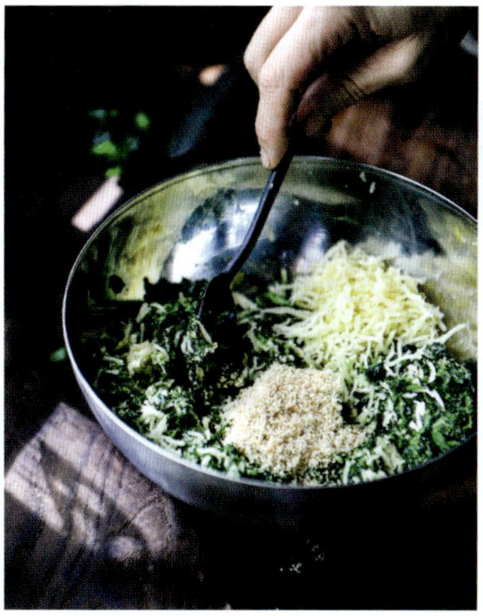
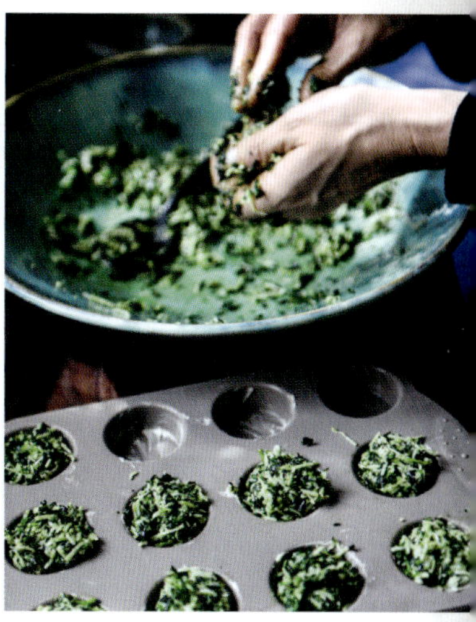

mini cheesy muffins

✓ keto

- **3½ oz (100 g) grated Comté cheese (or Gruyère)**
- **2 oz (50 g) nut flour**
- **1 egg**
- **3½ oz (100 g) fresh organic spinach (see tip)**

Preheat the oven to 350 °F (180 °C). Coarsely chop the spinach with the egg in a food processor. Put the mixture in a bowl and mix in the nut flour and cheese. Season generously with black pepper and a little bit of salt. Fill 10 small molds (ramekins or muffin tins) with the batter and bake in the oven for 10 minutes.

TIP: ORGANIC SPINACH

Organic spinach is thicker and sturdier and contains less moisture, which works better for these muffins.

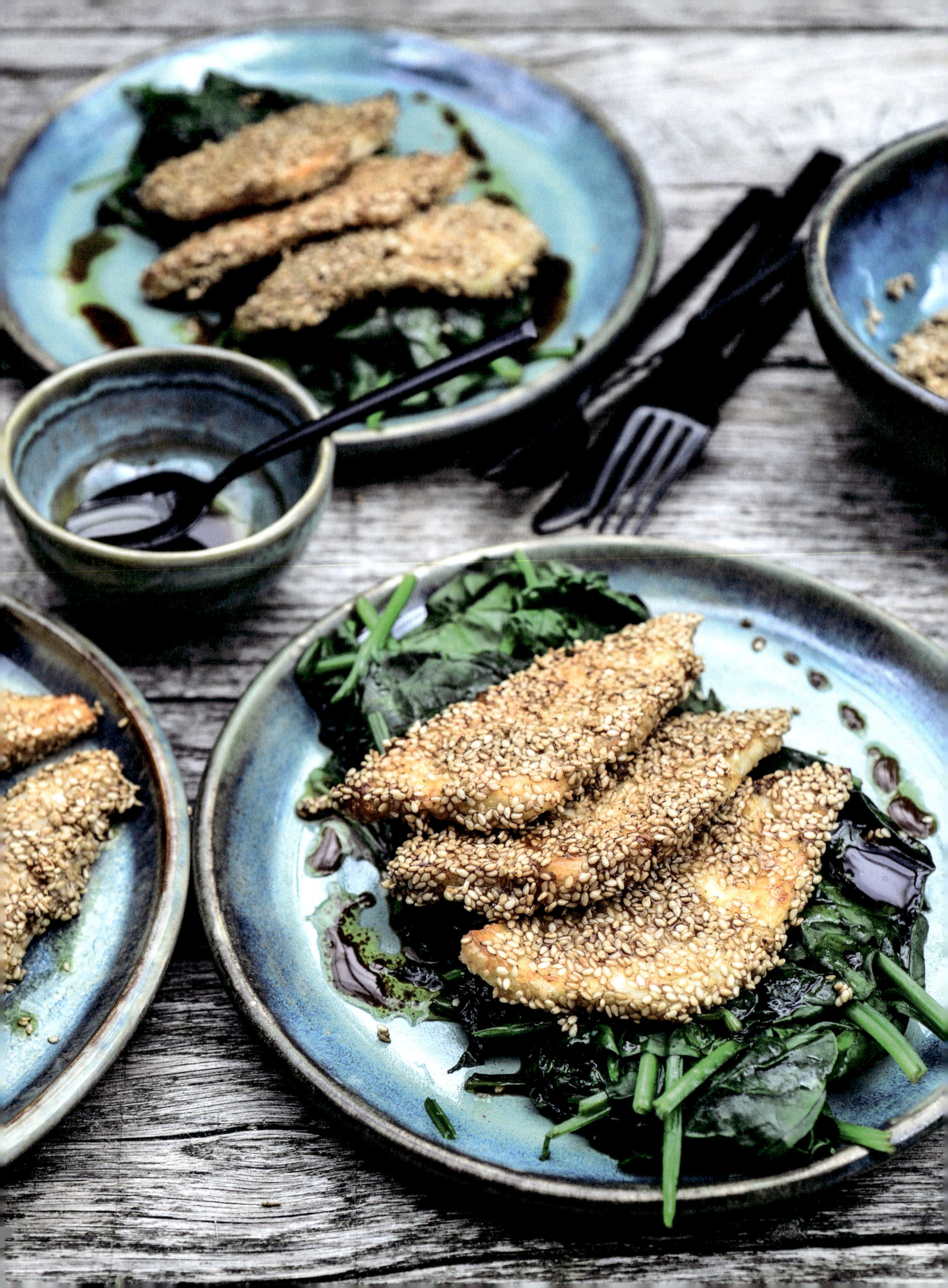

This tastes so good! You can serve the halloumi in smaller pieces as a snack.

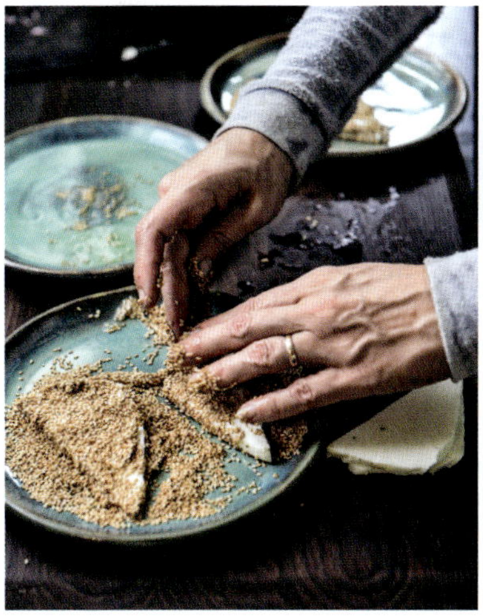

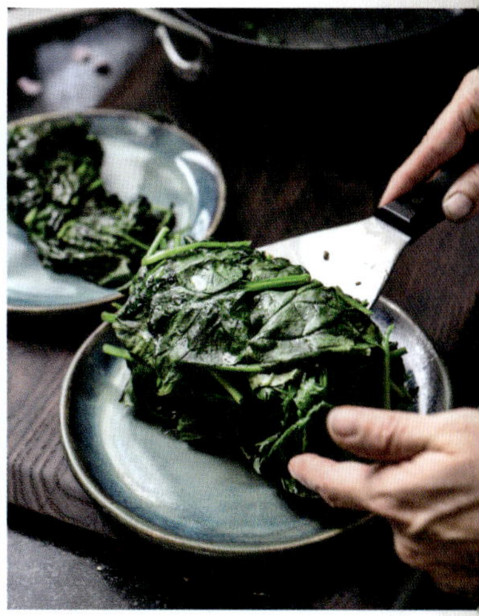

halloumi

✓ keto

in a crispy sesame seed crust with spinach

- **1 package halloumi**
- **roasted sesame seeds**
- **1 egg white**
- **10½ oz (300 g) spinach**

– soy sauce –
– butter or coconut oil –

Slice the halloumi and cut each slice again on the diagonal to form triangles. Put the lightly beaten egg white in a deep dish and the sesame seeds on a separate plate. Heat plenty of butter or coconut oil in a skillet. Coat the cheese slices first with the egg white and then the sesame seeds. Fry them for one minute on each side in the hot oil, or until the sesame seeds start to brown. In a separate pan, sauté the spinach with some olive oil and season with salt and pepper.
Spoon the spinach onto a plate and arrange the cheese slices on top.
Combine 3 tablespoons of soy sauce with 4 tablespoons of olive oil and spoon the sauce over the top.

TIP: HALLOUMI
Traditional halloumi from Cyprus is made with sheep's milk and this soft, curd-like cheese is rennet-free. It's the perfect cheese for frying because it browns without melting.

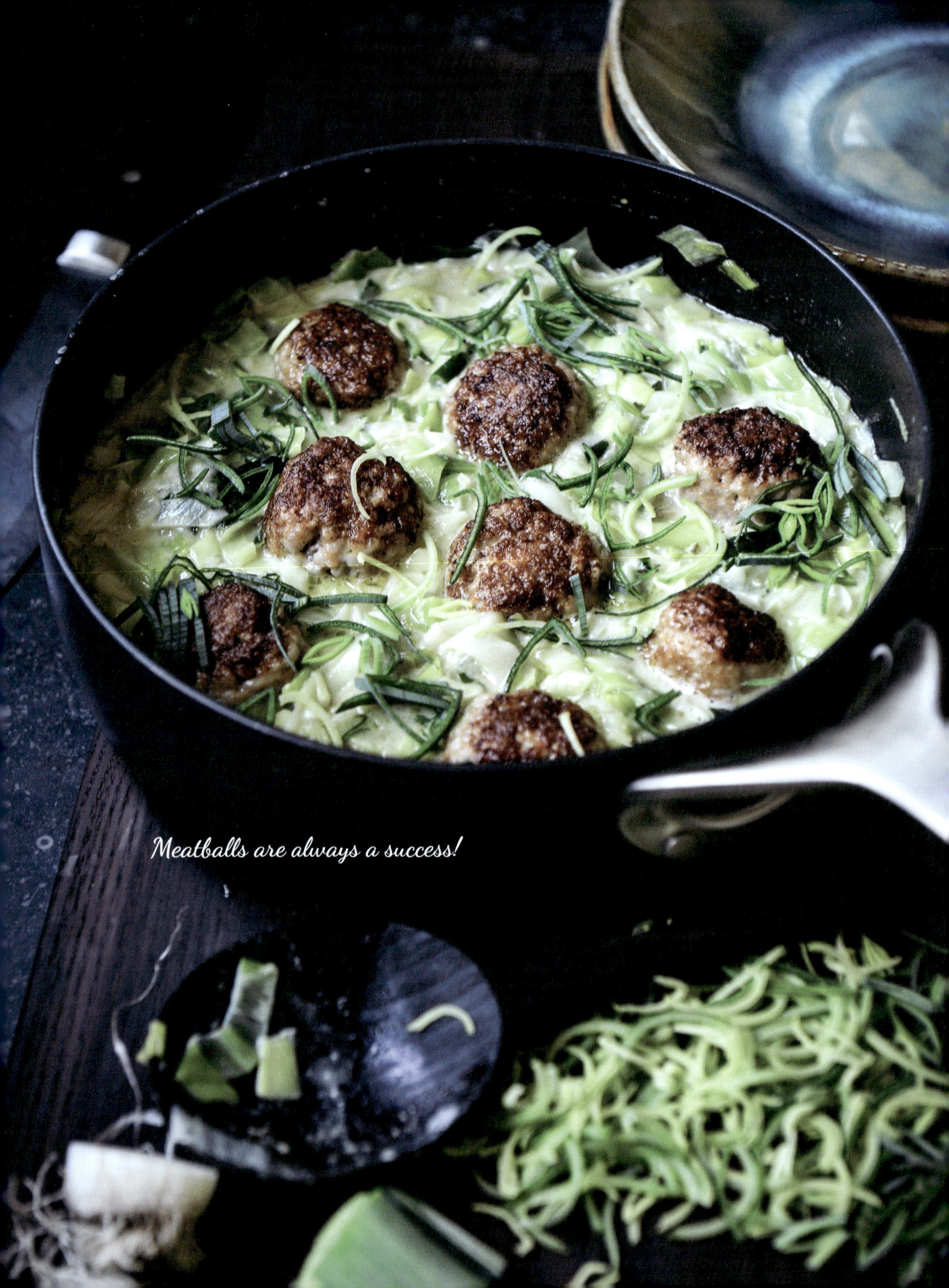
Meatballs are always a success!

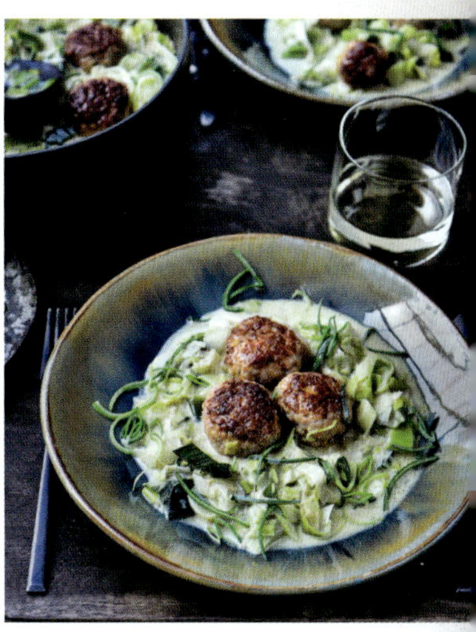

✓ keto

curried chicken meatballs

with leek

- **10½ oz (300 g) ground chicken**
- **2 tablespoons green curry paste (see tip)**
- **7 fl oz (200 ml) coconut milk**
- **2 leeks**

Season the ground chicken with salt and pepper, shape into meatballs and fry them in butter or olive oil until browned.
Meanwhile, slice the leeks into rings and set some of the green leaves aside for the garnish.
Remove the meatballs from the pan; they don't need to be cooked through, only browned.
Don't pour off the dripping and fat unless it's burnt. Put the leek into the pan, add a generous splash of water and then cover. Sauté the leeks for about 6 minutes until tender.
Stir in the coconut milk and 2 tablespoons of green curry paste. Season with salt and pepper, then add the meatballs. Allow to simmer until the meatballs are cooked through.
Serve in a deep dish and garnish with some finely chopped leek greens.

TIP: GREEN CURRY PASTE
Always be careful with curry paste. Taste the curry first to see how spicy it is; you can always add more to taste.

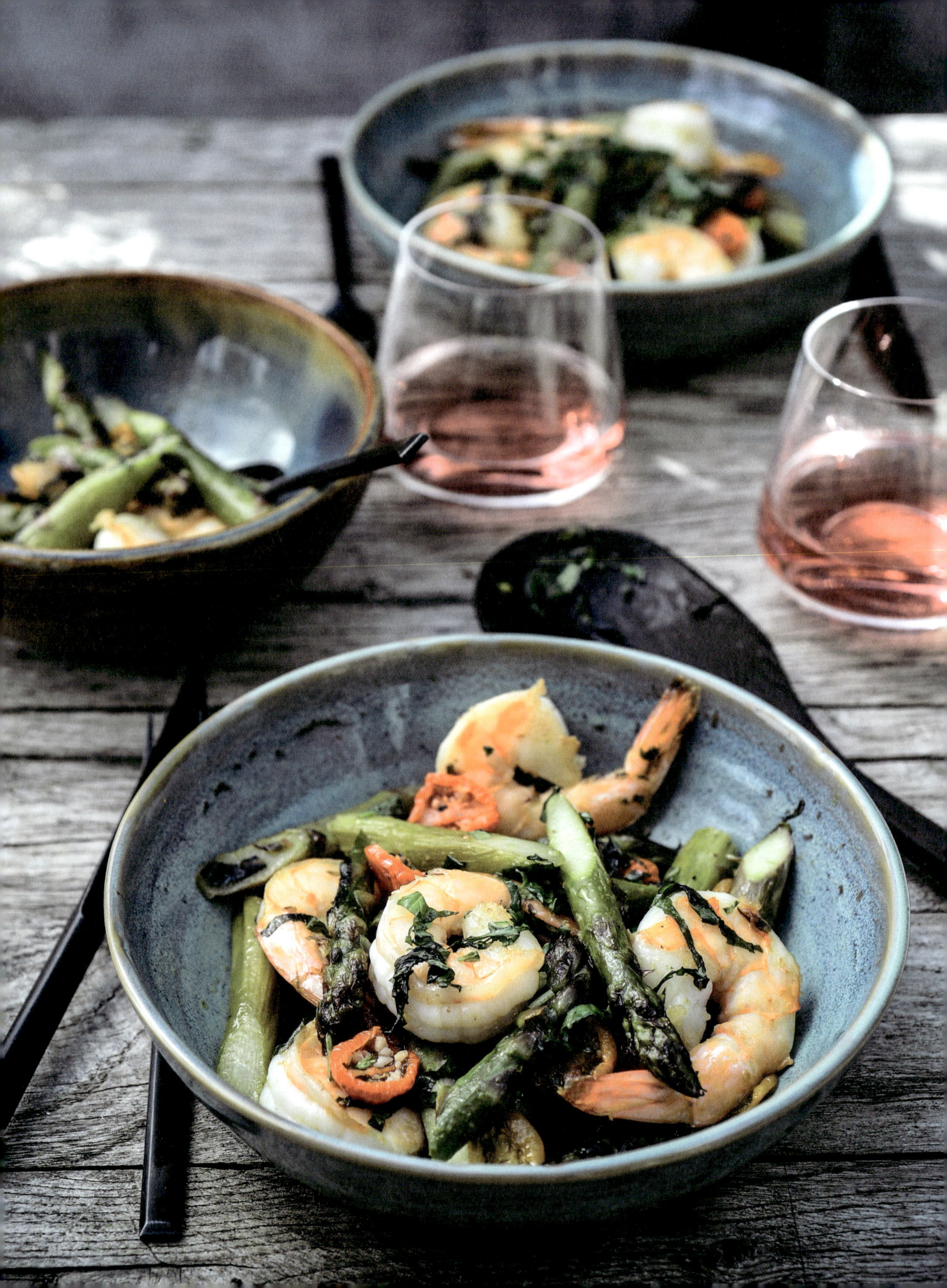

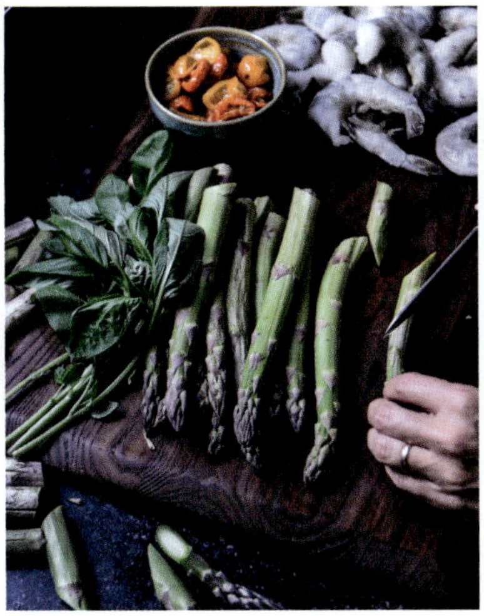
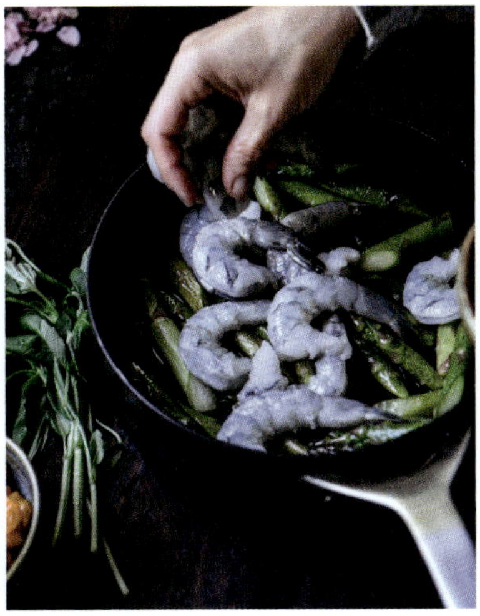
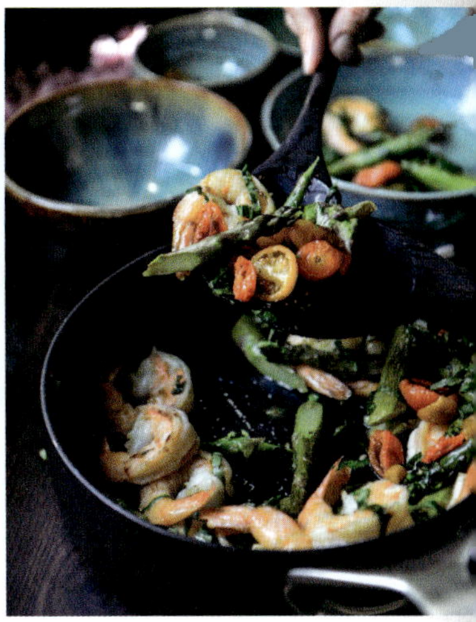

large shrimp ✓ keto

with asparagus and sundried tomatoes

- **1 lb (450 g) large shrimp, peeled (frozen - see tip)**
- **1½ bunches of green asparagus**
- **3½ oz (100 g) sundried tomatoes**
- **¾ oz (20 g) basil**

- soy sauce -

Cut off the hard ends of the asparagus and slice the asparagus into pieces.

Put them in a pan with plenty of olive oil and a small amount of water. Cover the pan and cook for about six minutes. Add the frozen shrimp, cover the pan once more and stir occasionally. Add the sundried tomatoes and the finely chopped basil once the shrimp turns pink (keep a few basil leaves aside for the garnish).

Season with plenty of black pepper and a little bit of salt and add a generous splash of soy sauce. Cook for an additional 2 minutes. Serve in a deep dish and garnish with some fresh basil.

TIP: SHRIMP

Some frozen shrimp contains a lot of moisture, but that creates a lovely broth.

You may have more or less moisture depending on which shrimp you use. Whichever you use, it will always taste good.

Cooking the carrots together with the beets gives them a lovely red color.

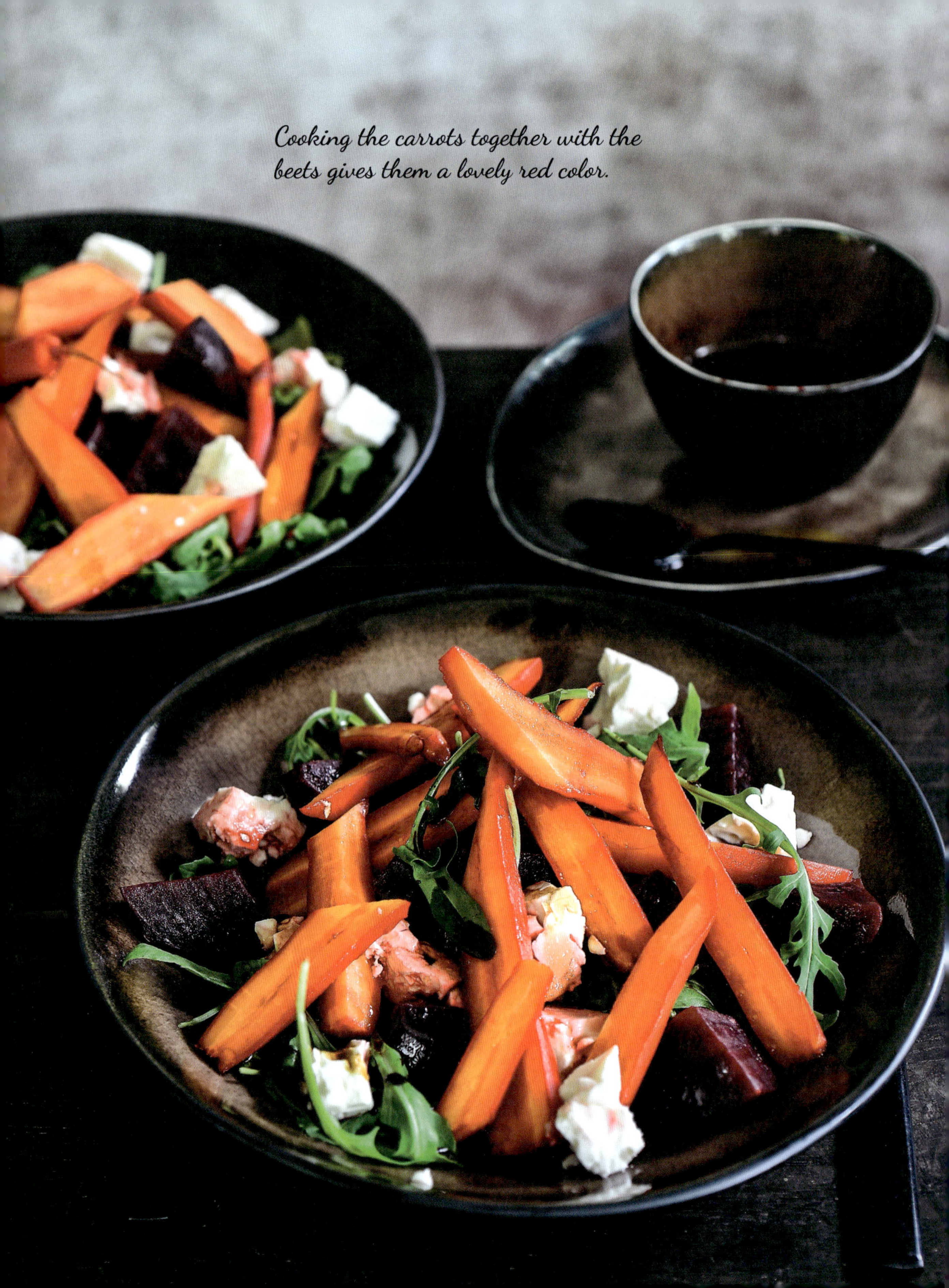

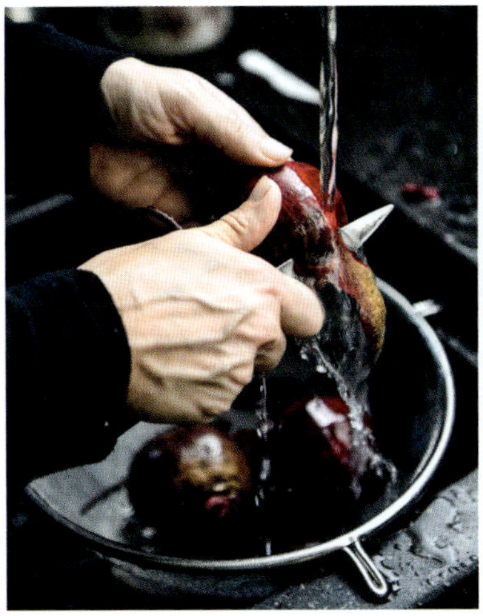

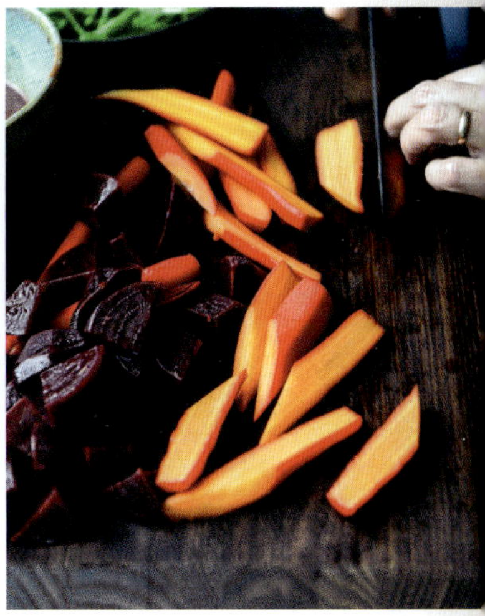

keto

cooked vegetable salad
with feta

- 7 oz (200 g) feta
- 10½ oz (300 g) carrots
- 10½ oz (300 g) red beets
- 3½ oz (100 g) arugula

– soy sauce –
– balsamic vinegar –

Peel the carrots so they can soak up the red color from the beets. Peel the beets under running water so you won't get red fingers. Dice the beets but leave the carrots whole. Cook them together in water with a generous splash of olive oil for about 10 to 13 minutes until tender. Season with salt and pepper. Drain off the water, or perhaps not (see tip). Divide the arugula evenly between the plates. Slice the carrots into pieces and put them, together with the beets, on top of the arugula. Crumble the feta over the top.
Combine 3 tablespoons of olive oil with 1 tablespoon of soy sauce and 1 tablespoon of balsamic vinegar. Serve the sauce separately.

TIP: COOKING LIQUID
The remaining cooking liquid has such a gorgeous red color, I can't bring myself to pour it down the drain. I reduce the liquid and serve it as a soup. You'll be surprised at how good it tastes. This explains why it's important to cook the vegetables with a generous splash of olive oil. Fat provides flavor. You can also add a couple of tablespoons of the liquid to your sauce. Delicious.

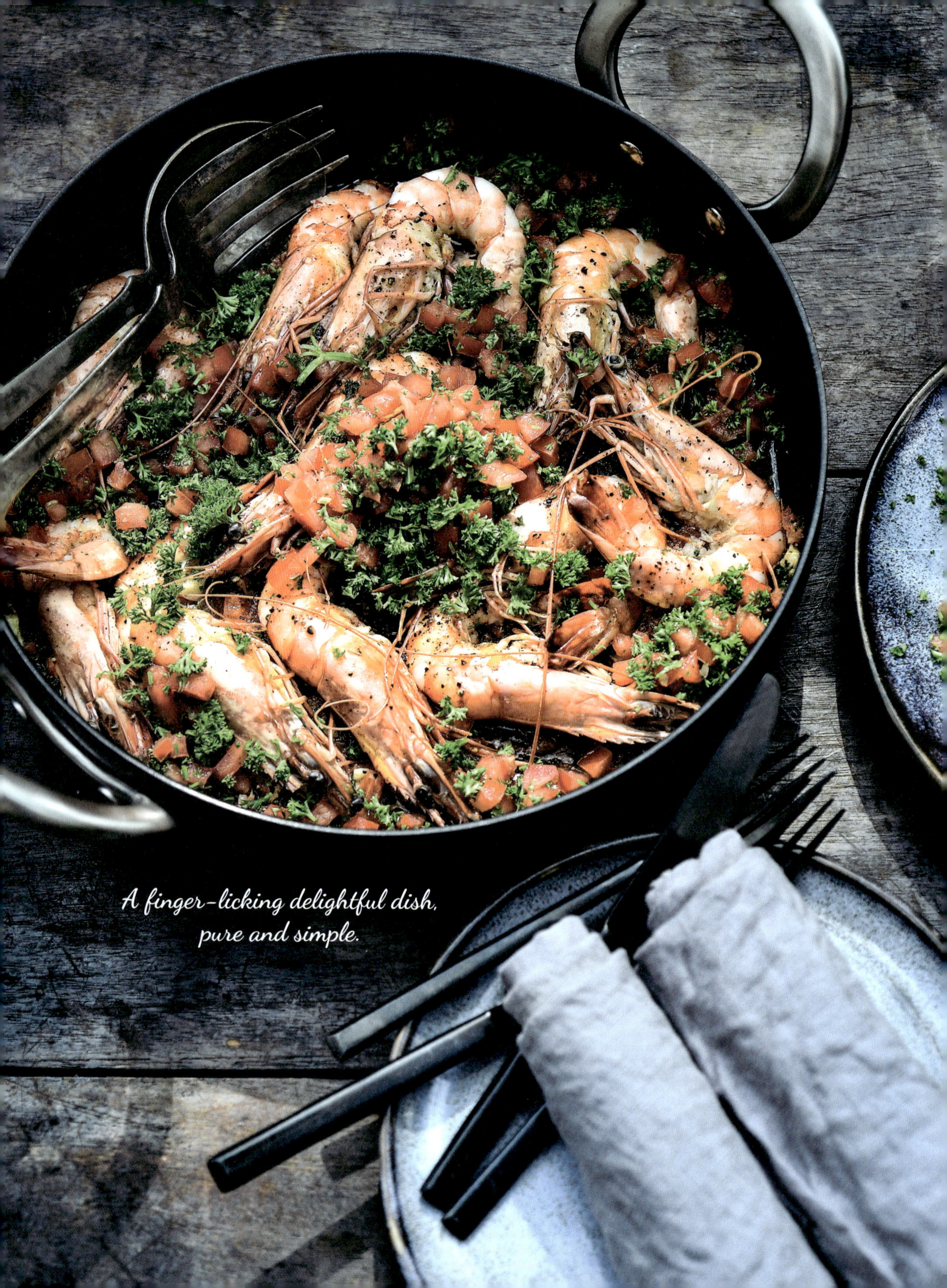

*A finger-licking delightful dish,
pure and simple.*

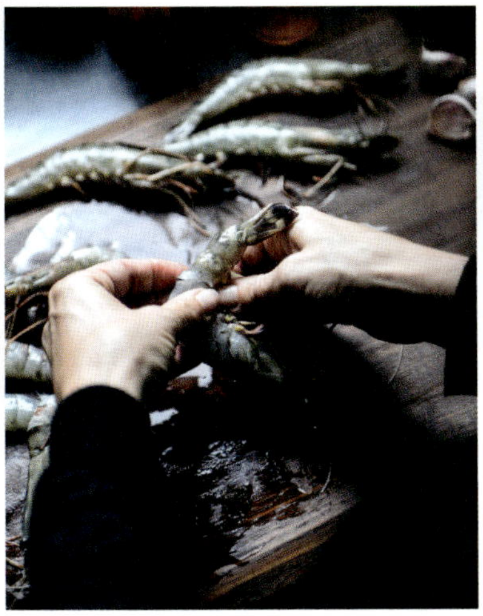

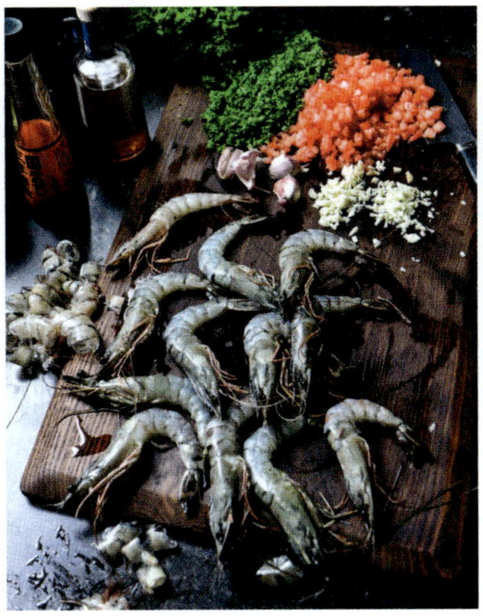

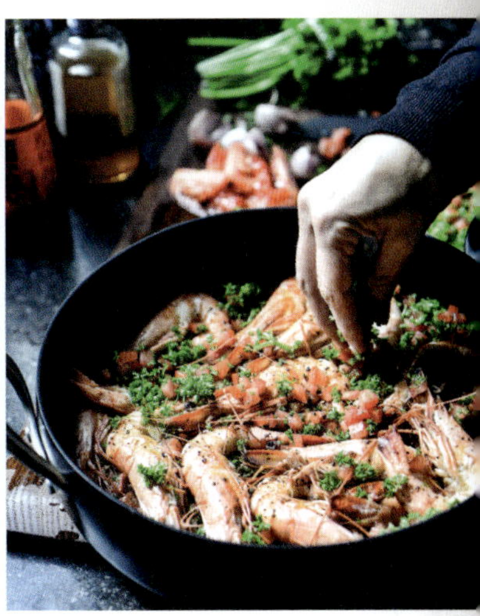

large shrimp

keto

with tomatoes and spring onions

- **10 large shrimp, with head and tail**
- **4 tomatoes**
- **6 spring onions**
- **a handful of curly-leaf parsley**

- fresh garlic -

Peel the shrimp but leave the head and tail attached. Finely chop 2 cloves of garlic and the parsley. Quarter the tomatoes, remove the seeds and dice the flesh. Slice the spring onions into small pieces. Pour a generous splash of olive oil into a pan and briefly sauté the garlic. After 30 seconds, add half the diced tomatoes, half the spring onions and half the parsley. Season with salt and pepper. Cook for about 2 minutes. Stir the sauce and add the shrimp to the pan. Drizzle a bit more olive oil over the top. Cover the pan and cook for 1 minute. Turn the shrimp over and cook for another minute until cooked through.

Just before serving, stir in the remaining diced tomatoes, spring onions and parsley. Finish with some extra olive oil, black pepper and a little bit of salt if necessary before serving.

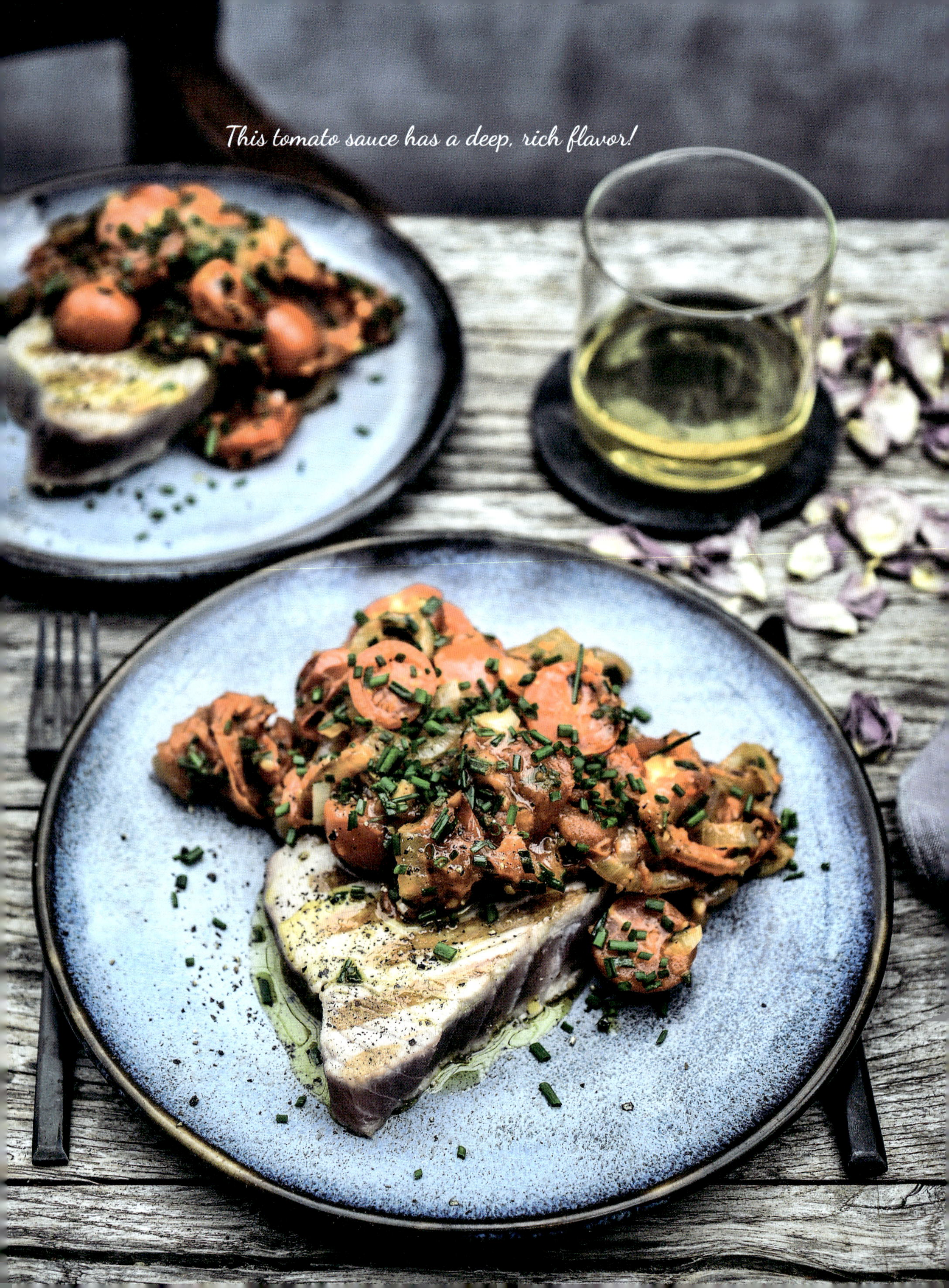

This tomato sauce has a deep, rich flavor!

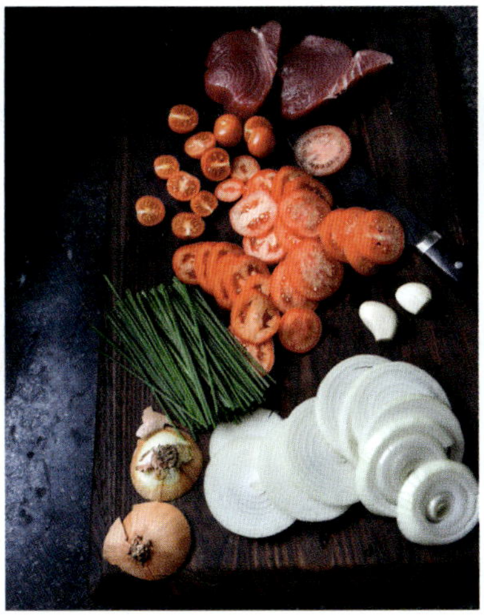
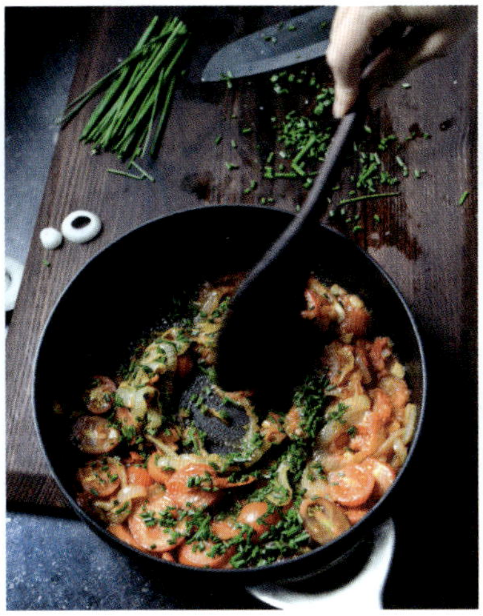
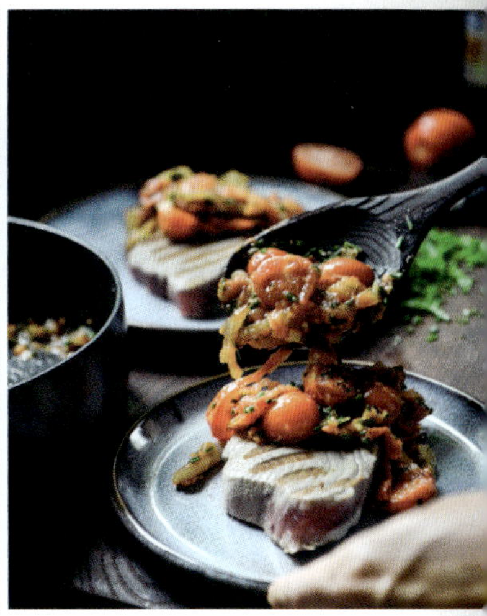

tuna
keto

with chunky tomato sauce

- **2 tuna fillets (with MSC label - see tip)**
- **10½ oz (300 g) various types of tomatoes (large and small)**
- **1 large onion**
- **1 bunch of chives**

- *fresh garlic* -

Slice the onions into rings and sauté them in plenty of olive oil. Slice the large tomatoes and cut the small tomatoes in half. After 4 minutes of cooking time, add three quarters of the tomatoes to the onions. Finely chop 2 cloves of garlic and add them to the pan. Let the vegetables sauté for another four minutes. Grill or fry the tuna for 1 minute on each side. Remove the onions and tomatoes from the heat and add the remaining tomatoes.

Finely chop the chives and mix three quarters of them into the sauce. Season with salt and pepper. Arrange the tuna onto the plates and spoon the sauce over half the fillet. Garnish with the remaining chives, some black pepper and a drizzle of olive oil.

TIP: MSC LABEL

The MSC label guarantees that the fish is caught with respect for the environment and fish populations. The label is managed by the Marine Stewardship Council, an independent non-profit organization for the promotion of sustainable fishing practices.

The label is found on wild-caught fish.

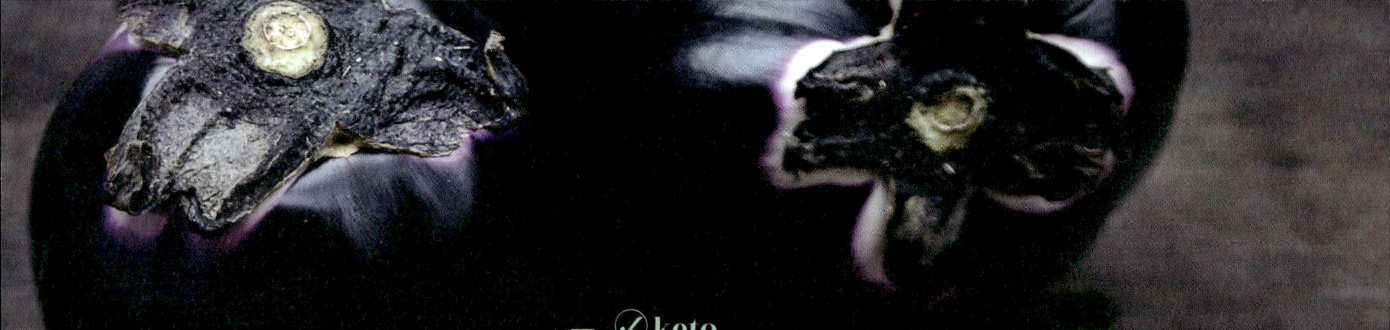

✓ keto

sautéed eggplant

with lamb

- 2 small eggplants (see tip)
- 2 lamb fillets
- 2 spring onions
- 4 sprigs of rosemary

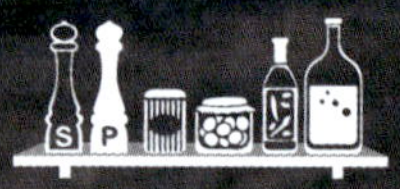

- fresh garlic -

Slice the eggplant into thick strips. Rub them with plenty of olive oil, season with salt and sauté them, covered, in a pan (see tip). Stir regularly to make sure they don't burn. Season towards the end with black pepper. Remove the rosemary leaves from the stems. Finely chop 2 cloves of garlic. Splash some olive oil into a pan and add the garlic and rosemary.
Sear the lamb for 2 minutes on each side, leaving the inside pink. Finely chop the spring onions. Place the lamb meat with the herbs on a plate and arrange the eggplant next to the meat. Garnish with the spring onions.

TIP: SAUTÉING EGGPLANT

Eggplant soaks up a lot of oil. You can just keep pouring it on, but the trick is not to use too much oil. That's why it's handy to use a non-stick pan and to stir regularly to make sure the eggplant doesn't burn. This takes about 10 minutes, but the result is definitely worth it.
Eggplant is available in different colors and shapes. I always like to experiment with them. The taste doesn't change much, but the shape does. I buy large eggplants whenever I see them. I also use them as decoration. How fun is it that you can eat your decorations?

I will admit that not everyone loves eggplant as much as I do. Some people do not react well to certain substances found in vegetables in the nightshade family, which includes eggplant. If you're not sure, start off with a small serving. You can also sprinkle some coarse sea salt over the pieces of raw eggplant and then leave them for 10 minutes to remove the moisture. This makes them easier to digest. Make sure to rinse the salt off of the eggplant afterwards.

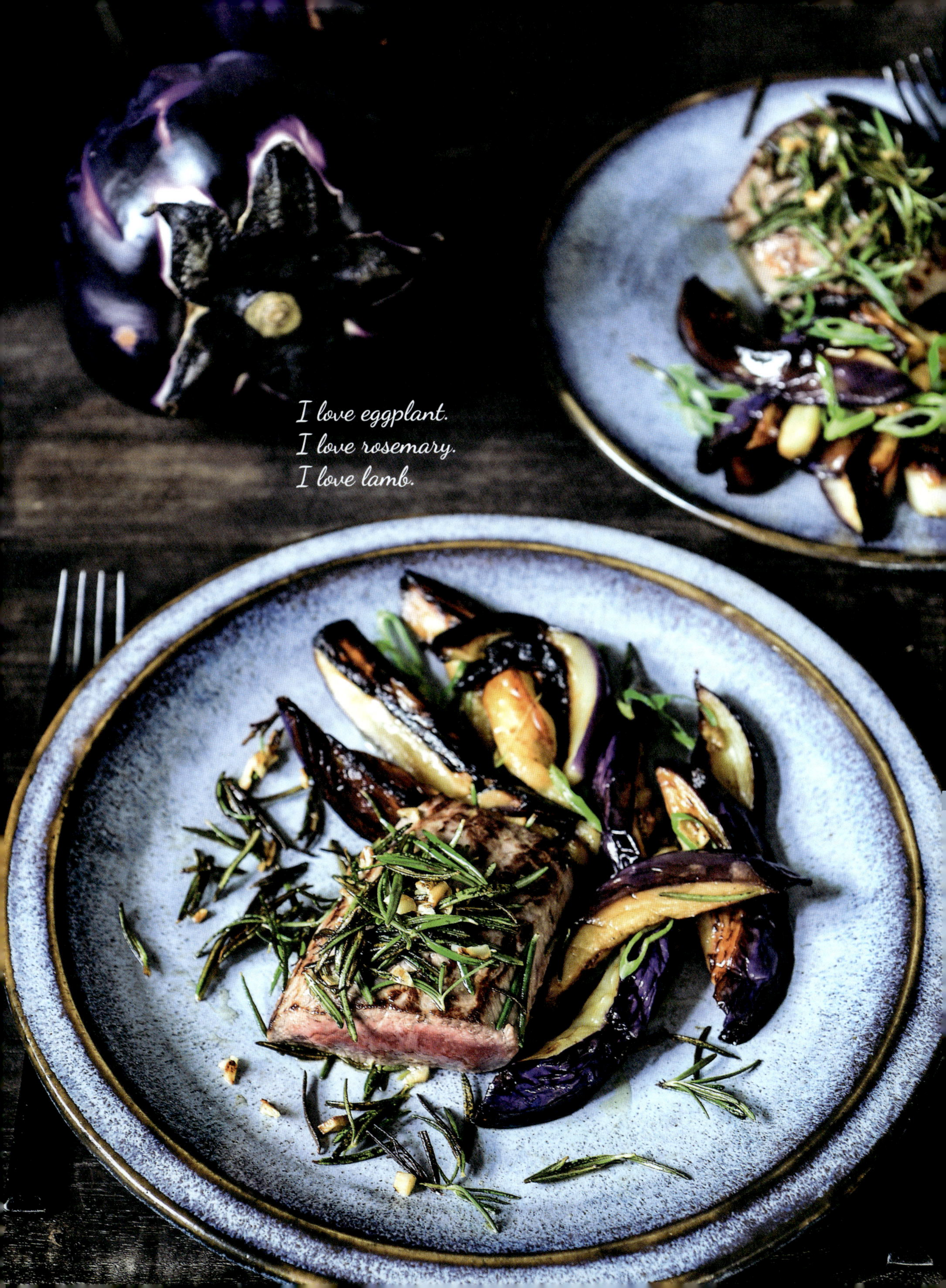

I love eggplant.
I love rosemary.
I love lamb.

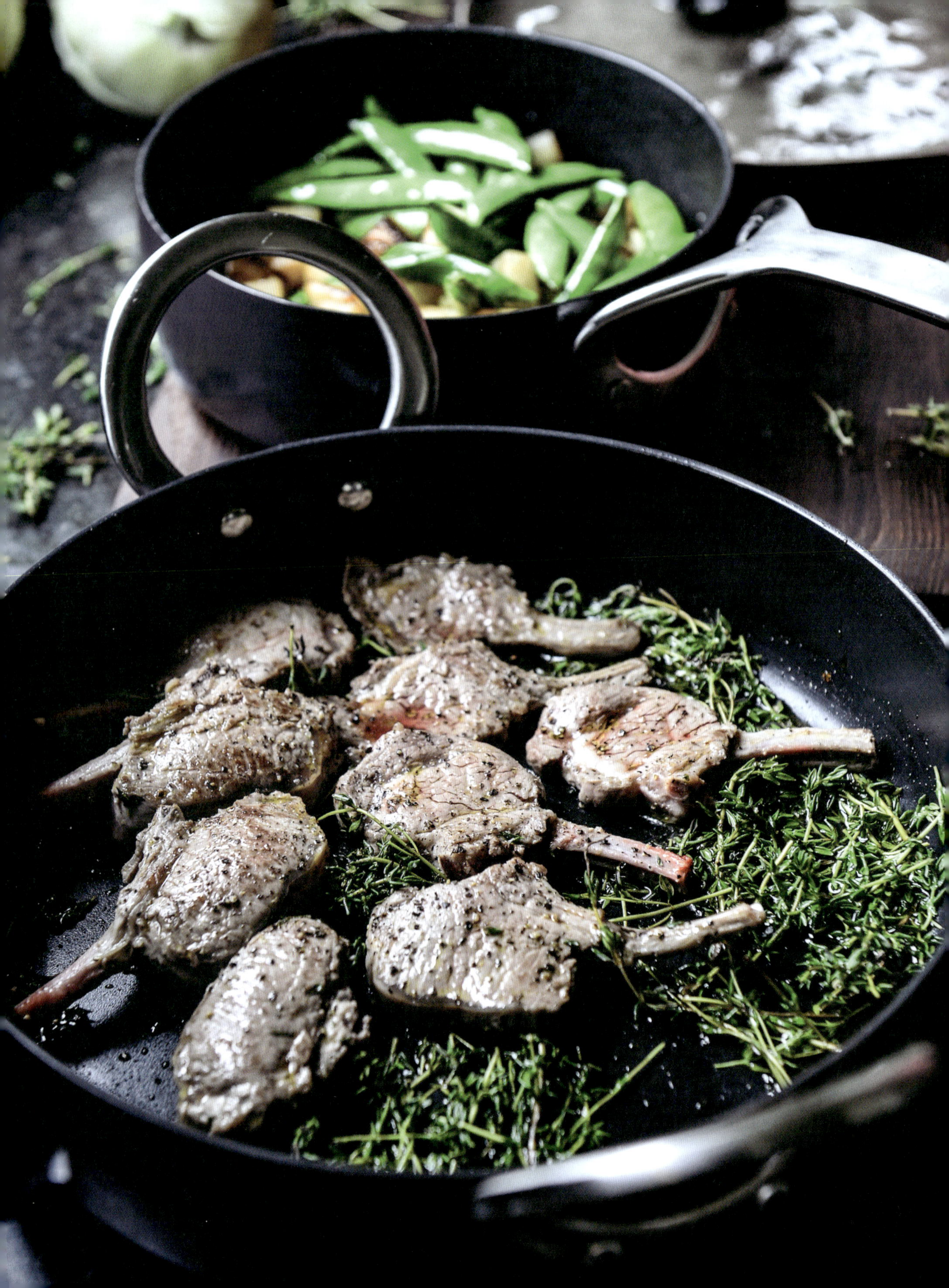

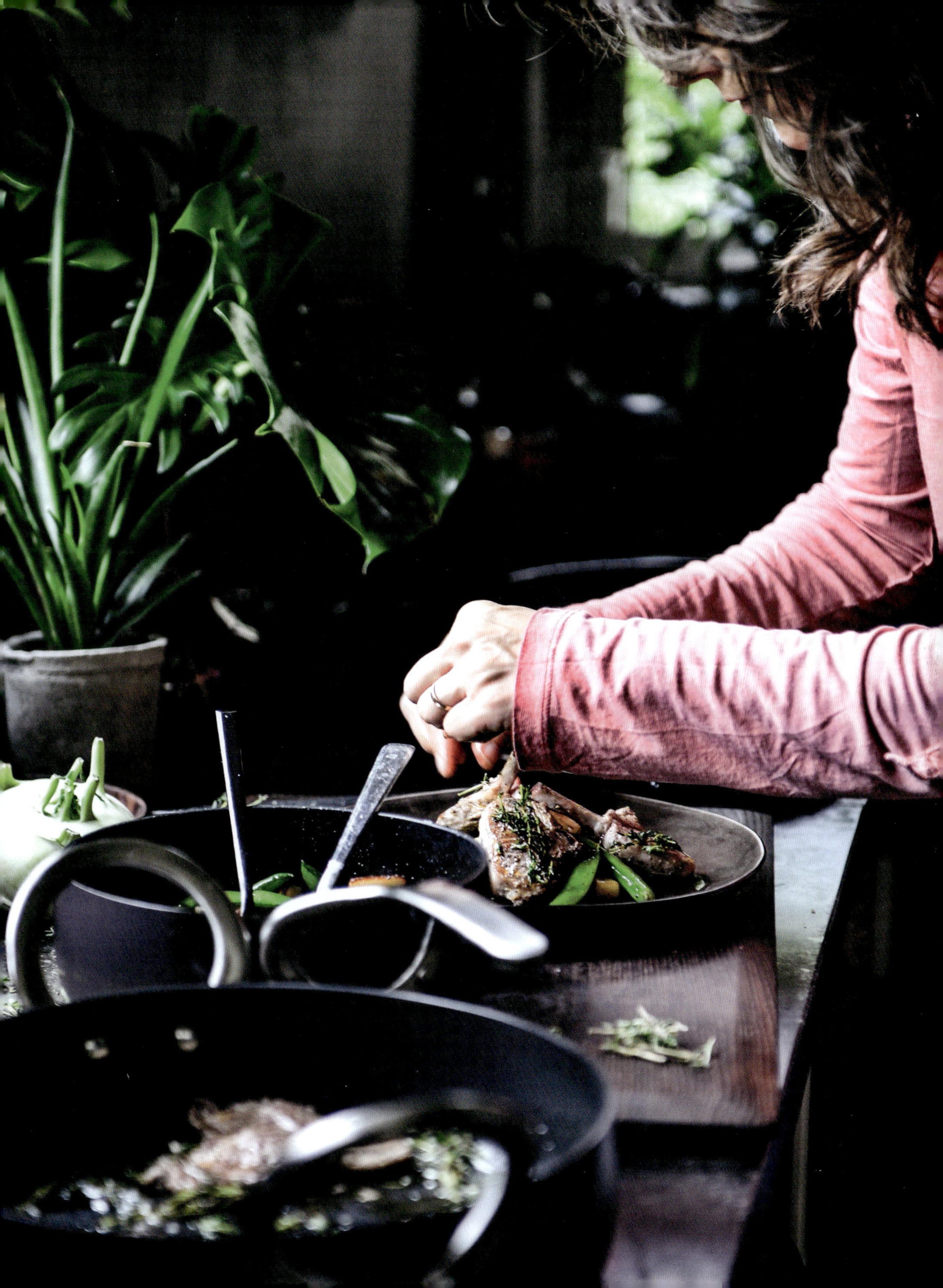

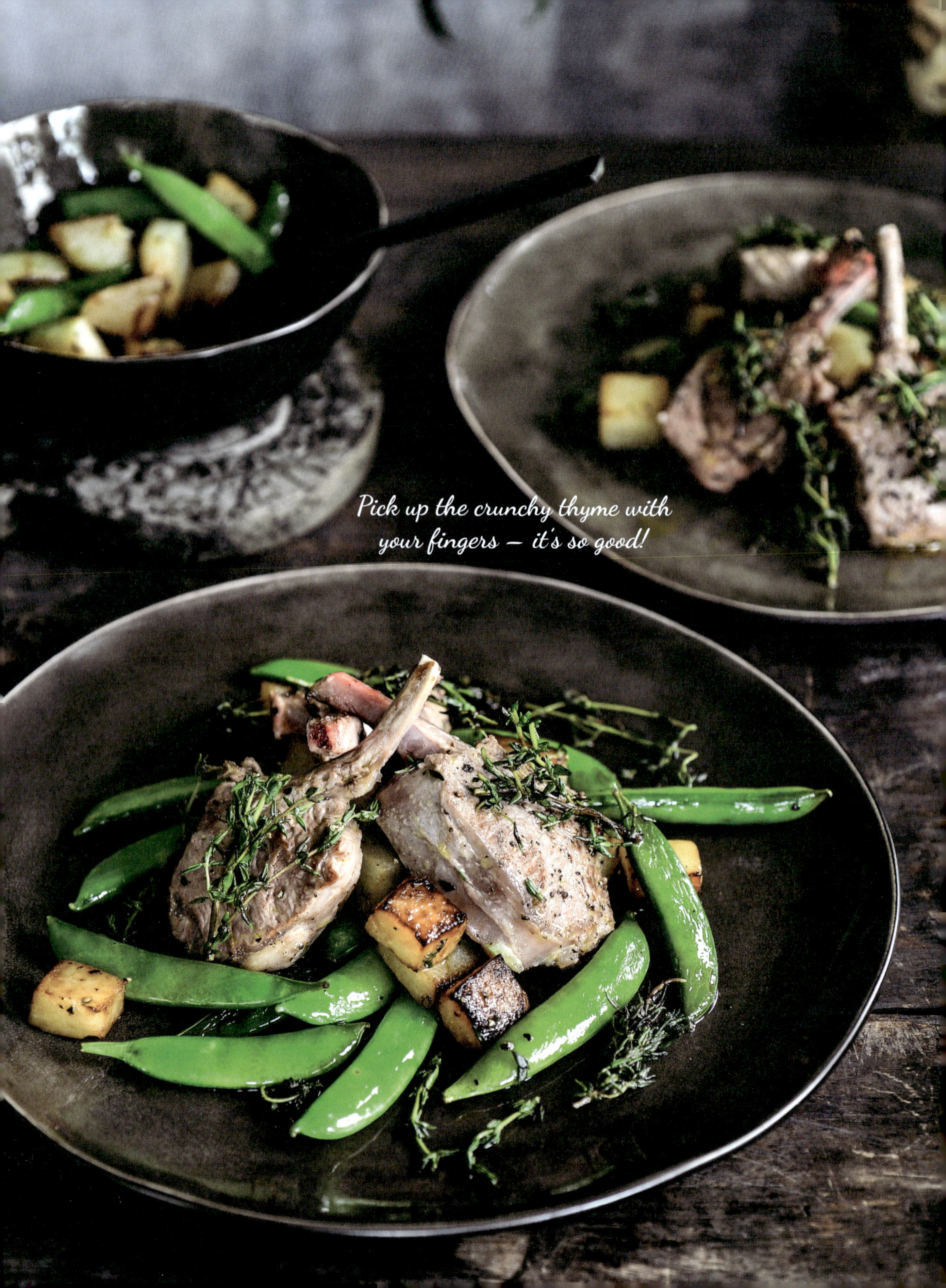

Pick up the crunchy thyme with your fingers – it's so good!

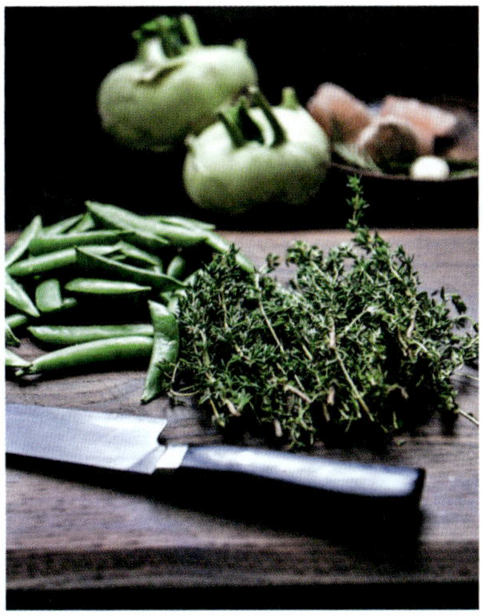 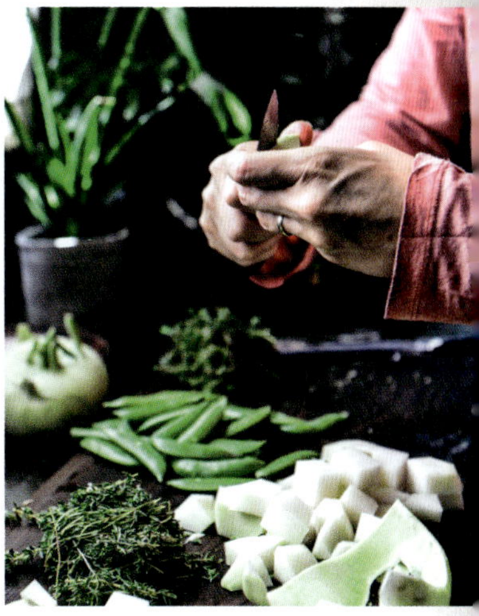

lamb ✓keto

with kohlrabi and sugar snap peas

- **1 rack of lamb**
- **2 kohlrabi (21 oz/600 g)**
- **7 oz (200 g) sugar snap peas**
- **1 bunch of fresh young thyme (¾ oz/20 g)**

Peel the kohlrabi and chop into large pieces. Sauté the kohlrabi in plenty of olive oil with a small glass of water. Season with salt and pepper.

Meanwhile, slice the rack of lamb into chops, cutting between the bones.

Finely chop the soft part at the top of the thyme sprigs and remove the leaves from the harder stem at the bottom.

Add the sugar snap peas to the kohlrabi as soon as it is almost tender and stir-fry for a few more moments. Season with salt and pepper.

In a separate pan, sear the lamb chops over a high heat and immediately add the thyme.

Two minutes per side should be enough; the meat should remain nice and pink on the inside. Season with salt and pepper.

Spoon the vegetables onto a plate and arrange the lamb on top with the bones pointing upwards. Garnish with the crunchy thyme.

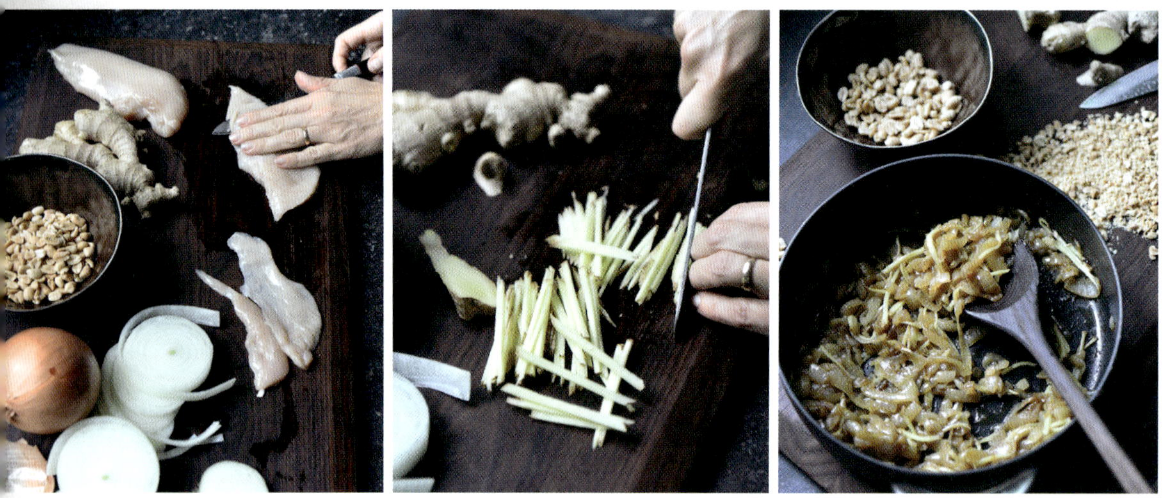

chicken

keto

with caramelized onion and ginger

- **2 chicken breasts**
- **2-inch (5 cm) ginger root**
- **2 large yellow onions**
- **a handful of peanuts**

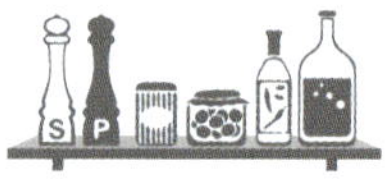

– soy sauce –

Thinly slice the onions and put them in a pan with plenty of olive oil.

Slice the ginger into matchsticks, leaving the skin on, and add to the onions.

Cook the onion and ginger for 15 to 20 minutes over a low heat until the onion is brown and caramelized. Cover the pan for the first 10 minutes to speed up the cooking process and stir regularly to make sure the onions don't burn. Season with salt and pepper.

Slice the chicken horizontally into thin slices. Don't worry if they're not perfectly even, they'll look fine after they're cooked. Coarsely chop the peanuts.

Brown the chicken slices in a separate pan. Season with salt and pepper.

Place the chicken slices on a plate, arrange the onions next to the chicken and sprinkle some chopped peanuts over the top. Make a sauce with 2 tablespoons of olive oil and 2 tablespoons of soy sauce and finish the dish with the sauce.

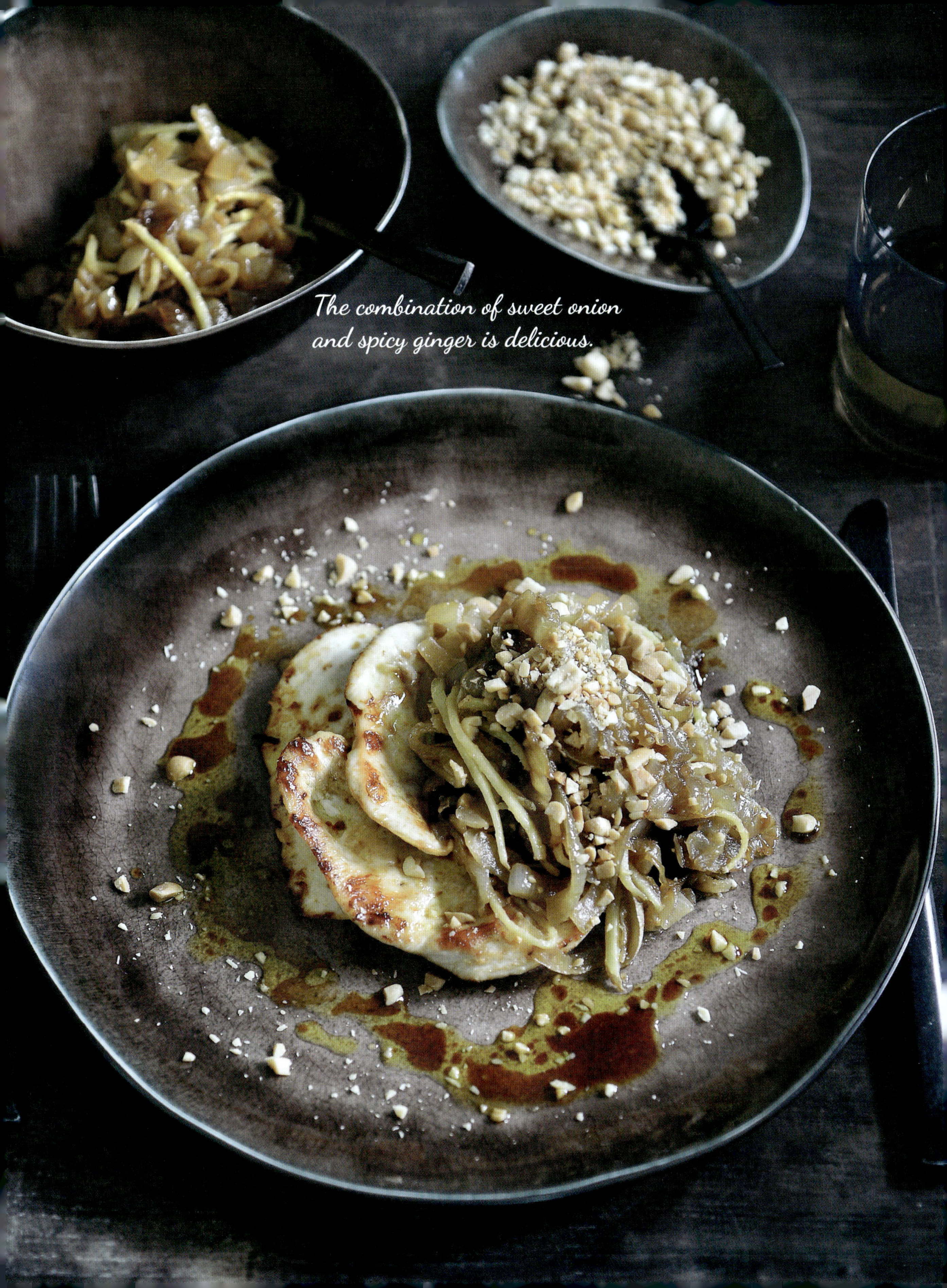
The combination of sweet onion
and spicy ginger is delicious.

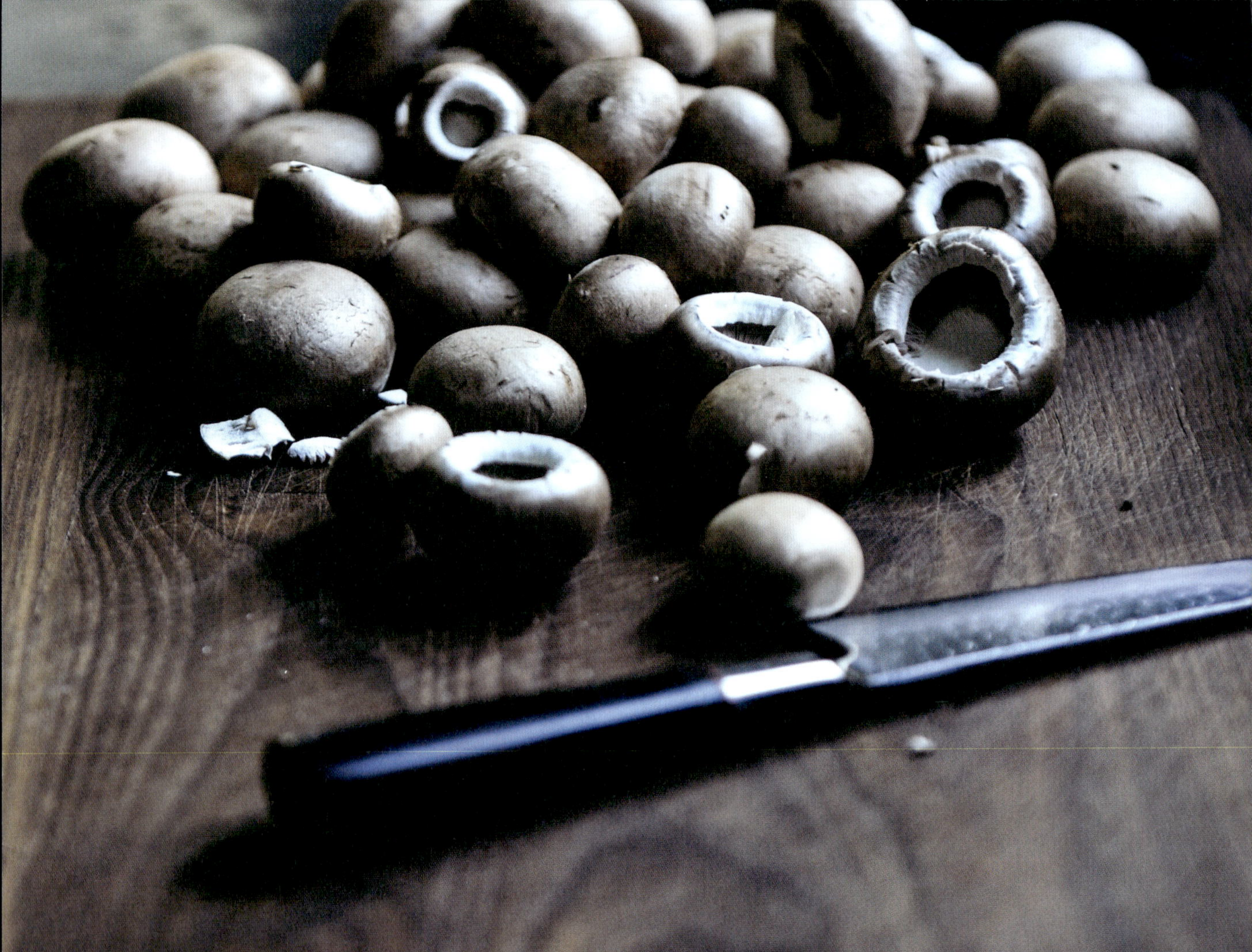

chicken ✓ keto

with mushroom cream sauce

- **a little over 1 lb (500 g) brown mushrooms**
- **2 small chicken breasts**
- **3½ oz (100 g) bacon, diced**
- **4½ fl oz (125 ml) cream**

Fry the chicken together with the bacon in some olive oil until brown on both sides. Remove the stems from the mushrooms and add the mushroom caps to the meat. Add a little olive oil if necessary. Season with salt and pepper, cover the pan and cook briefly until the mushrooms start to lose moisture. Add the cream and cook a little longer until the chicken is completely cooked through.

A timeless dish, always sure to please.

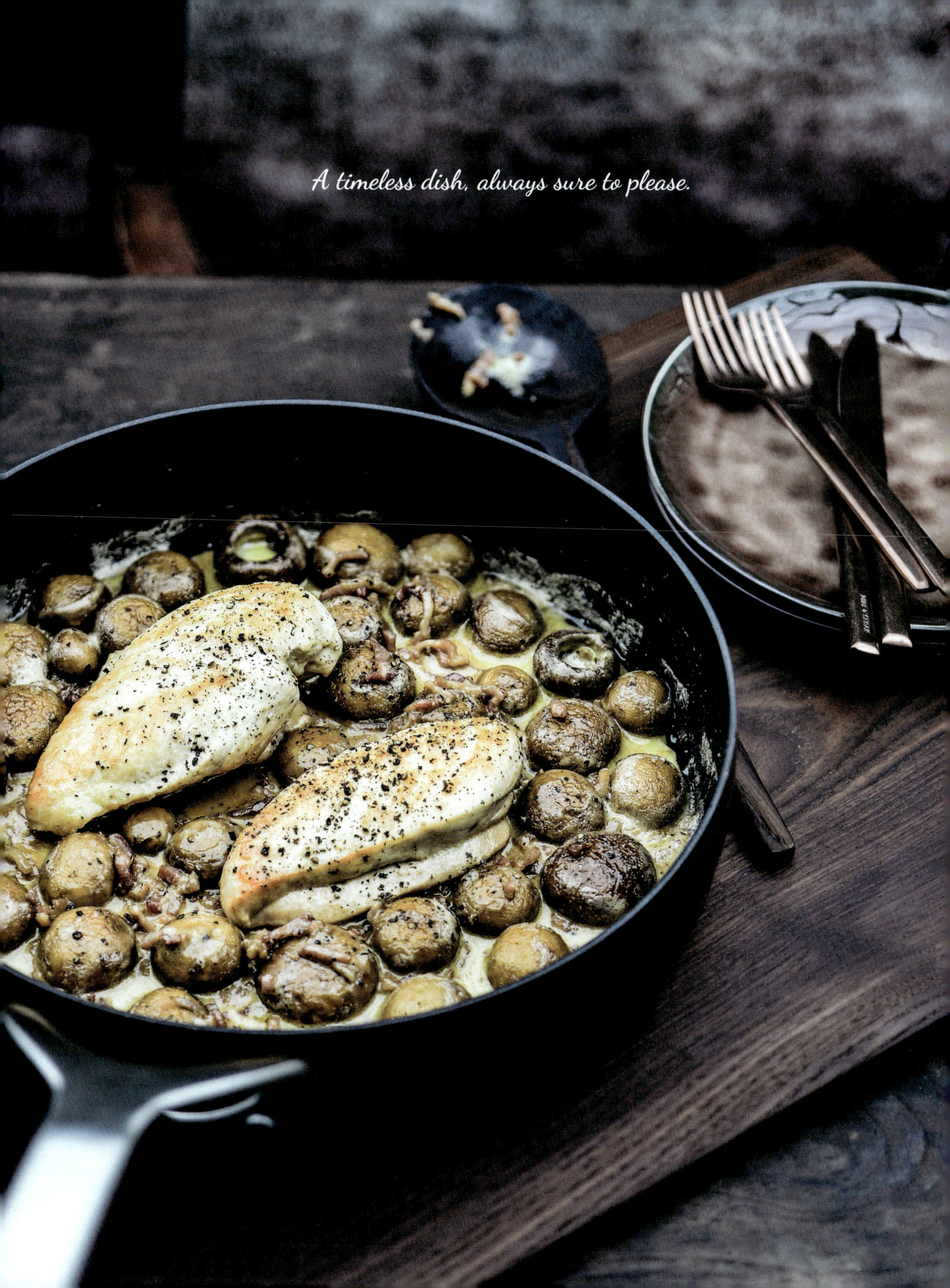

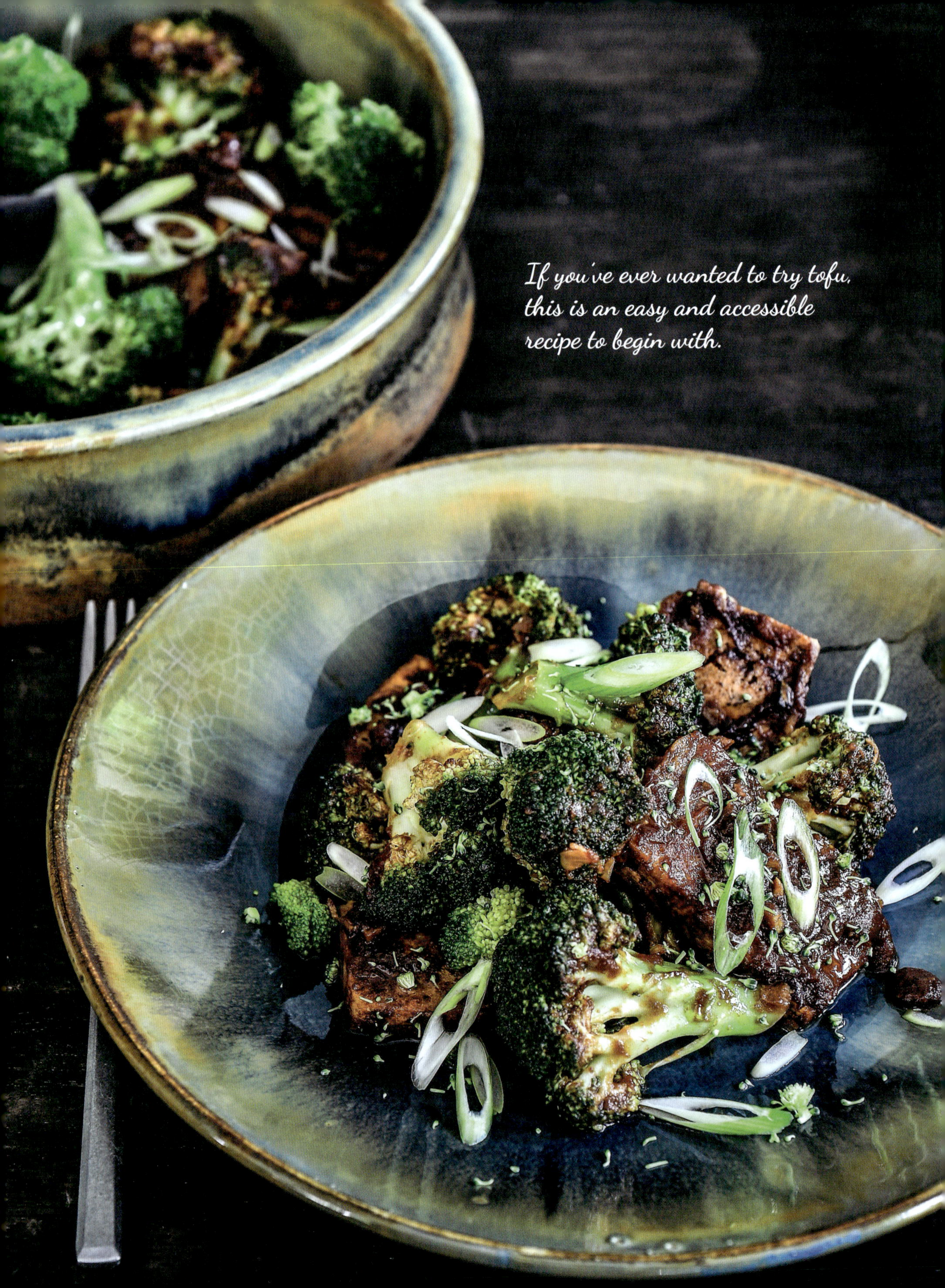

If you've ever wanted to try tofu, this is an easy and accessible recipe to begin with.

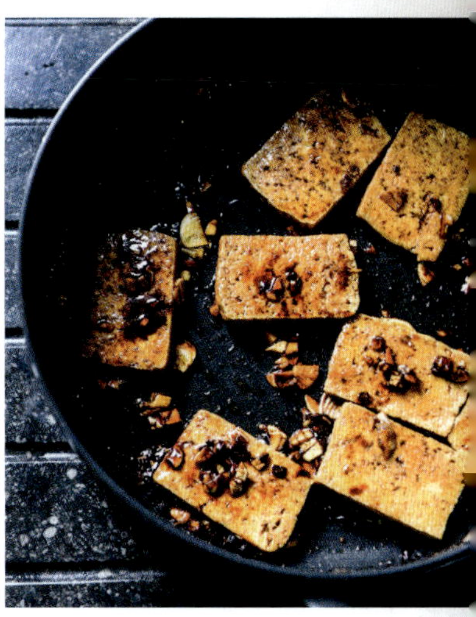

vegan

Chinese-style tofu

and broccoli

- **1 package tofu (about 350g - see tip)**
- **300 g passata**
- **1 broccoli**
- **2 spring onions, finely sliced**

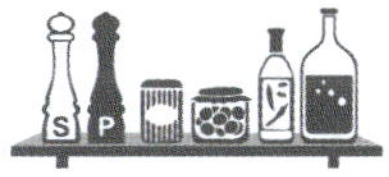

- soy sauce -
- balsamic vinegar -
- fresh garlic -

Cut the broccoli into florets and cook until tender in some water with a generous splash of olive oil. Slice the tofu into ¼-inch (0.5 cm) slices and fry them for 2 minutes on each side in plenty of olive oil until they turn light brown. Finely chop 3 cloves of garlic and add them to the pan. Add 2 tablespoons of soy sauce and 2 tablespoons of balsamic vinegar. Be careful as this may spatter; cover the pan to be on the safe side. After 1 minute, turn the tofu slices over and cook on the other side. Add the passata and cook for an additional 2 minutes. Stir in the broccoli florets just before serving and garnish with the finely chopped spring onions.

TIP: TOFU

Tofu comes from China. The first references to tofu date back to about two thousand years ago. Tofu was later introduced in Japan. It is made by curdling soymilk, a process that is also used in cheesemaking. Tofu is rich in proteins. I don't like to use the term "meat substitute", because nothing can replace meat. I see it more as an addition to my rich and diverse cuisine. Soy products are generally considered exceptionally healthy, but you sometimes hear conflicting messages about genetic modification and the fact that soybeans contain antinutrients. Fermented soy products such as miso, soy sauce and tempeh contain the lowest levels of antinutrients. Tofu itself is very bland, but it's an excellent absorber of other flavors. The tofu in this recipe is a great example of this.

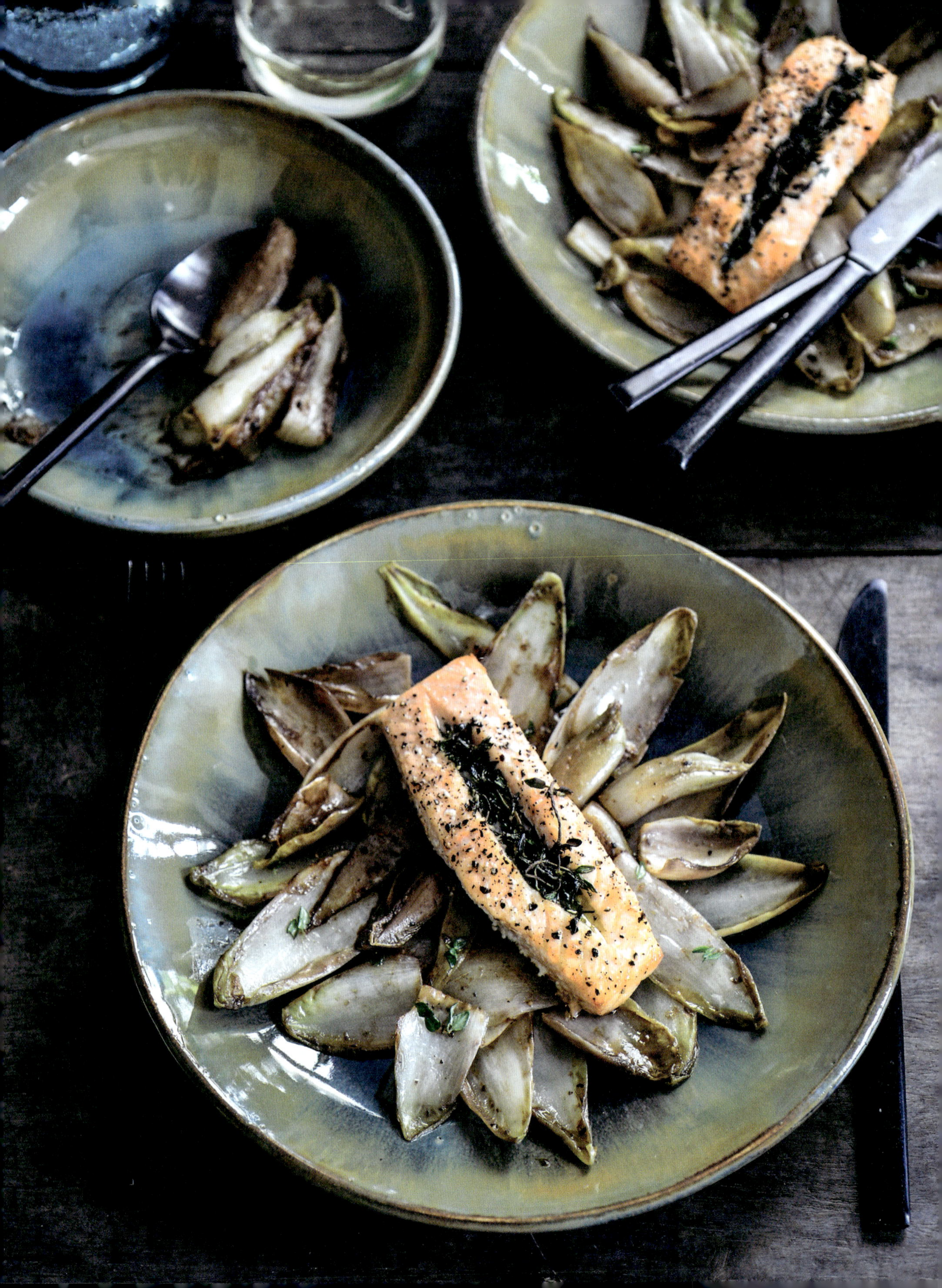

The miso instantly gives this recipe a deliciously intense flavor.

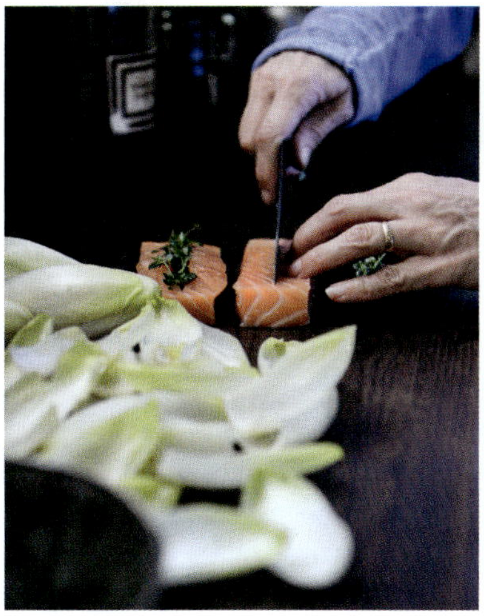

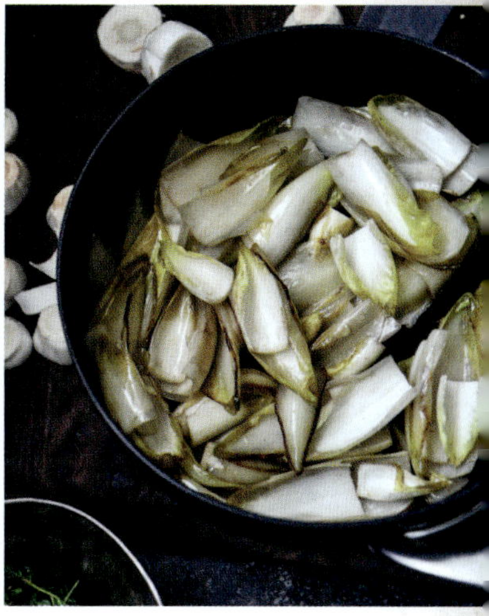

salmon

keto

with fresh thyme and endive in miso

- **2 salmon fillets**
- **about 5 sprigs fresh thyme**
- **10 to 12 endives**
- **1 tablespoon brown miso (see tip)**

– butter –

Preheat the oven to 400 °F (200 °C). Chop the soft tops of the fresh thyme and combine with a splash of olive oil. Season with salt and pepper. Score the salmon fillets lengthwise, making cuts about ¼ inch (0.5 cm) deep, and put the thyme inside the cuts. Place the salmon in a baking dish and bake for about 10 minutes in the oven. Put a pan with butter over the heat. Cut off the bottoms of the endives and separate the leaves. Put the leaves in the pan and stir constantly. Season with some pepper. The leaves you have put into the pan first will be soft and cooked through while the top leaves will remain crunchy. The different textures make this dish so delicious! Dissolve the miso in a little bit of water and pour it over the endive in the final moments of cooking. Season with salt and pepper. Spoon the endive onto a plate and arrange the salmon fillet on top.

TIP: BROWN MISO

Miso is a Japanese fermented soybean paste with a distinct umami flavor. Miso comes in different colors varying from light to dark. The darker the miso, the stronger and saltier the flavor. Miso is available in Asian specialty stores, but these days you can also find it on many supermarket shelves. For this recipe, use hatcho miso, genmai miso, or any other type of brown miso.

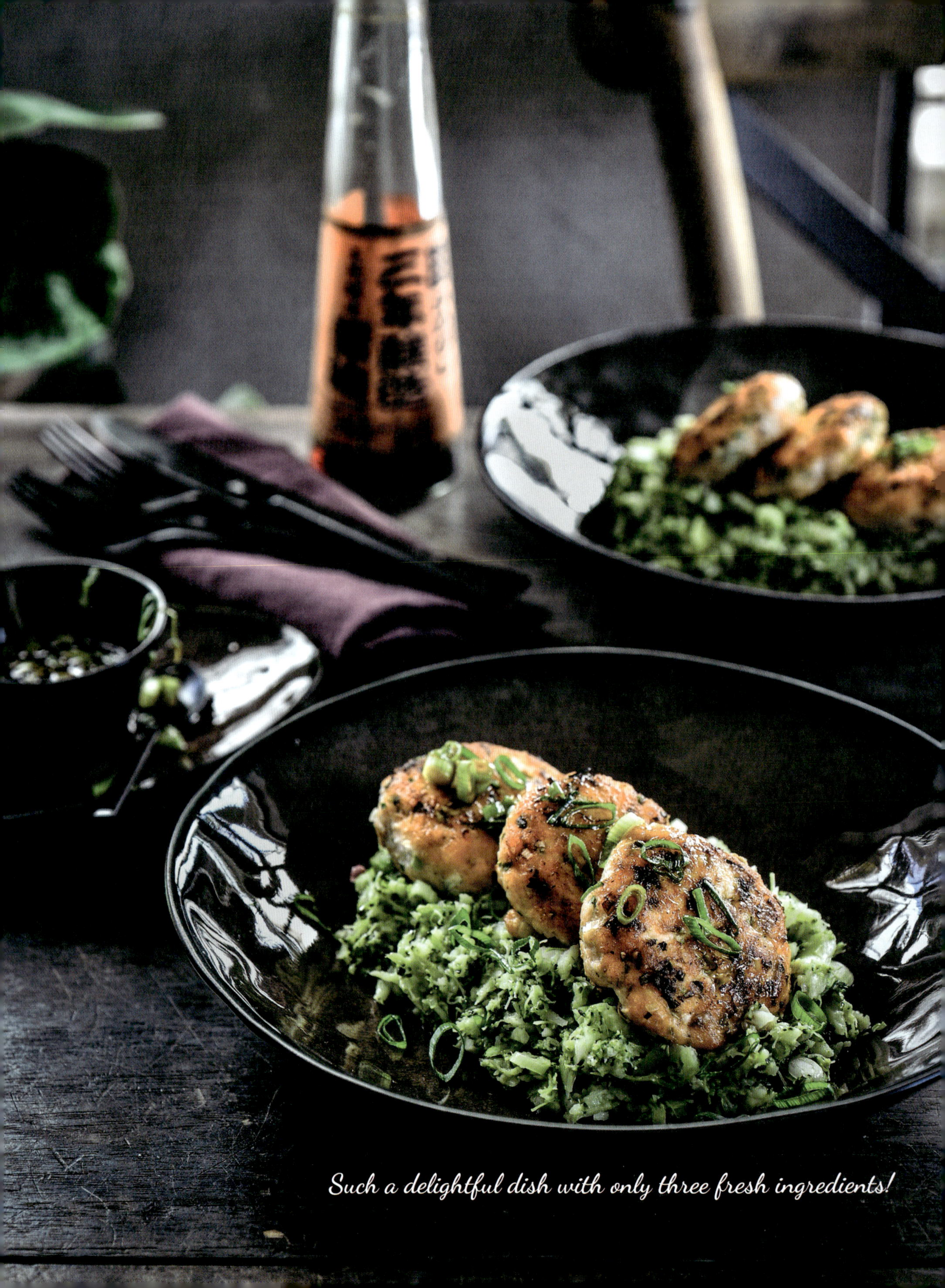
Such a delightful dish with only three fresh ingredients!

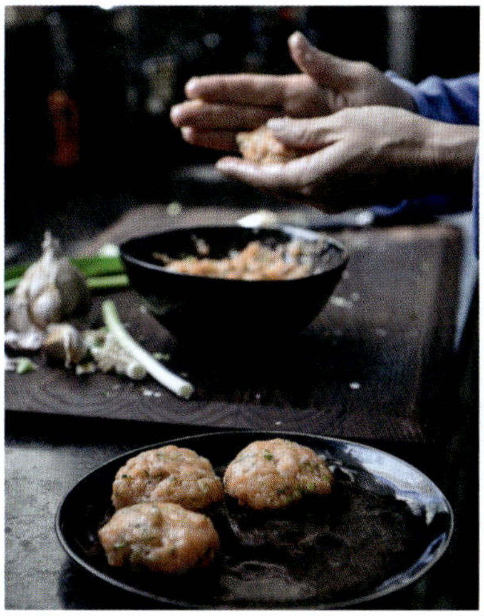

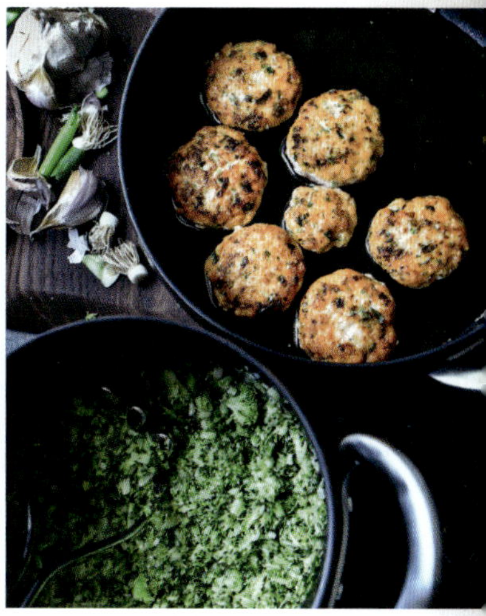

salmon burgers ✓ keto

with broccoli puree

- **2 salmon fillets, without skin**
- **1 head of broccoli**
- **8 spring onions**

– fresh garlic –
– soy sauce –

Finely chop 5 spring onions and cut the broccoli into florets. Sauté the spring onions with the broccoli in some water and a generous splash of olive oil until tender. Finely chop 2 cloves of garlic and 2 spring onions. Put them together with the salmon in a mixer, add some salt and pepper and mix the ingredients together.

Shape the ground salmon into burger patties and fry them for 2 minutes on each side in plenty of olive oil. Drain the broccoli, add a generous splash of olive oil and blend or mash the broccoli to a puree. Season with salt and pepper. Finely chop the remaining spring onion and make a sauce with 4 tablespoons of soy sauce, 2 tablespoons of olive oil and the finely chopped onion. Serve the broccoli puree on a plate, place a salmon burger on top and serve with the soy sauce.

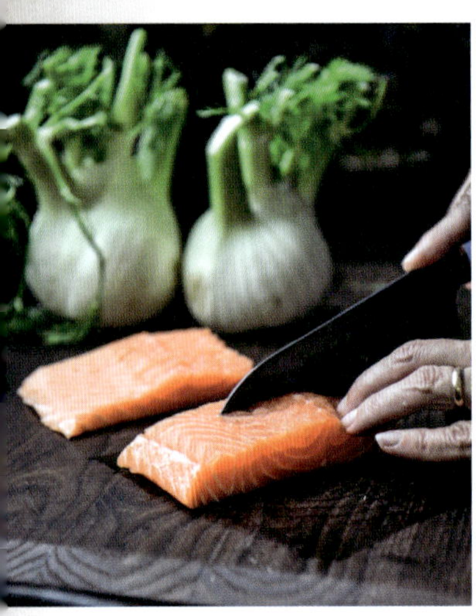

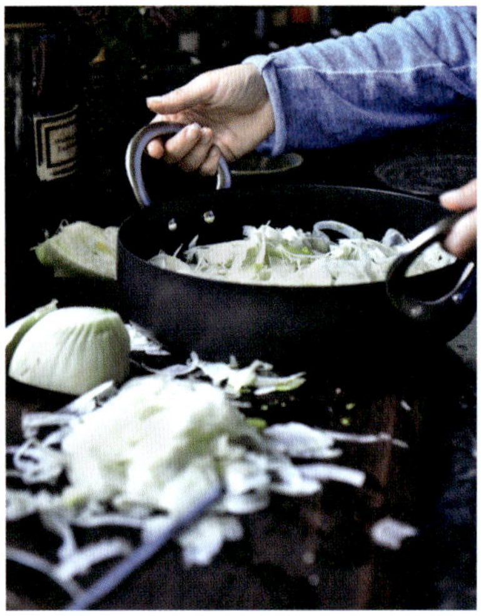

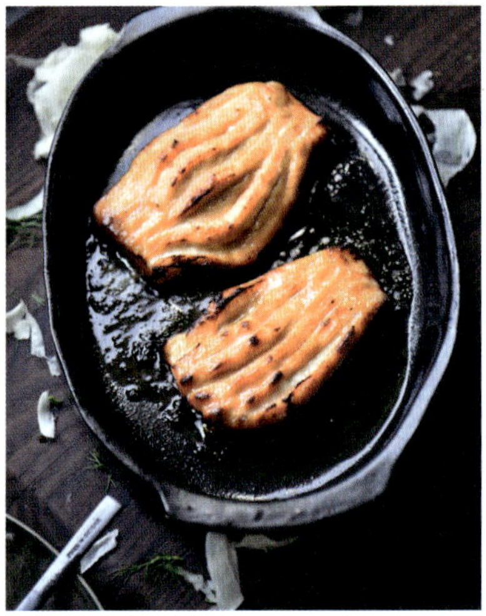

salmon
✓ keto

with miso and fennel

- **2 salmon fillets, without skin**
- **2 level tablespoons shiro miso (see tip)**
- **2 fennel bulbs**
- **roasted sesame seeds**

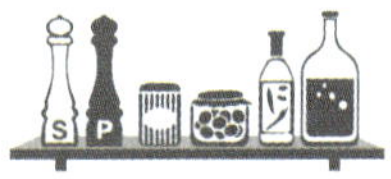

– *soy sauce* –

Preheat the oven to 400 °F (200 °C). Score the salmon with cuts measuring ¼ inch (0.5 cm) deep (see photo). Combine 2 tablespoons of miso with 2 tablespoons of soy sauce and coat the salmon with the mixture, making sure to rub it into the cuts as well. Place the salmon in a baking dish and bake for about 10 minutes in the oven.
Slice the fennel into thin slices. Save some of the fluffy green tops from the fennel to use as garnish. Cook the fennel, covered, in a pan with some olive oil and a small amount of water for about 8 minutes. Stir occasionally to make sure the fennel colors without burning. Season with salt and pepper. Place the fennel on the plates and arrange the salmon fillets on top. Garnish with some of the fennel tops and sprinkle some sesame seeds over the dish.

TIP: SHIRO MISO
Miso is a Japanese paste made from fermented soybeans, rice or barley. The color indicates how long the miso has been fermented. The shorter the fermentation period, the lighter the color and the milder and sweeter the taste. The longer the fermentation period, the more intense and saltier the flavor.
For this recipe, I used shiro miso; a lightly fermented, white miso with a mild, sweet taste. This paste goes well with fish, root vegetables and ginger and is even delicious in desserts.
One spoonful of shiro miso is about 10 grams and contains 1/10 of an ounce (2.8 g) of carbohydrates. This recipe also works well in a keto diet because you use so little of the miso paste.

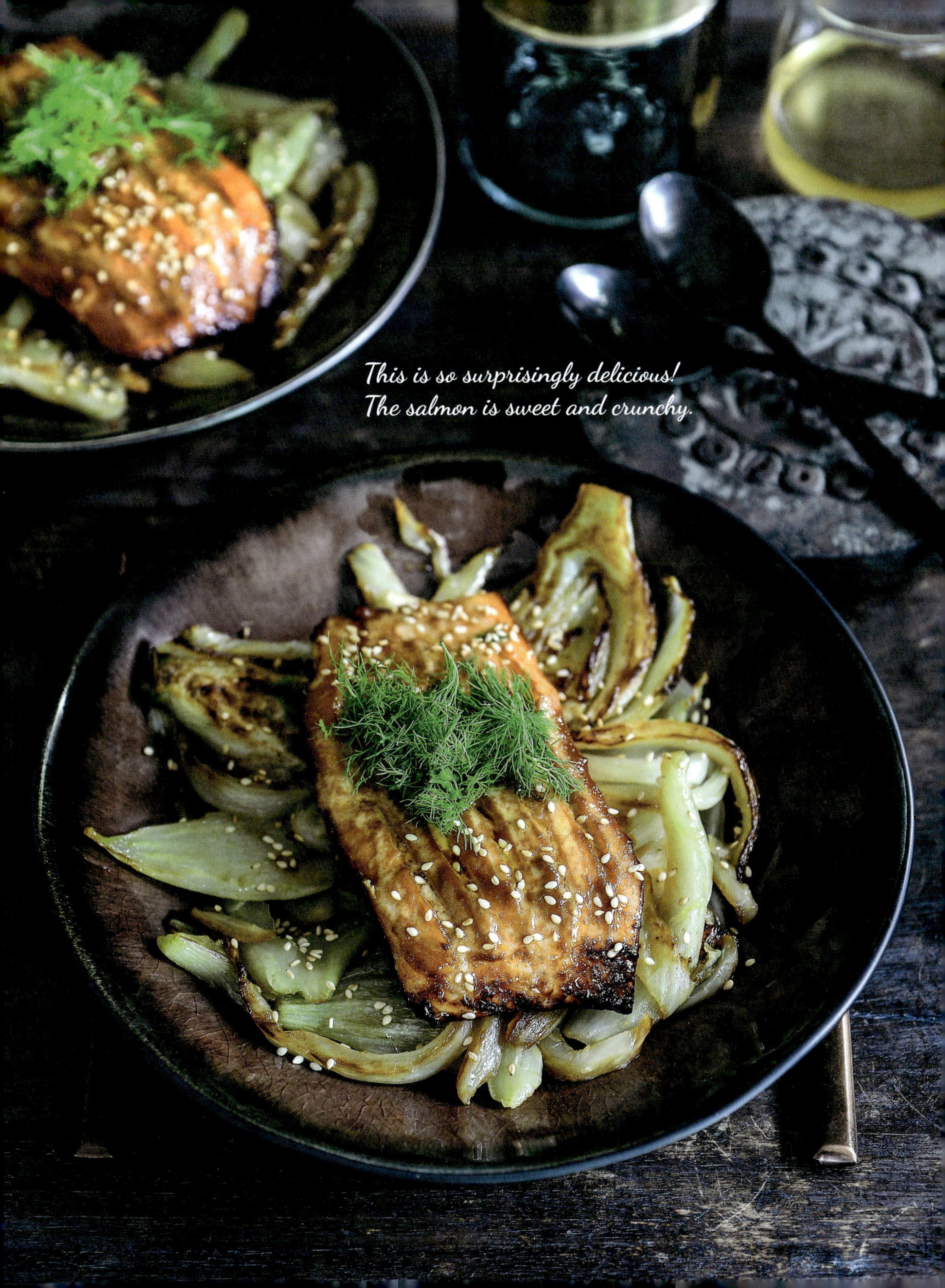
This is so surprisingly delicious!
The salmon is sweet and crunchy.

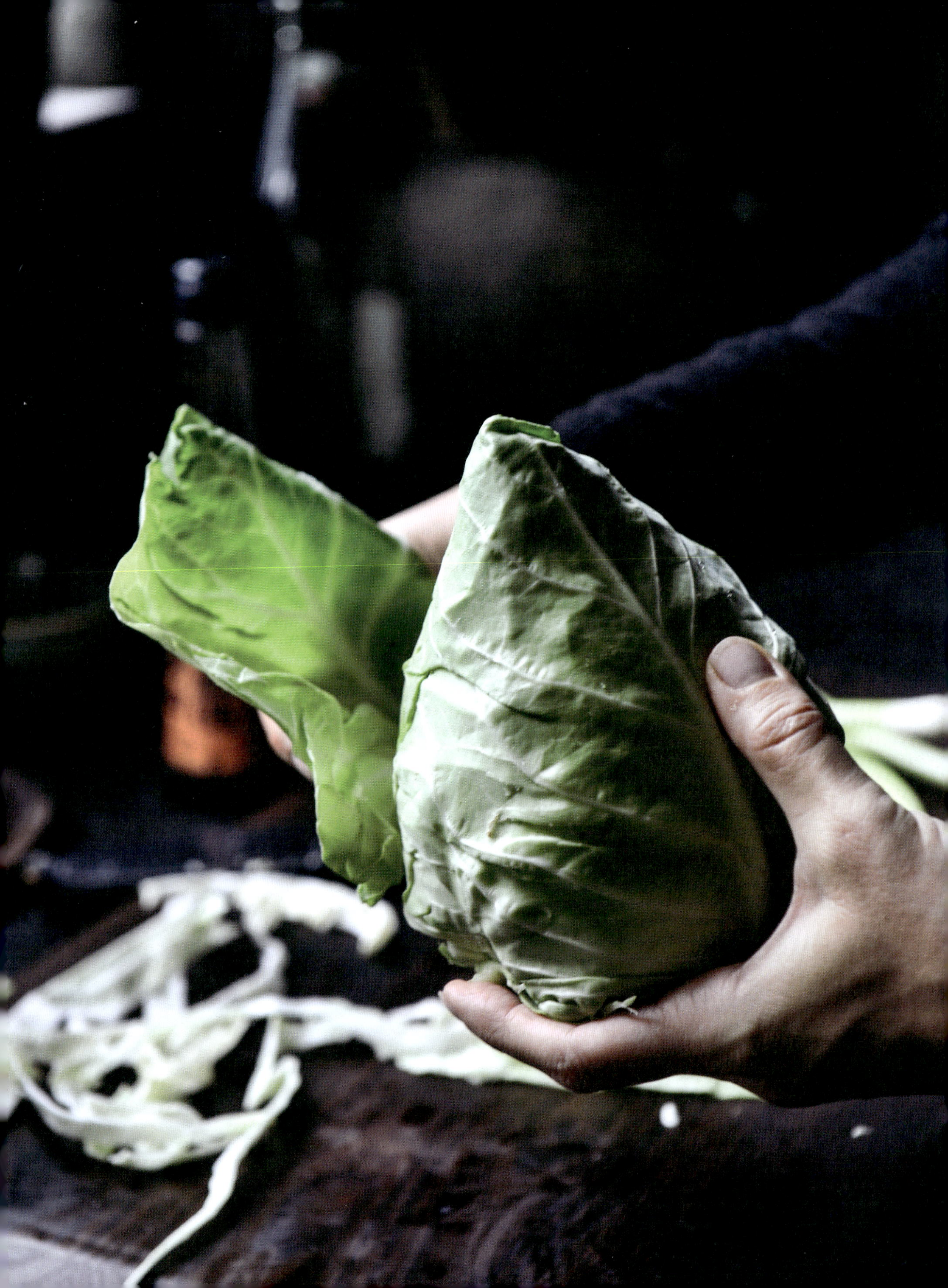

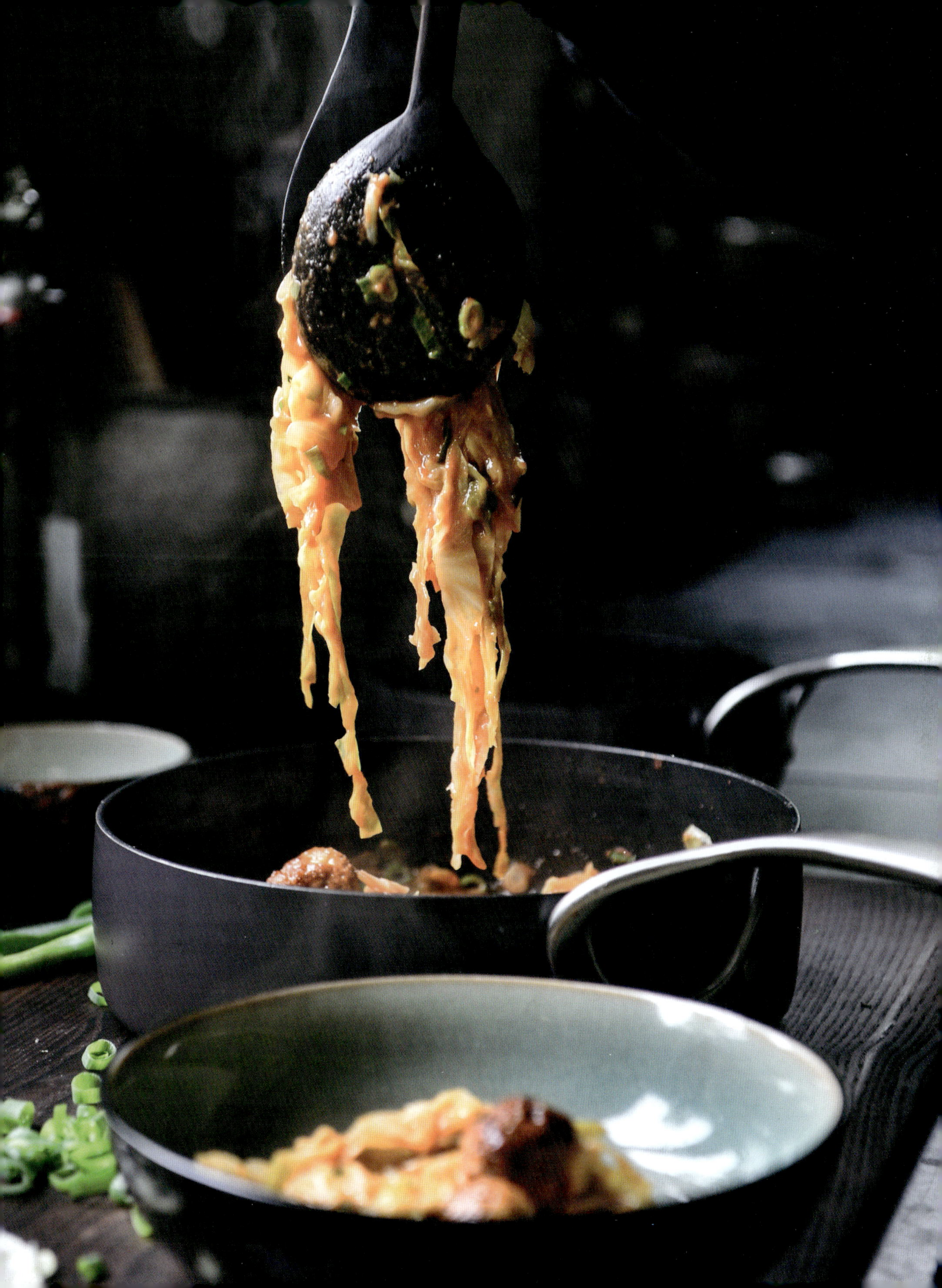

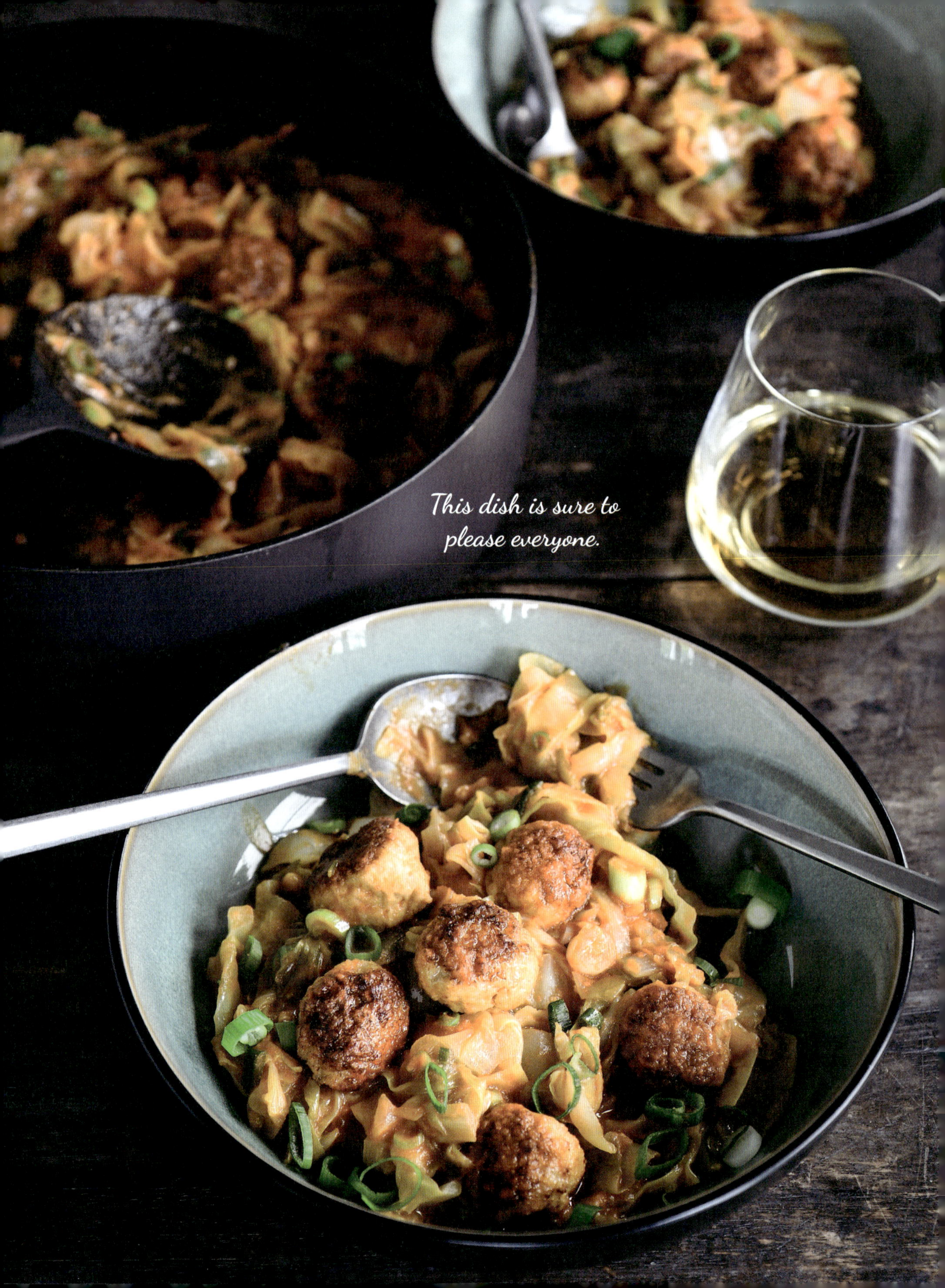

This dish is sure to please everyone.

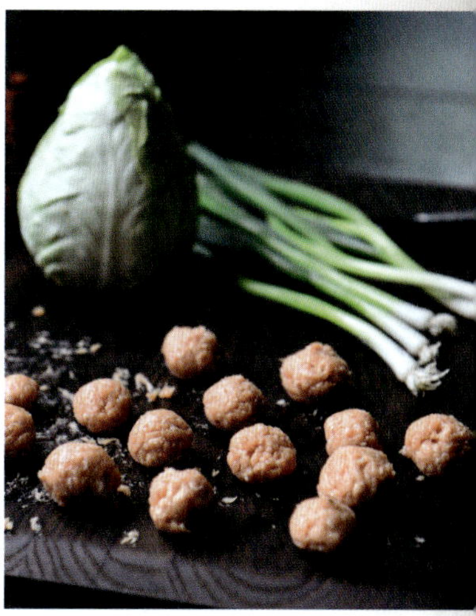

✓ keto

pointed cabbage spaghetti

with meatballs in tomato sauce

- 1 pointed (or Napa) cabbage
- 7 oz (200 g) strained tomatoes or tomato puree (see tip)
- 7 to 10½ oz (200 to 300 g) chicken, ground
- 2 spring onions, finely chopped

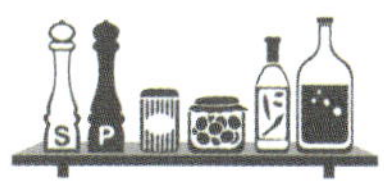

– mild mustard –

– soy sauce –

Slice the cabbage into long strips, starting from the top. Cook the cabbage in plenty of olive oil and half a glass of water, covered, until it is almost tender. This will take about five minutes.

Season the ground chicken with salt and pepper if it hasn't been seasoned already. Shape the chicken into meatballs and brown them in plenty of olive oil. Add the tomato sauce to the cabbage together with 2 tablespoons of mustard and 5 tablespoons of soy sauce. Carefully stir the sauce into the cabbage and cook for a little longer. Add the meatballs. Serve and garnish with finely chopped spring onion.

TIP: STRAINED TOMATOES OR TOMATO PUREE

Strained tomatoes or tomato puree is tomato sauce from strained raw tomatoes, without the skin and seeds. I love the taste and texture. You can also use fresh tomatoes when they're in season. The sauce will have a different flavor and texture but will taste equally delicious.

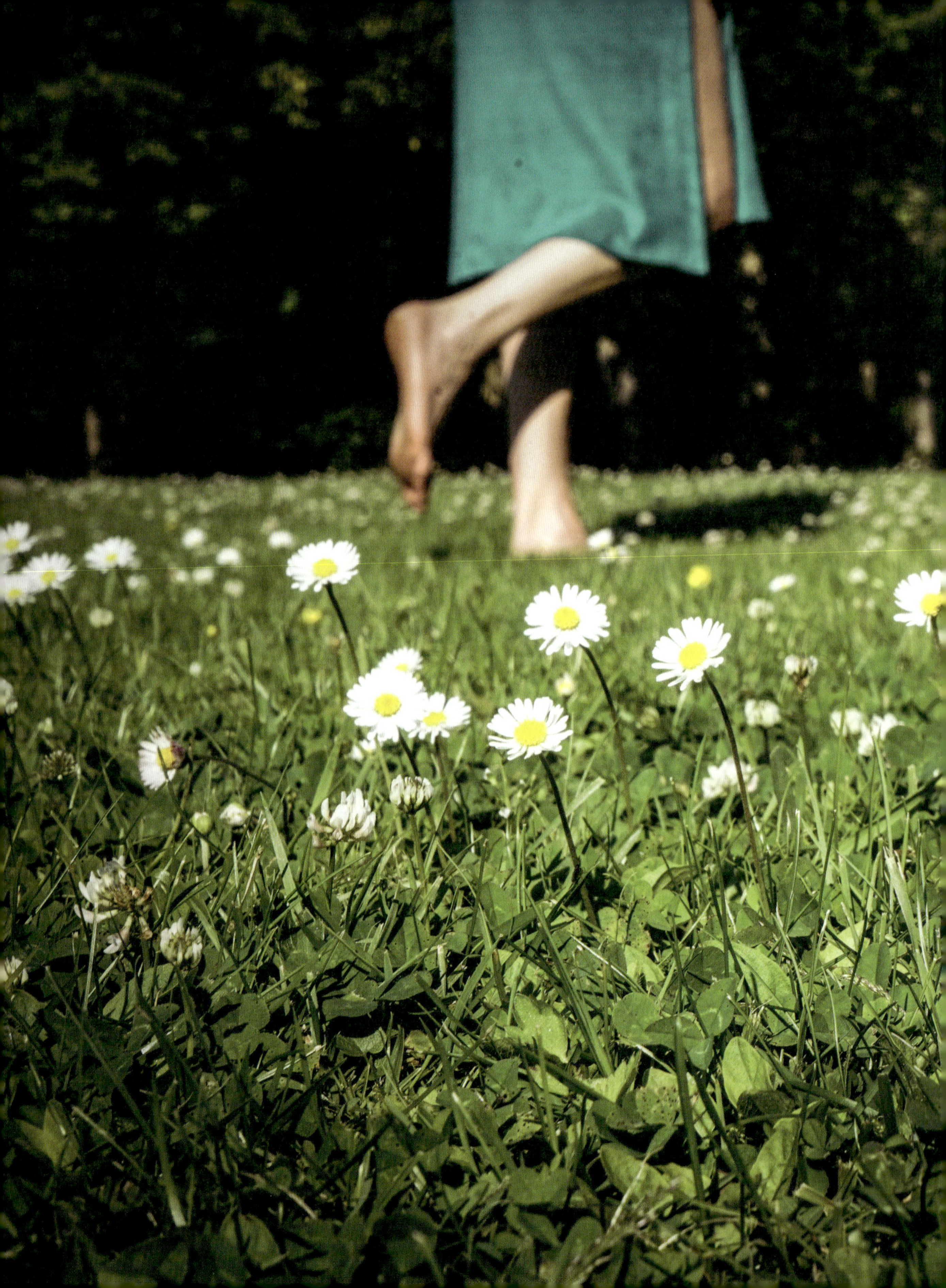

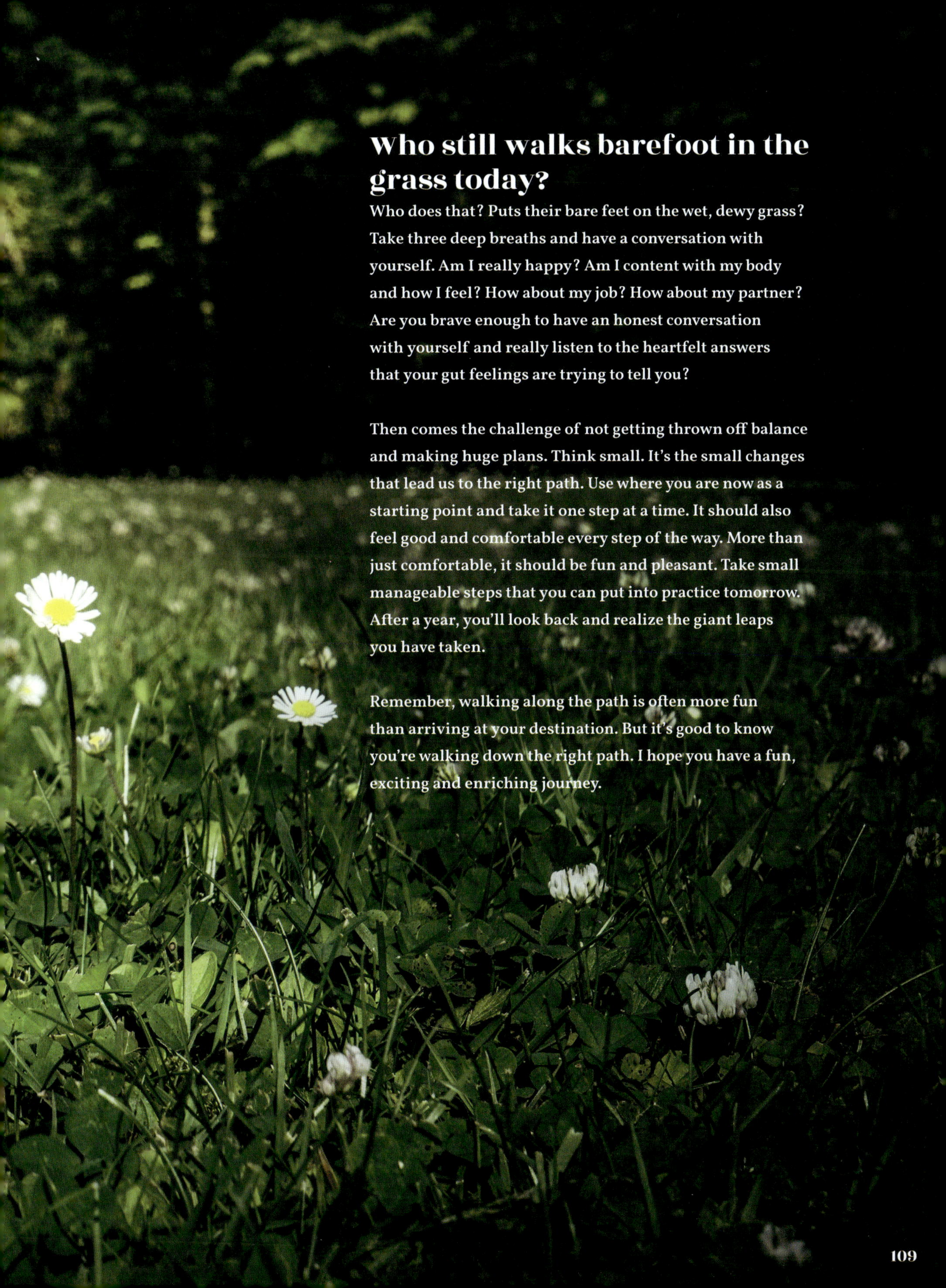

Who still walks barefoot in the grass today?

Who does that? Puts their bare feet on the wet, dewy grass? Take three deep breaths and have a conversation with yourself. Am I really happy? Am I content with my body and how I feel? How about my job? How about my partner? Are you brave enough to have an honest conversation with yourself and really listen to the heartfelt answers that your gut feelings are trying to tell you?

Then comes the challenge of not getting thrown off balance and making huge plans. Think small. It's the small changes that lead us to the right path. Use where you are now as a starting point and take it one step at a time. It should also feel good and comfortable every step of the way. More than just comfortable, it should be fun and pleasant. Take small manageable steps that you can put into practice tomorrow. After a year, you'll look back and realize the giant leaps you have taken.

Remember, walking along the path is often more fun than arriving at your destination. But it's good to know you're walking down the right path. I hope you have a fun, exciting and enriching journey.

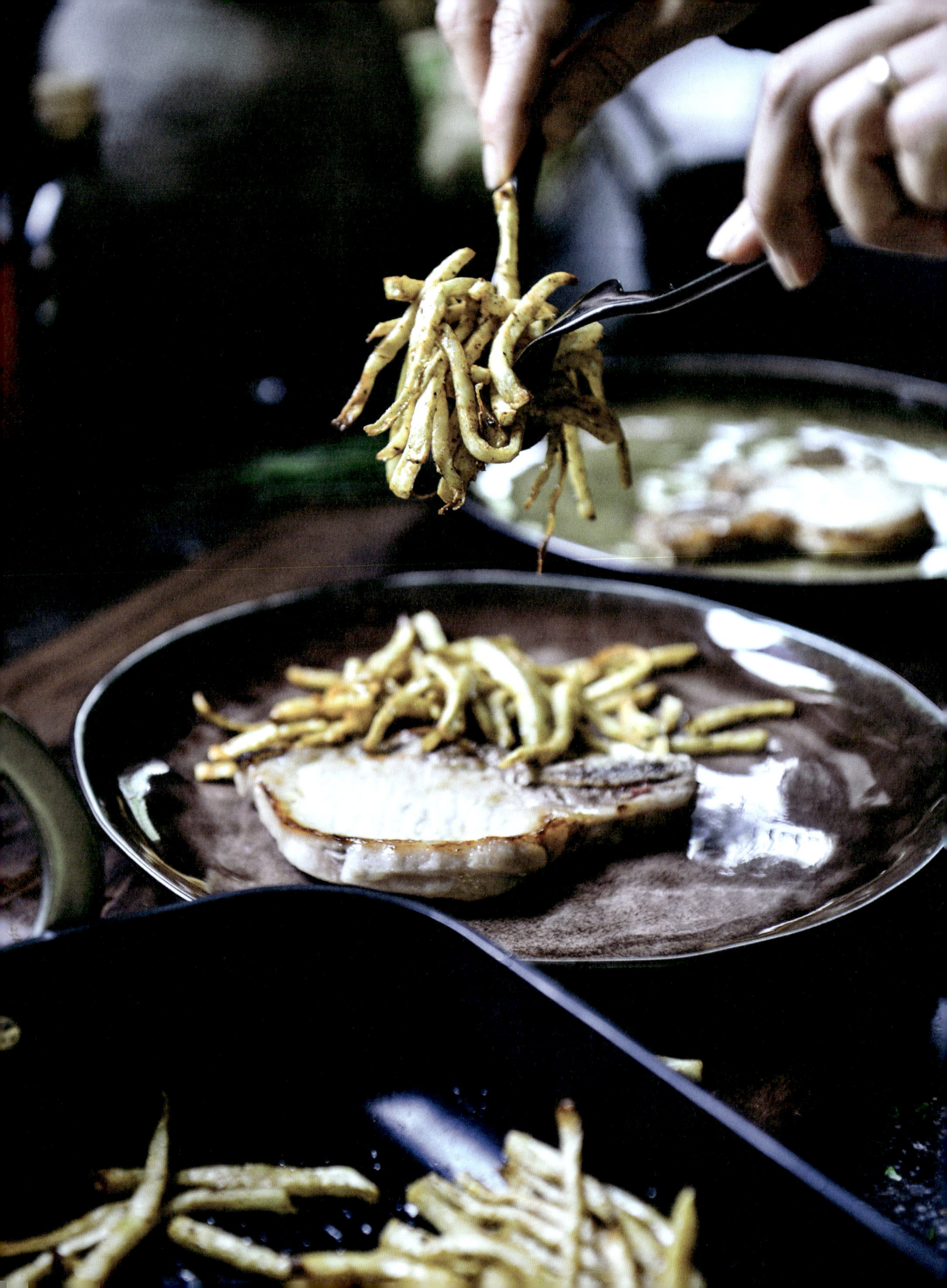

ready in
25 minutes

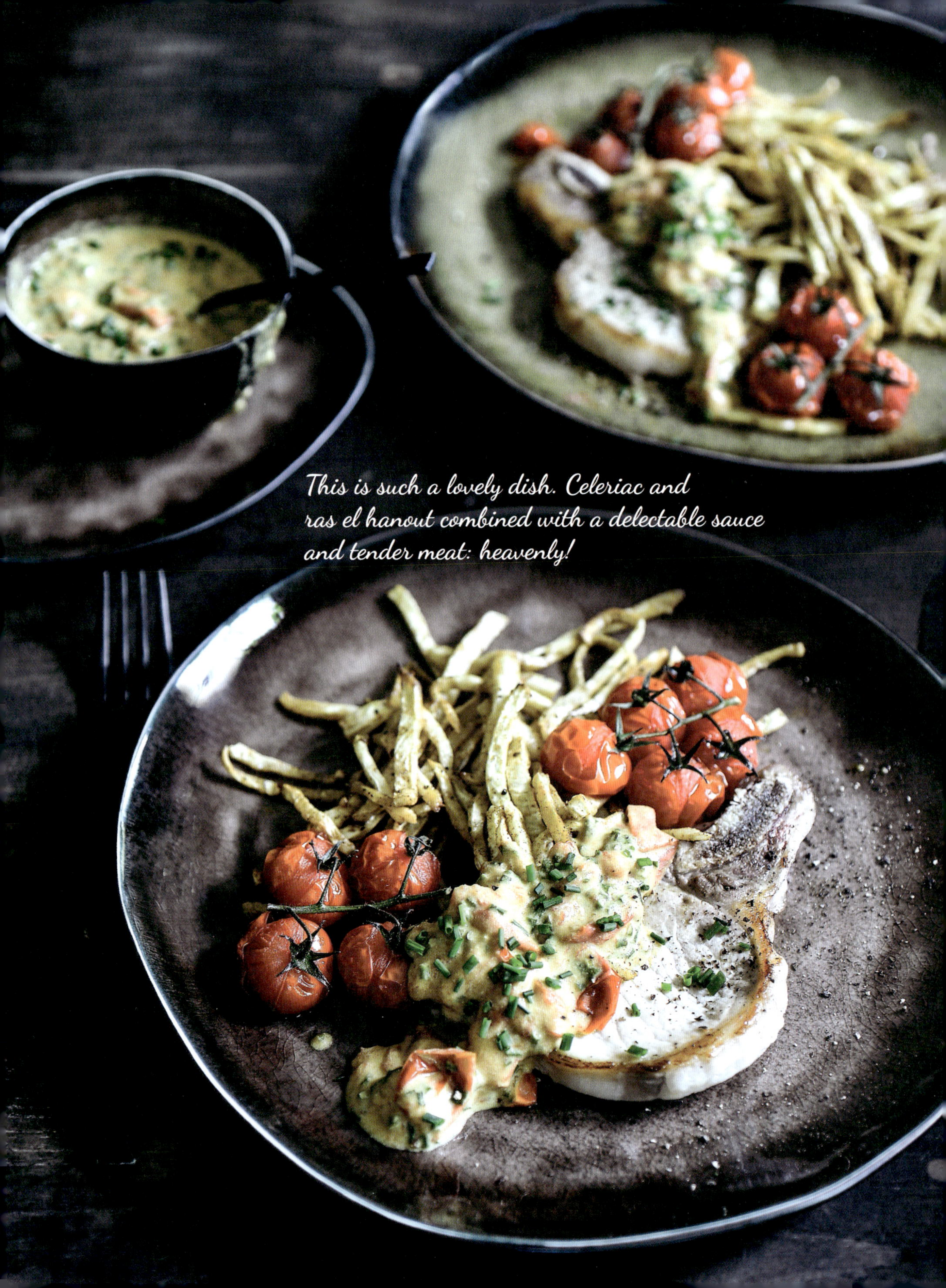

This is such a lovely dish. Celeriac and ras el hanout combined with a delectable sauce and tender meat: heavenly!

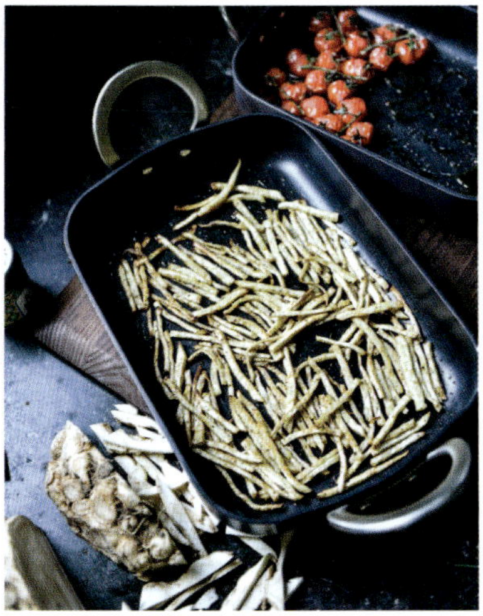
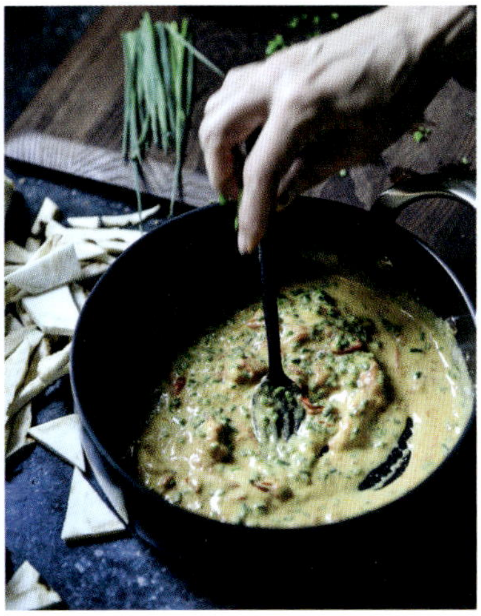
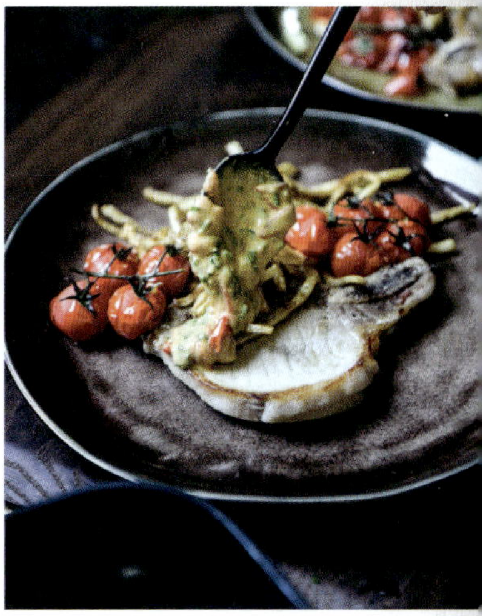

pork loin

keto

with celeriac and tomato-mustard sauce

- **2 pork loin chops**
- **14 oz (400 g) celeriac**
- **about 30 cherry tomatoes, on the vine**
- **¾ oz (20 g) chives**

– mustard (see tip) –
– ras el hanout –

Preheat the oven to 350 °F (180 °C). Slice the celeriac into thin slices and then again into matchsticks. Put them in a baking dish, sprinkle salt, 1 teaspoon of ras el hanout, and a drizzle of olive oil over the top. Toss everything together well to make sure the spices and oil are distributed evenly over the celeriac. Halve about ten tomatoes and leave the rest on the vine as they are. Put all the tomatoes next to the celeriac or use a separate baking dish. Season with salt and pepper and pour some olive oil over the top. Bake in the oven for 15 to 20 minutes. Fry the meat for 2 to 3 minutes on each side. Season with salt and pepper. Finely chop the chives. For the sauce, put 3 large tablespoons of mustard in a pan and add the halved, cooked tomatoes. Crush the tomatoes to get all the moisture out and mix well. Season with salt and pepper and three quarters of the chives. Add a generous splash of olive oil and some water until you have a nice, thick sauce. Serve the pork loin with the celeriac and pour the sauce over the top. Arrange the cherry tomatoes on the vine next to the pork loin and garnish with the remaining chives.

TIP: MUSTARD
Use mild mustard. Change the amount if you use a spicier mustard. The key here is to keep tasting.

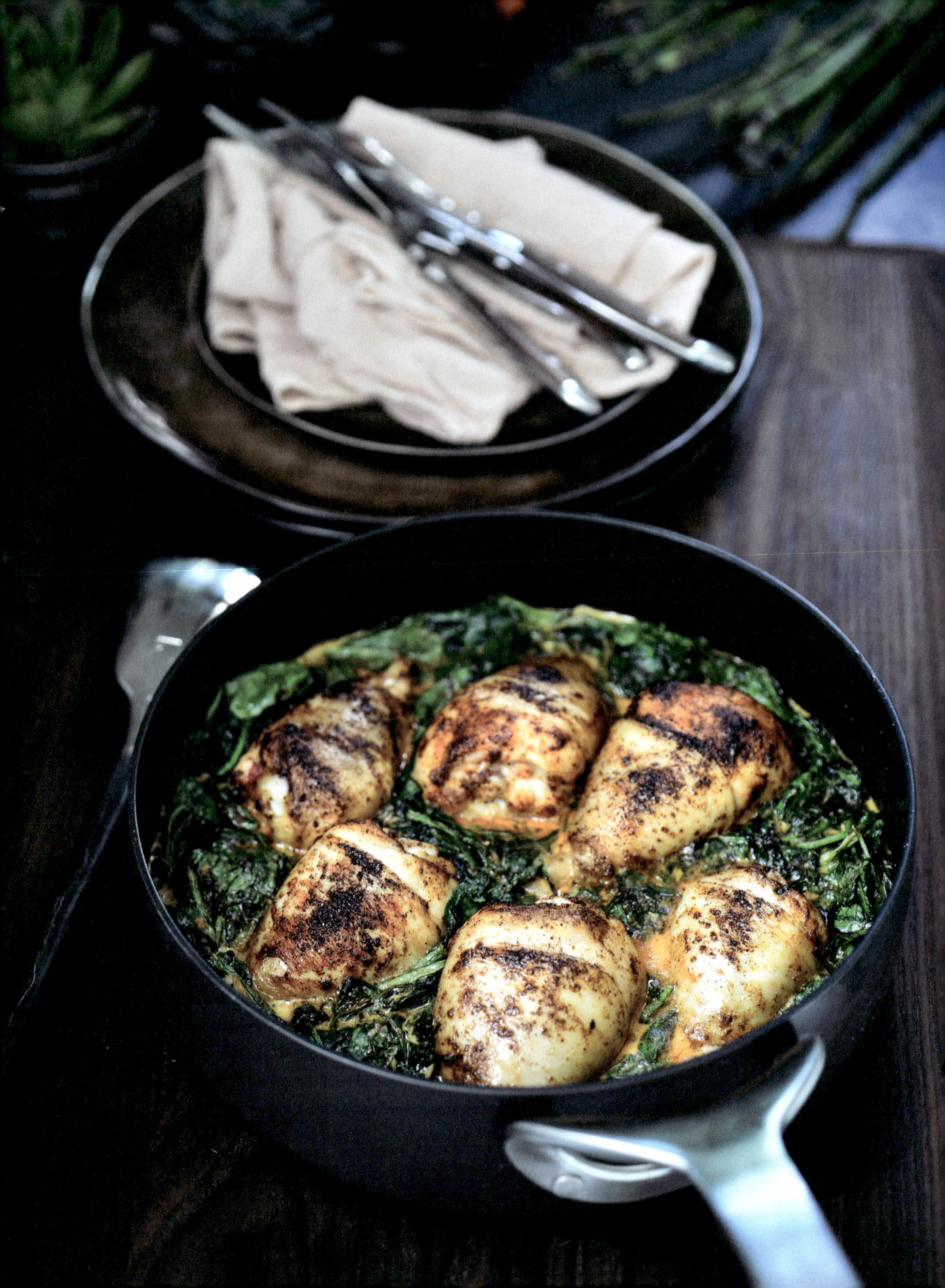

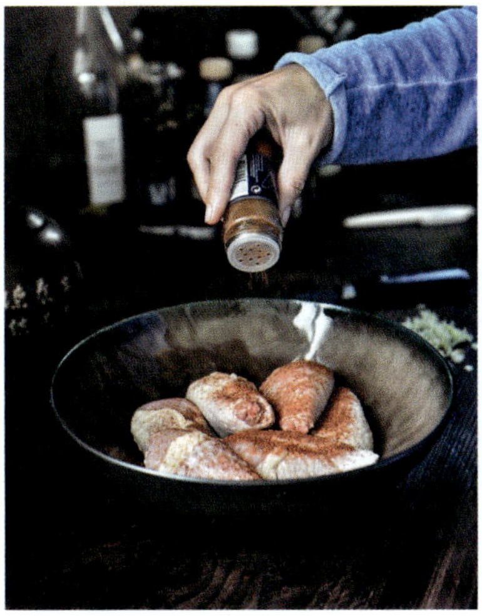

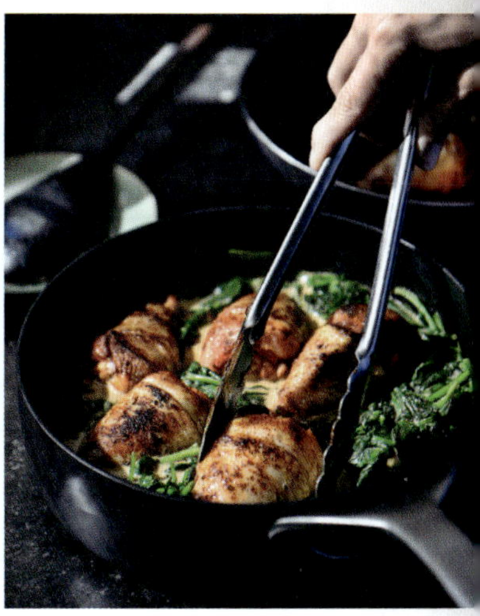

The paprika gives a beautiful red color and intense flavor to this dish.

chicken

✓ keto

with cream and spinach

- **6 chicken drumsticks**
- **10½ oz (300 g) spinach**
- **7 fl oz (200 ml) cream or coconut milk**
- **sweet paprika powder**

– fresh garlic –
– butter –

Preheat the oven to 350 °F (180 °C). Coat the chicken drumsticks with plenty of paprika powder (I use about 2 heaped tablespoons) and some salt and pepper. Make sure the drumsticks are completely covered. Fry the chicken in plenty of butter until brown, about four minutes. Make sure that the butter doesn't burn. If it does, pour it off and use fresh butter for the next step. Meanwhile, finely chop 2 cloves of garlic.

Remove the chicken from the pan, but leave the melted butter in. Add and briefly sauté the garlic. Then add the cream or coconut milk and spinach to the pan. Cover the pan so the spinach wilts quickly. Stir everything thoroughly and return the chicken drumsticks to the pan. Put the pan, uncovered, in the preheated oven for 15 minutes.

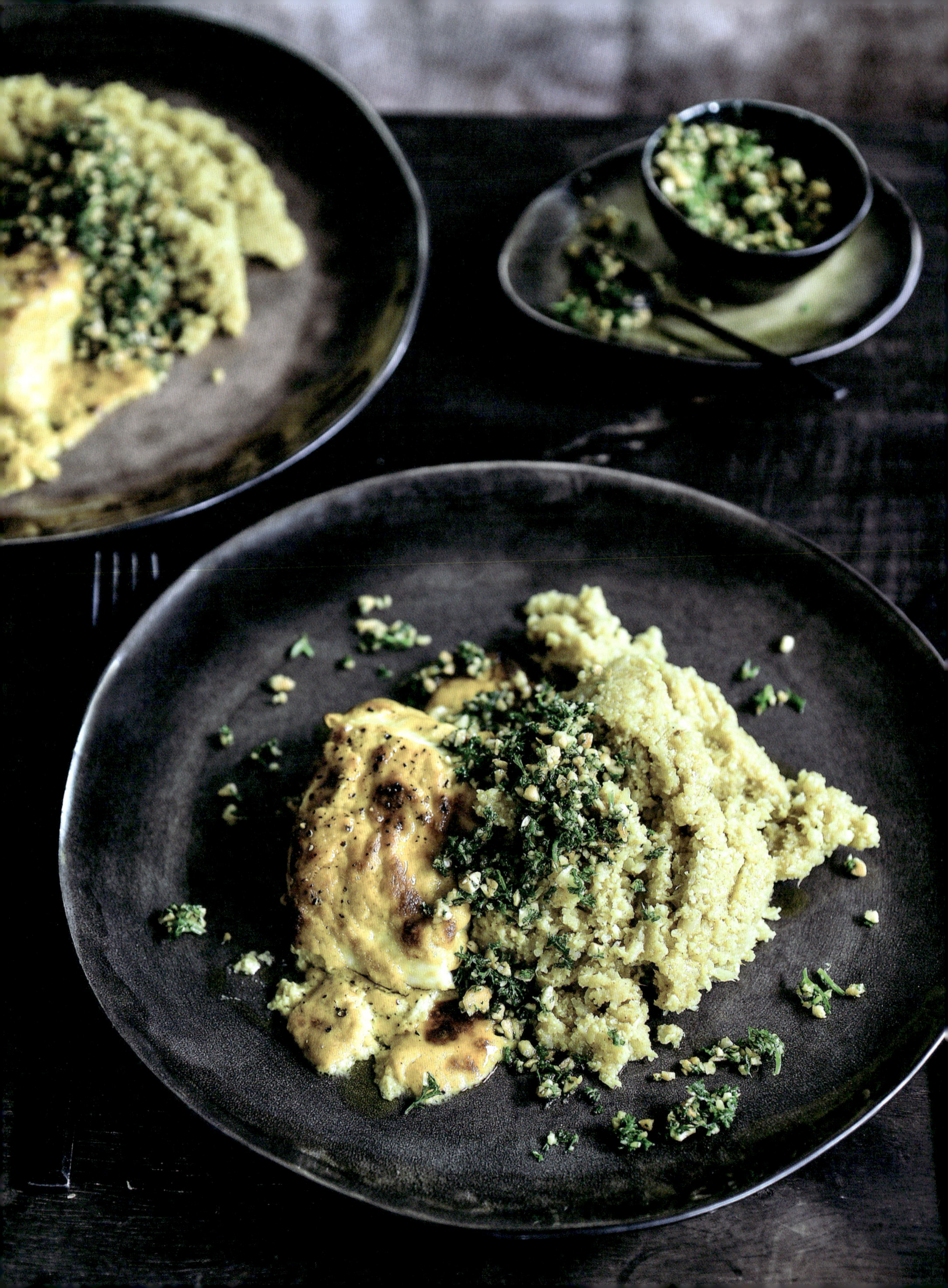

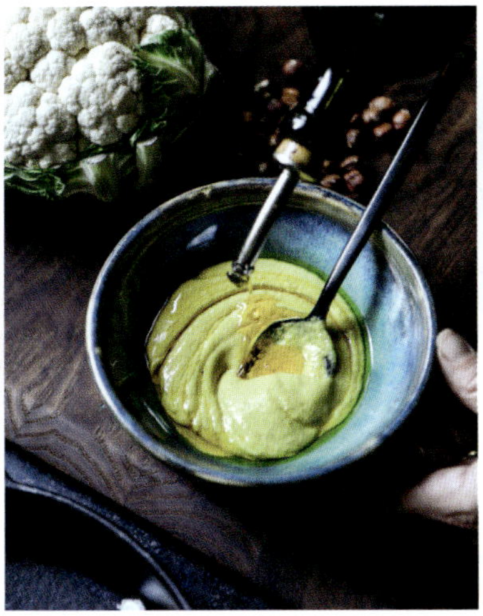 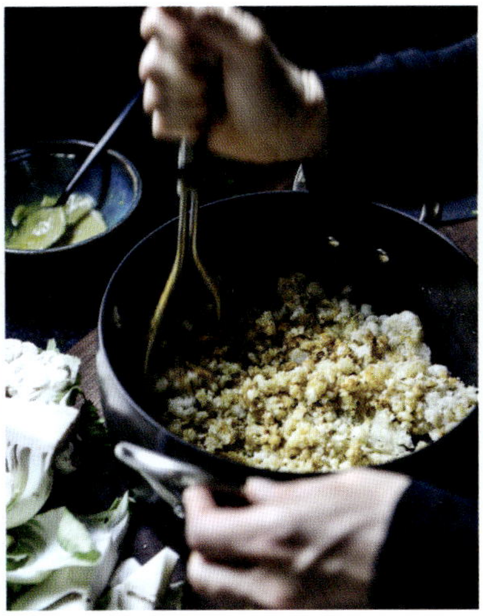 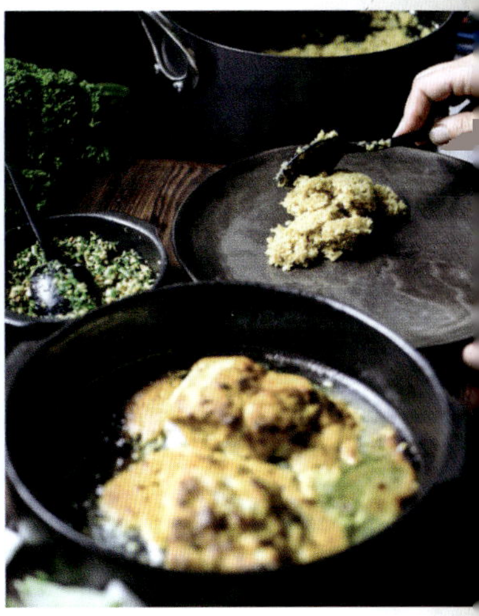

cod

keto

with mustard sauce and cauliflower puree

- **2 cod fillets**
- **½ cauliflower**
- **a handful of roasted hazelnuts**
- **a handful of curly-leaf parsley**

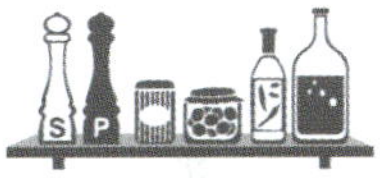

– mild mustard (see tip) –

– ras el hanout –

Cut the cauliflower into pieces and cook until tender in water with a generous splash of olive oil. Preheat the oven to 400 °F (200 °C). Put the cod fillets in a baking dish. Combine 4 tablespoons of mustard with 4 tablespoons of olive oil and coat the fish with the mixture (see tip). Bake in the oven for about 15 minutes.

Drain the cauliflower and return the pan to the heat. Add a generous splash of olive oil, sprinkle 1 tablespoon of ras el hanout over the top and season with salt and pepper. Mash everything together to a puree. Coarsely chop the nuts together with the parsley. Spoon the cauliflower puree onto a plate, arrange the fish next to it and garnish with the parsley-nut mixture.

TIP: MUSTARD SAUCE

Feel free to pour some mustard sauce next to the cod. The cod can become dry and the sauce makes it extra delicious.

TIP: MUSTARD

Use mild mustard. Change the amount if you use a spicier mustard. The key here is to keep tasting.

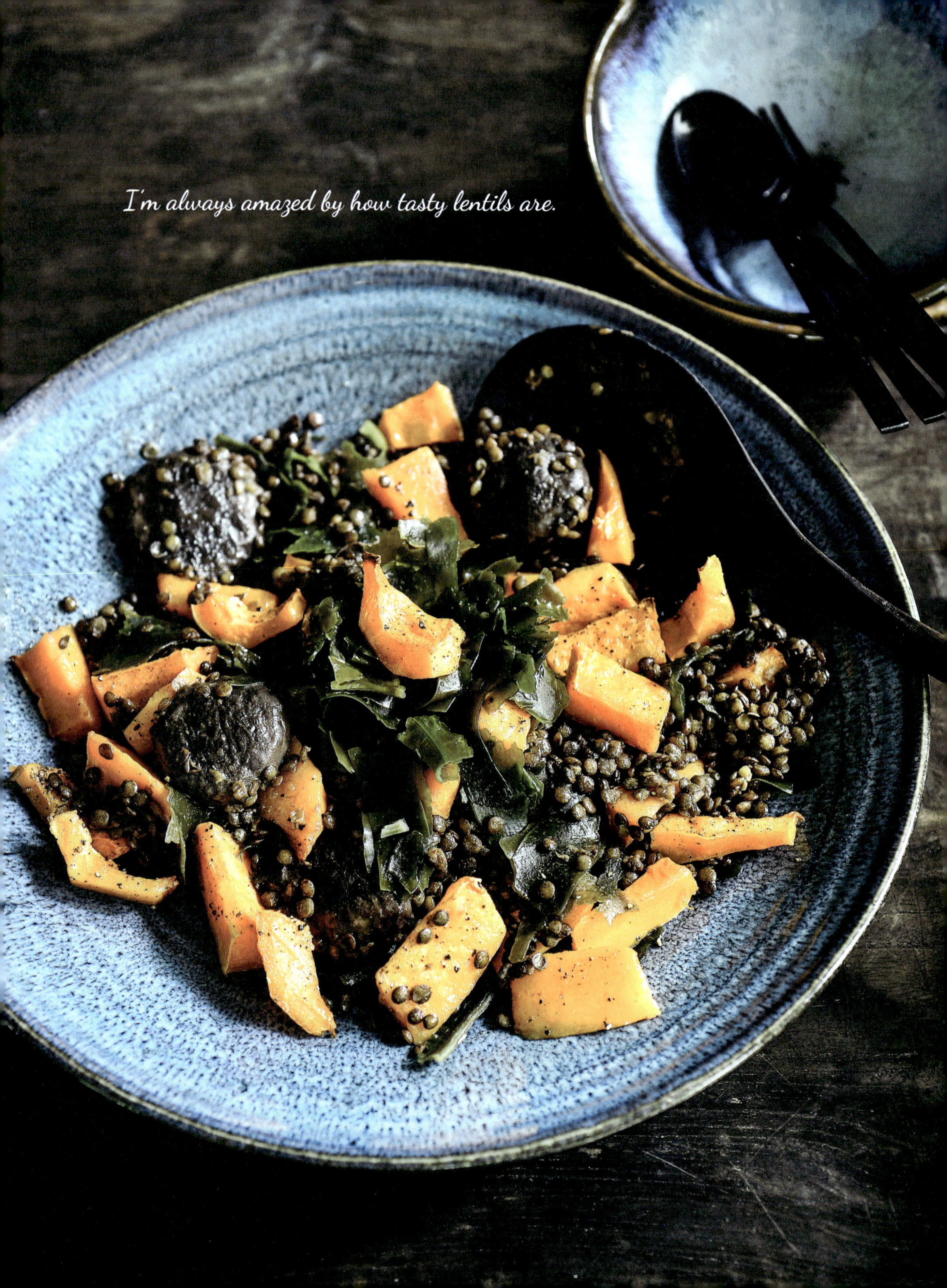

I'm always amazed by how tasty lentils are.

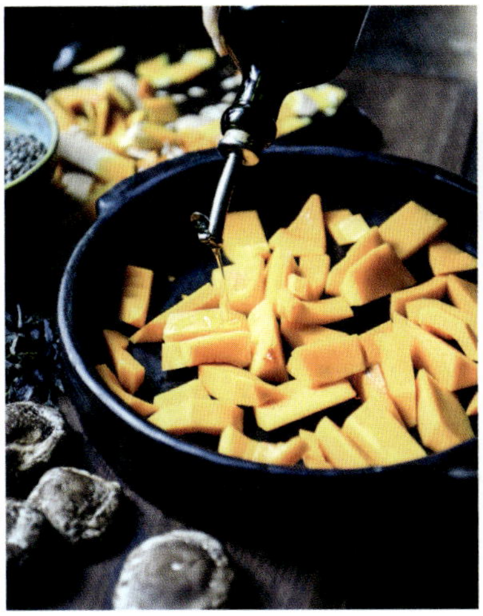

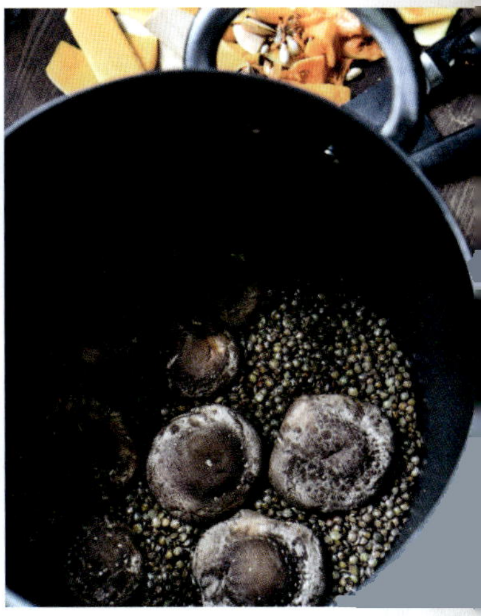

vegan

lentils

with pumpkin, shiitake mushrooms and wakame

- **3½ oz (100 g) dried green lentils**
- **9 oz (250 g) shiitake mushrooms**
- **a little over 1 lb (500 g) butternut squash**
- **⅓ oz (10 g) dried wakame (seaweed)**

Rinse the lentils, put them in a pot and add four times the volume of water. Add a generous splash of olive oil and cook the lentils, covered, for about 20 minutes. Preheat the oven to 350 °F (180 °C). Peel and slice the butternut squash into medium-sized pieces. Place the butternut squash pieces in a baking dish, add a splash of olive oil, season with salt and pepper, and bake for about 20 minutes in the oven. Soak the wakame in lukewarm water and remove the hard pieces, if necessary. Add the shiitake mushrooms to the lentils during the final 6 minutes of cooking.

Make sure that the lentils don't dry out during cooking! The water should have been completely absorbed by the end of cooking time. If that's not the case, drain off the excess water. Just before serving, stir the butternut squash pieces and wakame into the lentils. Season with salt and pepper. Serve in a large bowl.

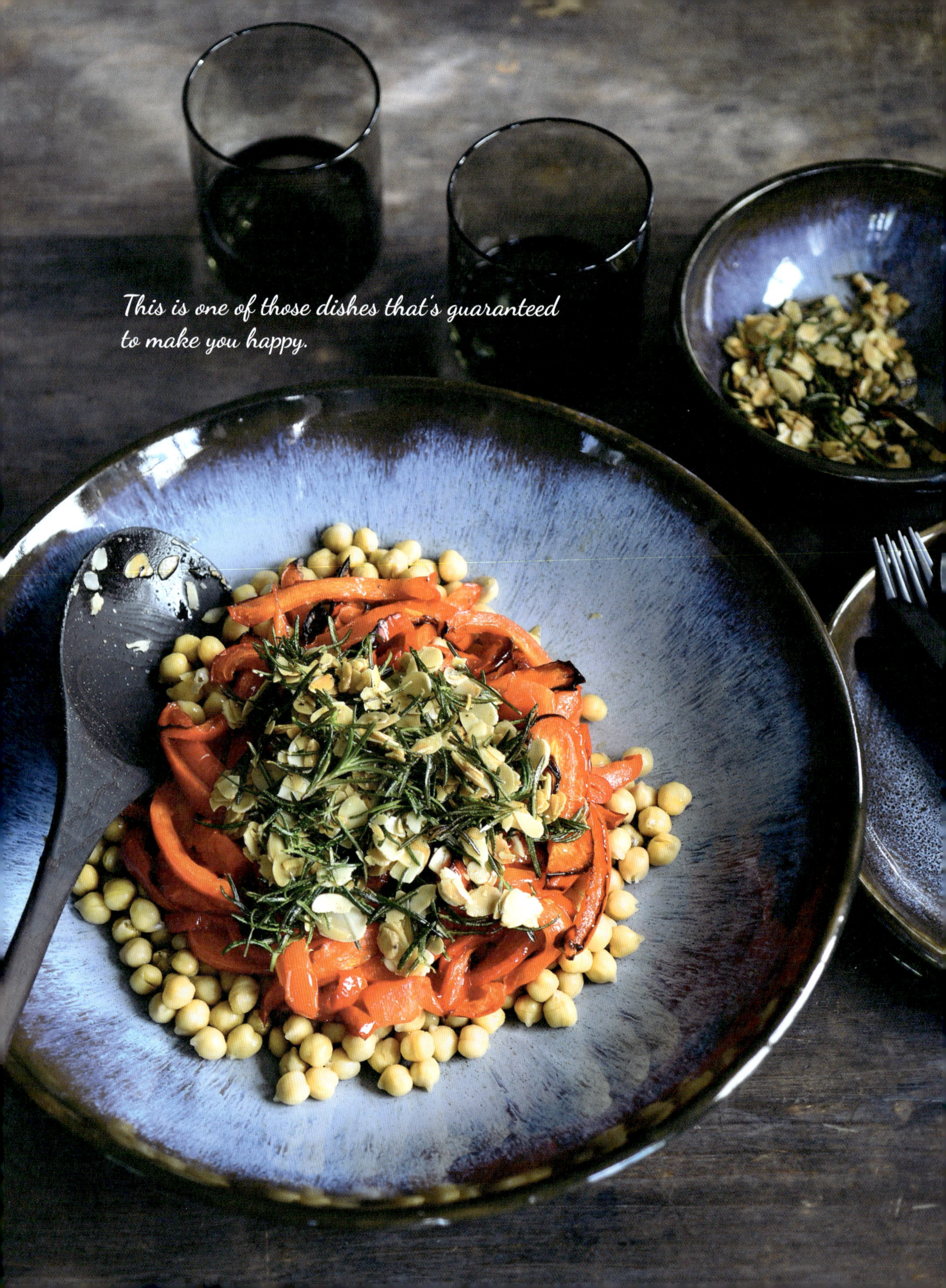

This is one of those dishes that's guaranteed to make you happy.

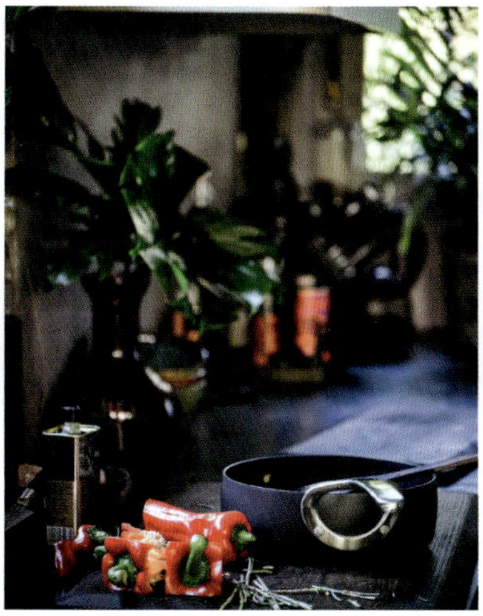

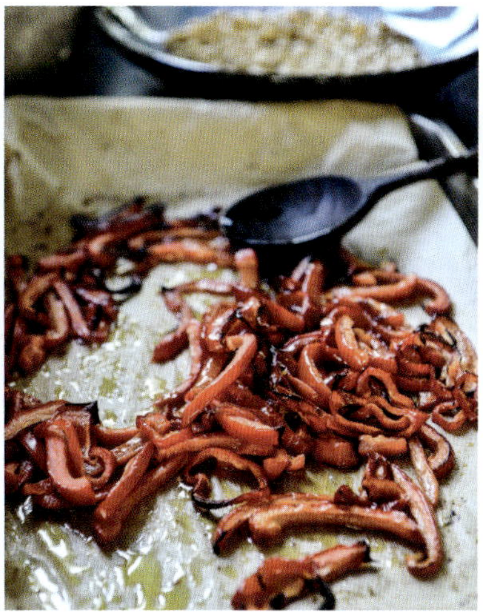

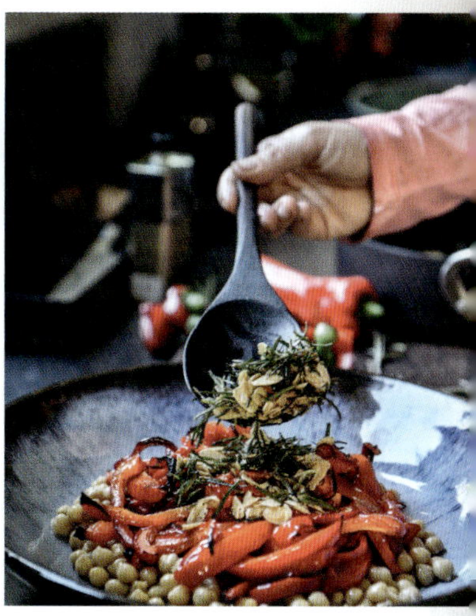

vegan

chickpeas

with paprika, sliced almonds and rosemary

- **9 oz (250 g) chickpeas (canned and drained, or soaked and cooked)**
- **3 red bell peppers**
- **5 sprigs of rosemary**
- **a handful of sliced almonds**

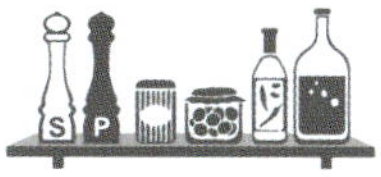

extra: parchment paper

Preheat the oven to 350 °F (180 °C).
Slice the red bell peppers into strips. Put them in a baking dish lined with parchment paper, drizzle some olive oil over the top and season with salt and pepper. Bake in the oven for 20 minutes. Sauté the sliced almonds in butter. Remove the leaves from the rosemary stems and add them to the almonds. Season with salt and pepper. Keep cooking the almonds until they turn crispy. Heat the chickpeas in a separate pan with a generous splash of olive oil. Place the chickpeas on a plate, spoon the sweet peppers next to them and garnish with the herbed sliced almonds.

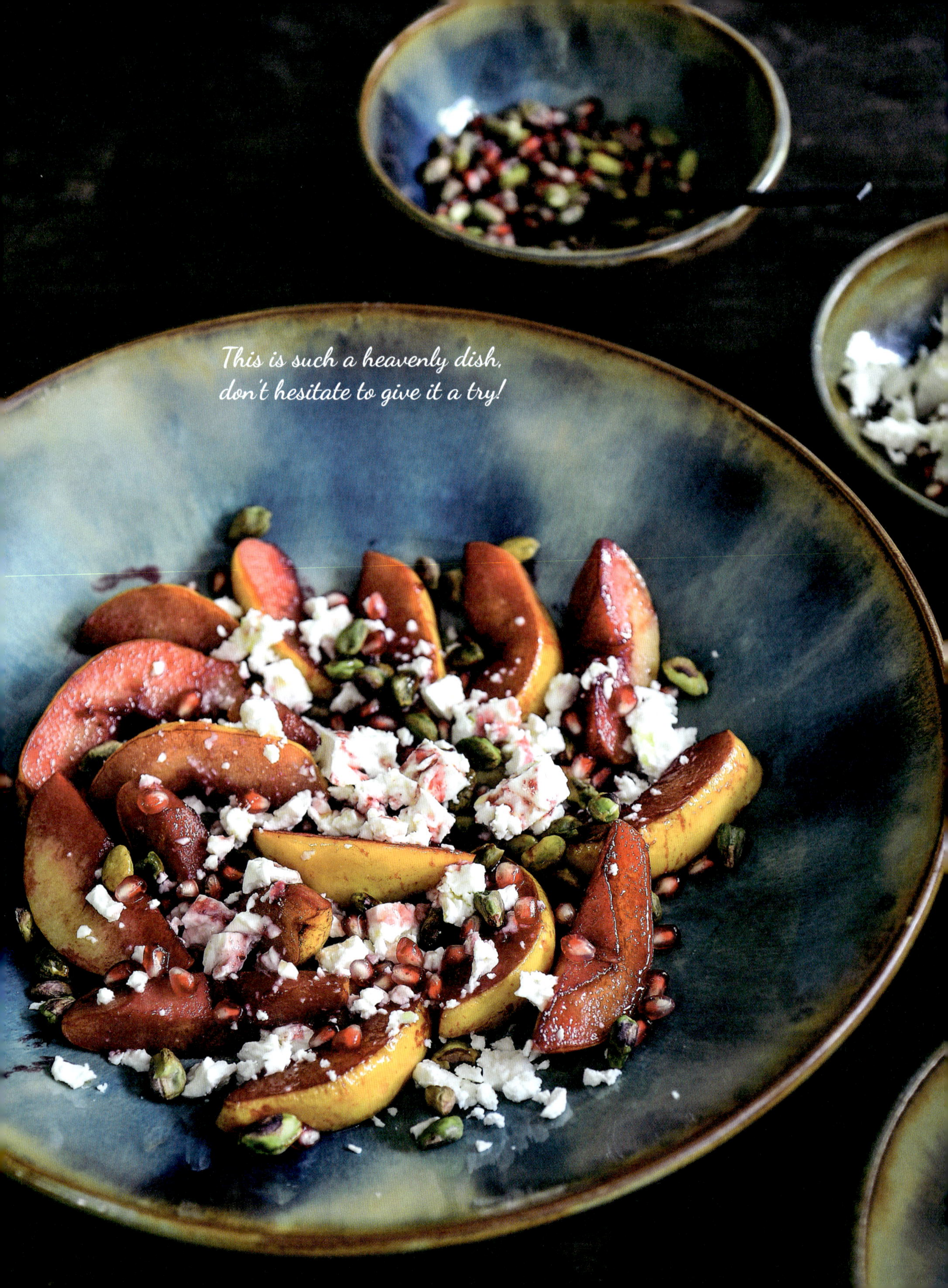
This is such a heavenly dish,
don't hesitate to give it a try!

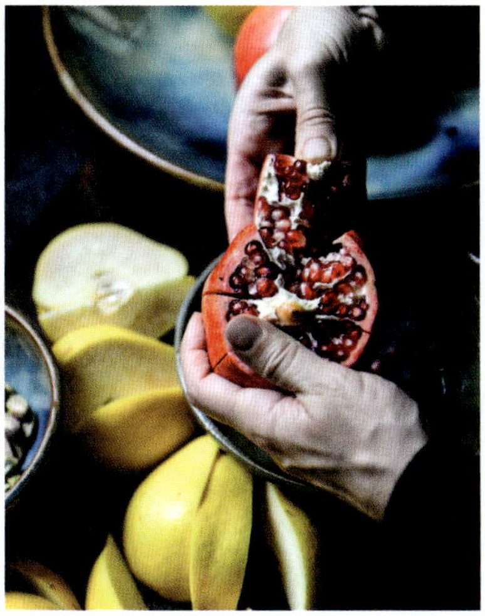

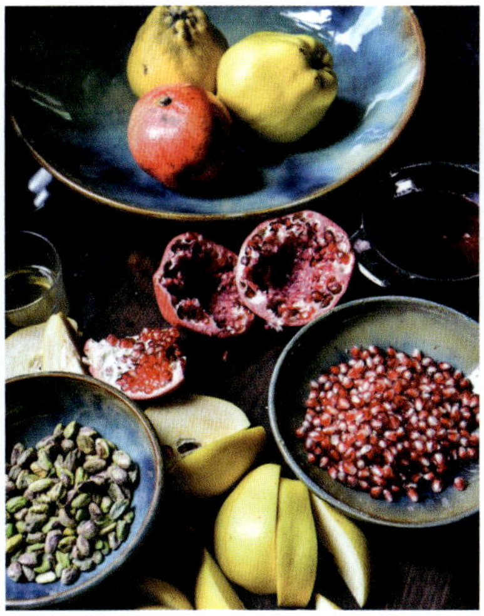

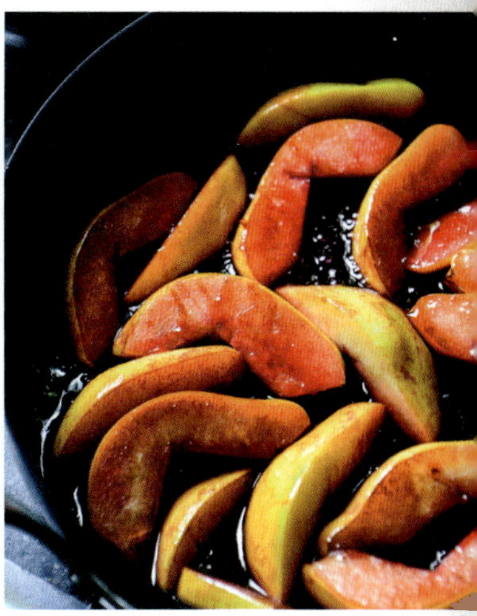

quinces
with feta, pistachios and pomegranate

- **2 quinces (see tip)**
- **a handful of pistachios**
- **7 oz (200 g) feta**
- **2 pomegranates**

- butter -

Slice the quinces in half. Put them cut side down and slice each quince half into three wedges. Remove the core. Cook the quinces in plenty of butter with a small amount of water. Cover the pan. Turn the wedges over after 10 minutes. Add a little more butter if necessary. Squeeze the juice from one pomegranate. While squeezing the juice, push on the pomegranate instead of twisting it. Remove the seeds from the other pomegranate (see tip). Pour the pomegranate juice over the quinces and cook, uncovered, for another five minutes, allowing the sauce to thicken. Season with black pepper.
Put the quinces in a dish, sprinkle the pomegranate seeds and pistachios over the top and crumble the feta on top as well. Finish with the delicious red sauce.

TIP: QUINCE
Quinces are truly a divine gift. They are lovely to look at, smell wonderful, taste amazingly delicious and keep for a very long time. I don't understand why we don't use them more often when we cook. Granted, they can be hard to slice because they are somewhat hard, but don't let that stop you!

TIP: POMEGRANATE
Read about how to remove the seeds from the pomegranate under the "Tips" header on page 40 (salad with paneer and peanut sauce).

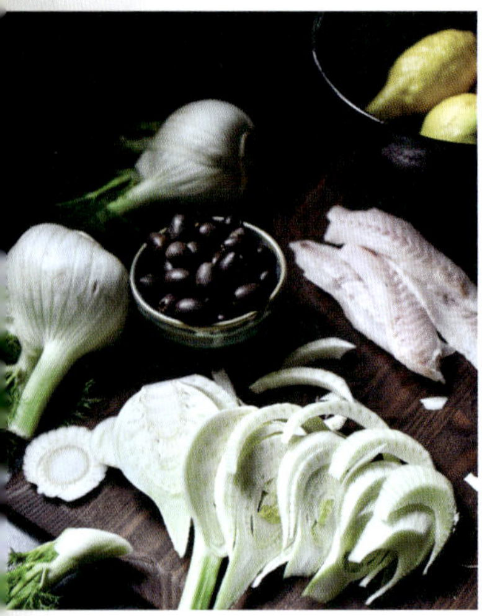

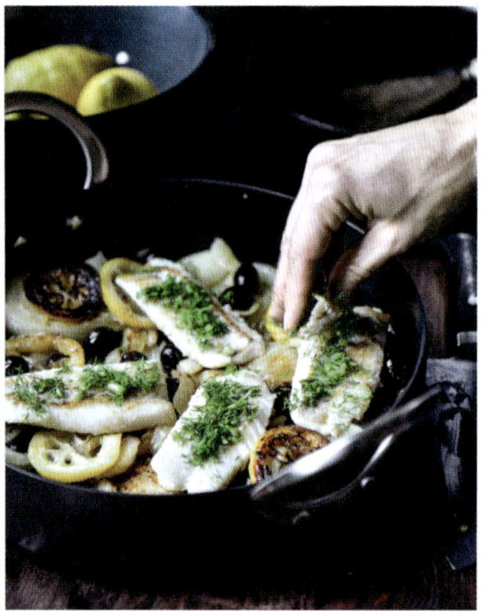

Remember to eat the browned lemon slices as well! They're almost sweet to the taste.

✓ keto

fish with fennel,

olives and lemon

- 10½ oz (300 g) white fish (e.g. redfish fillet)
- 2 fennel bulbs
- 7 oz (100 g) olives
- 2 organic lemons

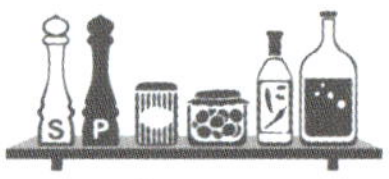

– butter –

Slice the fennel into thin slices and set the fluffy green tops aside. In a covered pan, sauté the fennel slices in plenty of butter with a small amount of water. Slice the lemon and add the slices. Cook for 20 minutes, stirring occasionally. Add the olives during the last 5 minutes of cooking and season with salt and pepper.

In a separate pan, cook the fish in some olive oil and season with salt and pepper.

Place the cooked fish on the fennel and garnish with the fennel tops.

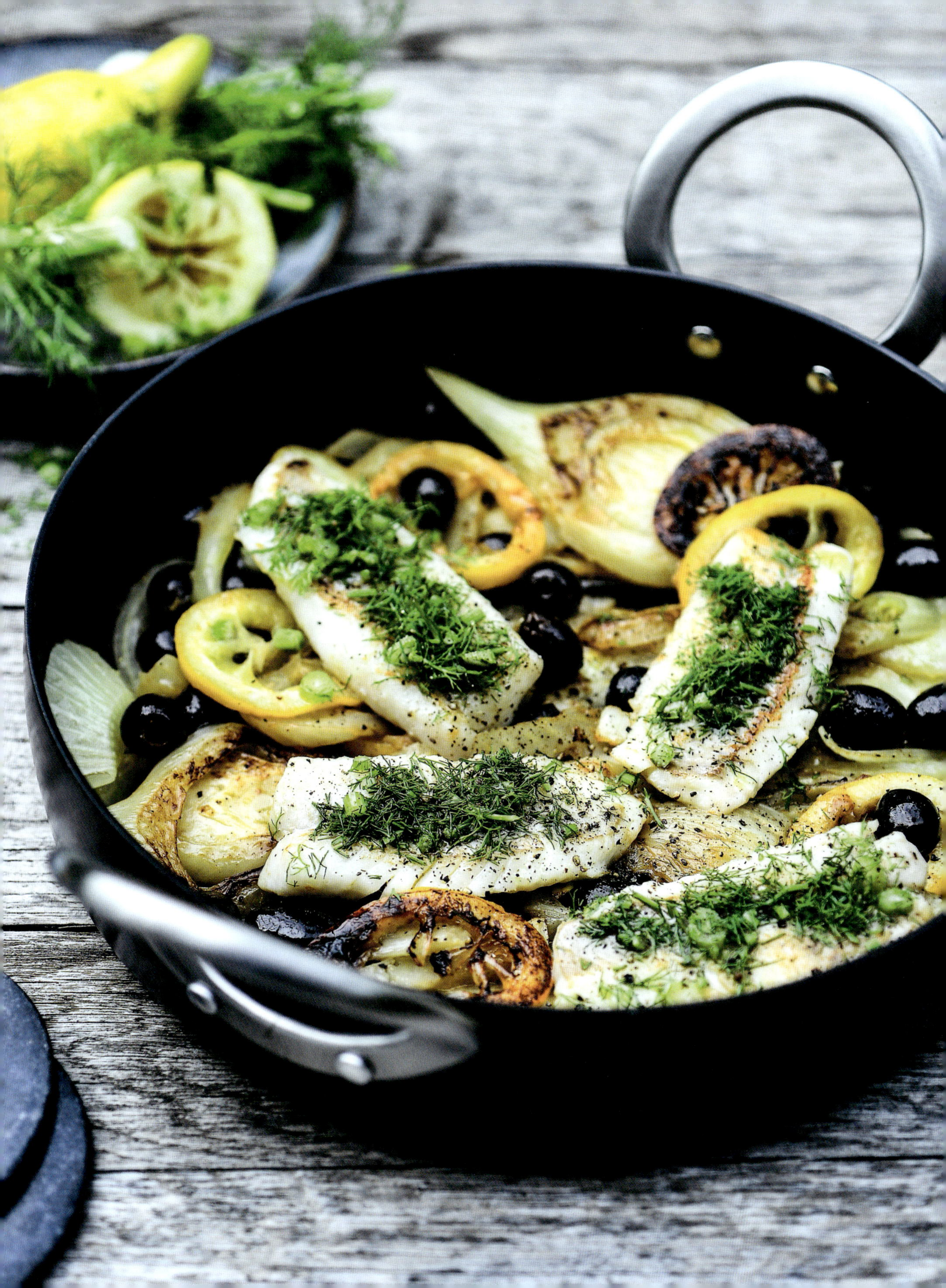

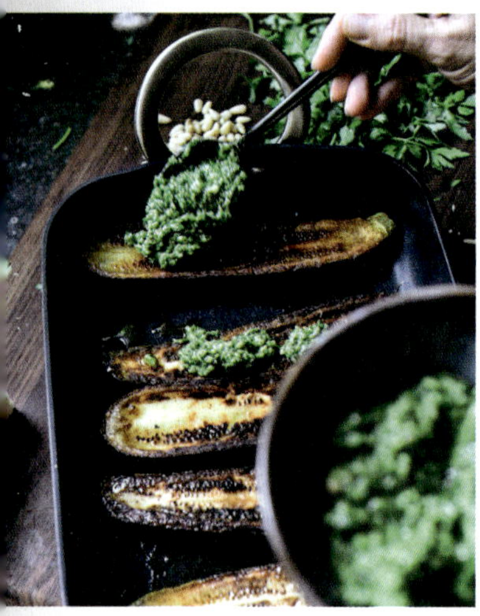

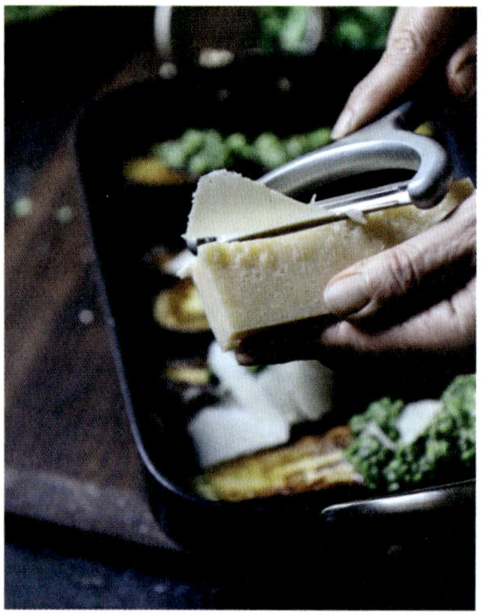

sautéed zucchini

✓ keto

with Parmesan cheese

- 3 zucchini (pick out the smaller ones)
- a handful of pine nuts
- 3½ oz (100 g) flat-leaf parsley
- 3 oz (70 g) Parmesan cheese

– cider vinegar –
– fresh garlic –

Cut the zucchini in half lengthwise and sauté them, cut side down, in a large pan with plenty of olive oil. Cover the pan and cook for about 13 minutes. Turn the zucchini over and cook for another 3 minutes. Put the pine nuts and flat-leaf parsley (set some of both aside for the garnish) in a blender. Add 1 clove of garlic, plenty of olive oil and a splash of cider vinegar. Add ¾ oz (20 g) Parmesan cheese and blend to form a pesto. Place the zucchini, cut side up, on a plate or dish. Spoon the pesto over the top and then garnish with some Parmesan cheese shavings followed by finely chopped flat-leaf parsley and a sprinkling of pine nuts.

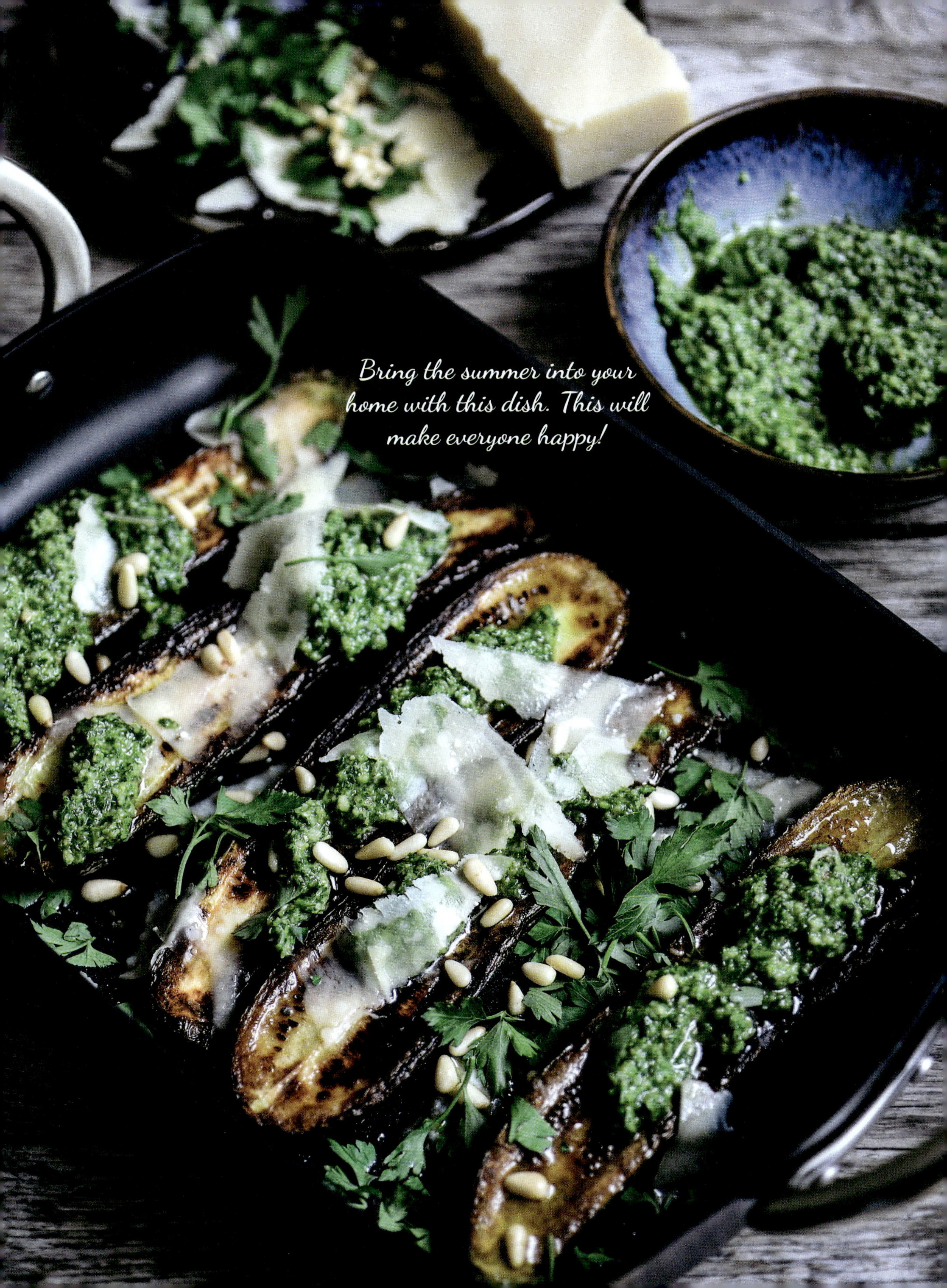
Bring the summer into your
home with this dish. This will
make everyone happy!

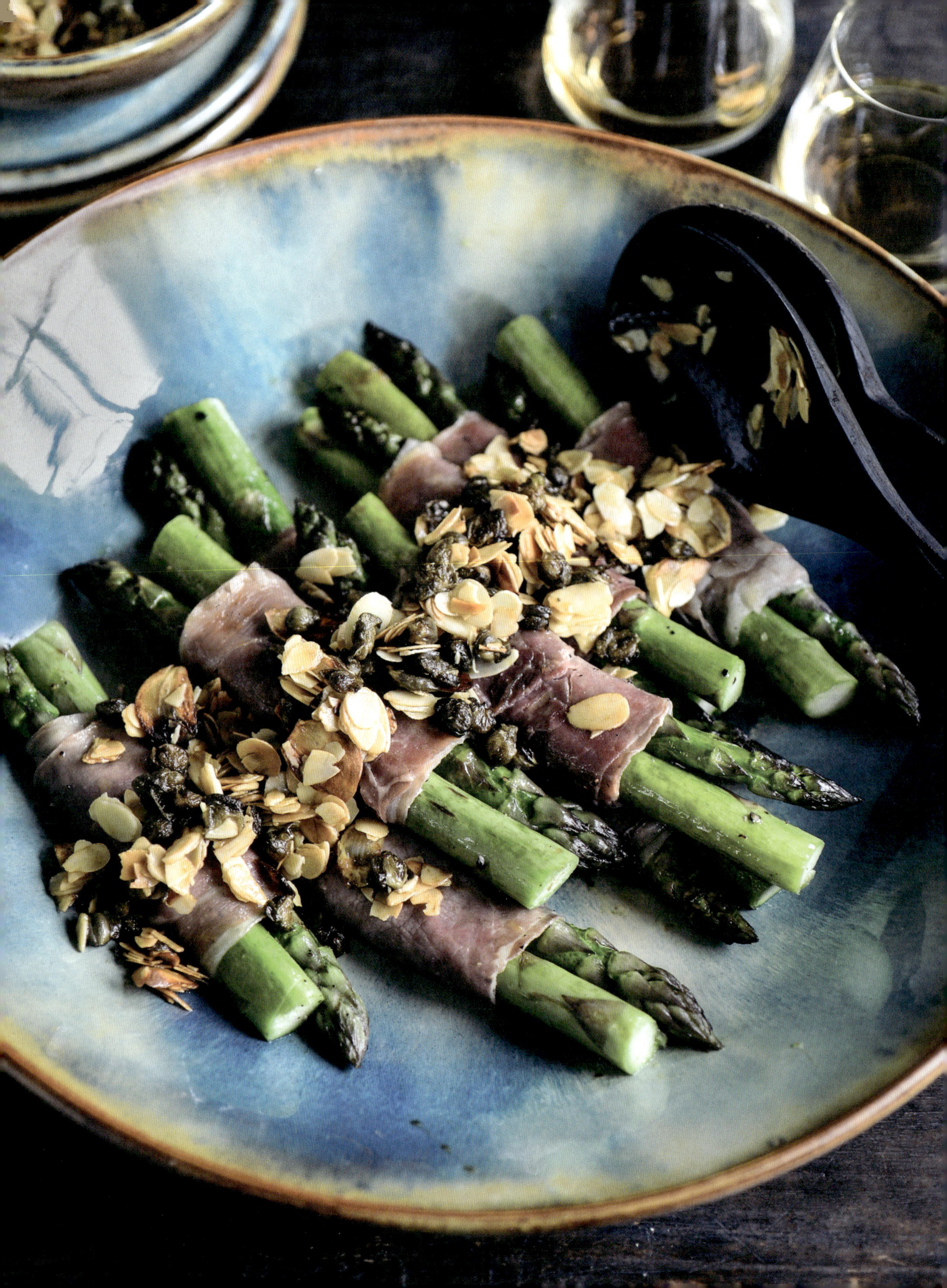

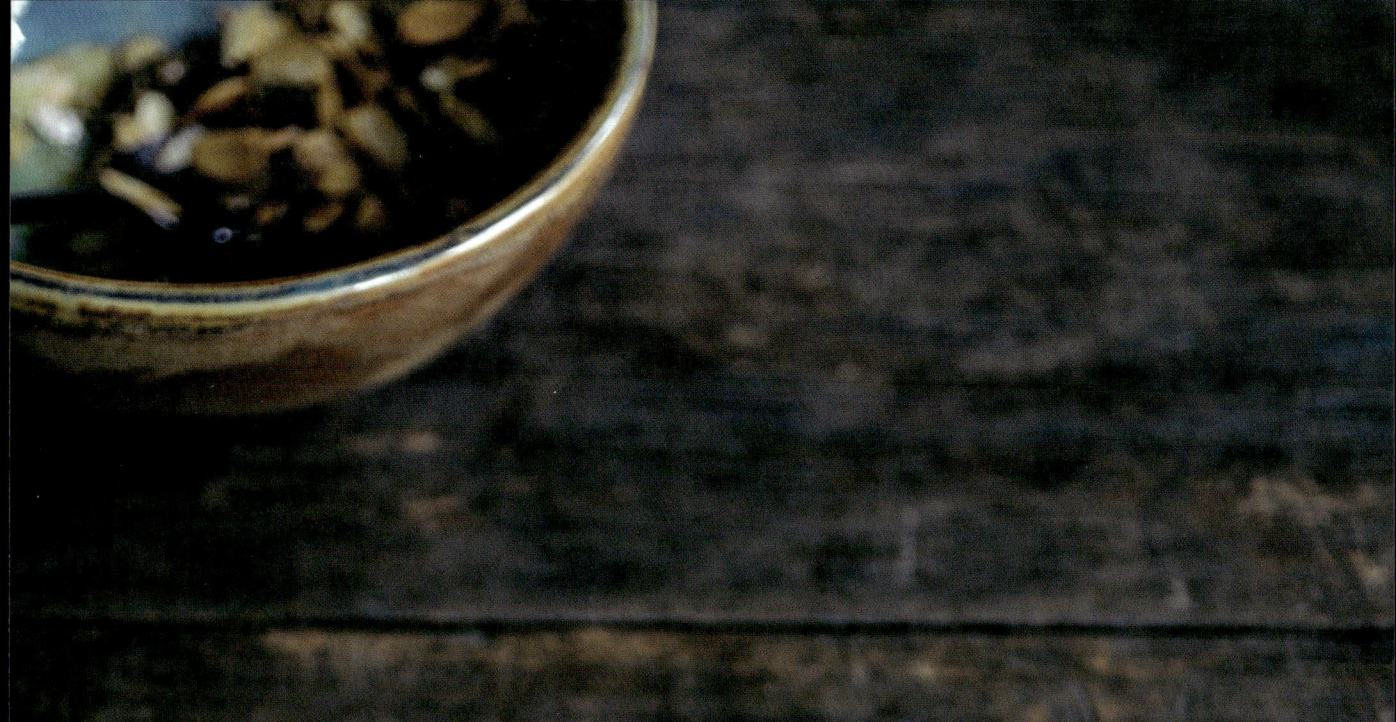

Ideal as an appetizer, a light lunch, or for when you feel like something different. This nut sauce is truly delectable.

green asparagus
with ham and almond-caper sauce

✓ keto

- **20 green asparagus spears**
- **20 slices of firm, dry-cured ham (suitable for rolling up)**
- **a handful of sliced almonds**
- **a handful of capers**

- soy sauce -
- fresh garlic -

Cut off the hard ends of the asparagus. Cook the asparagus al dente, covered, in plenty of olive oil and half a glass of water. Season with salt and pepper. Remove the asparagus from the pan.
Place two slices of ham on top of each other and wrap the asparagus, two at a time, in the ham slices. Put the ham rolls back in the pan and cook them for 1 minute on each side or until the ham turns brown. Place the capers between two paper towels and squeeze out the moisture.
Slice 3 cloves of garlic. Sauté the garlic, capers and sliced almonds in plenty of olive oil until the sliced almonds turn brown. Add a generous splash of soy sauce.
Place the asparagus rolls on a plate and spoon the sauce over the top.

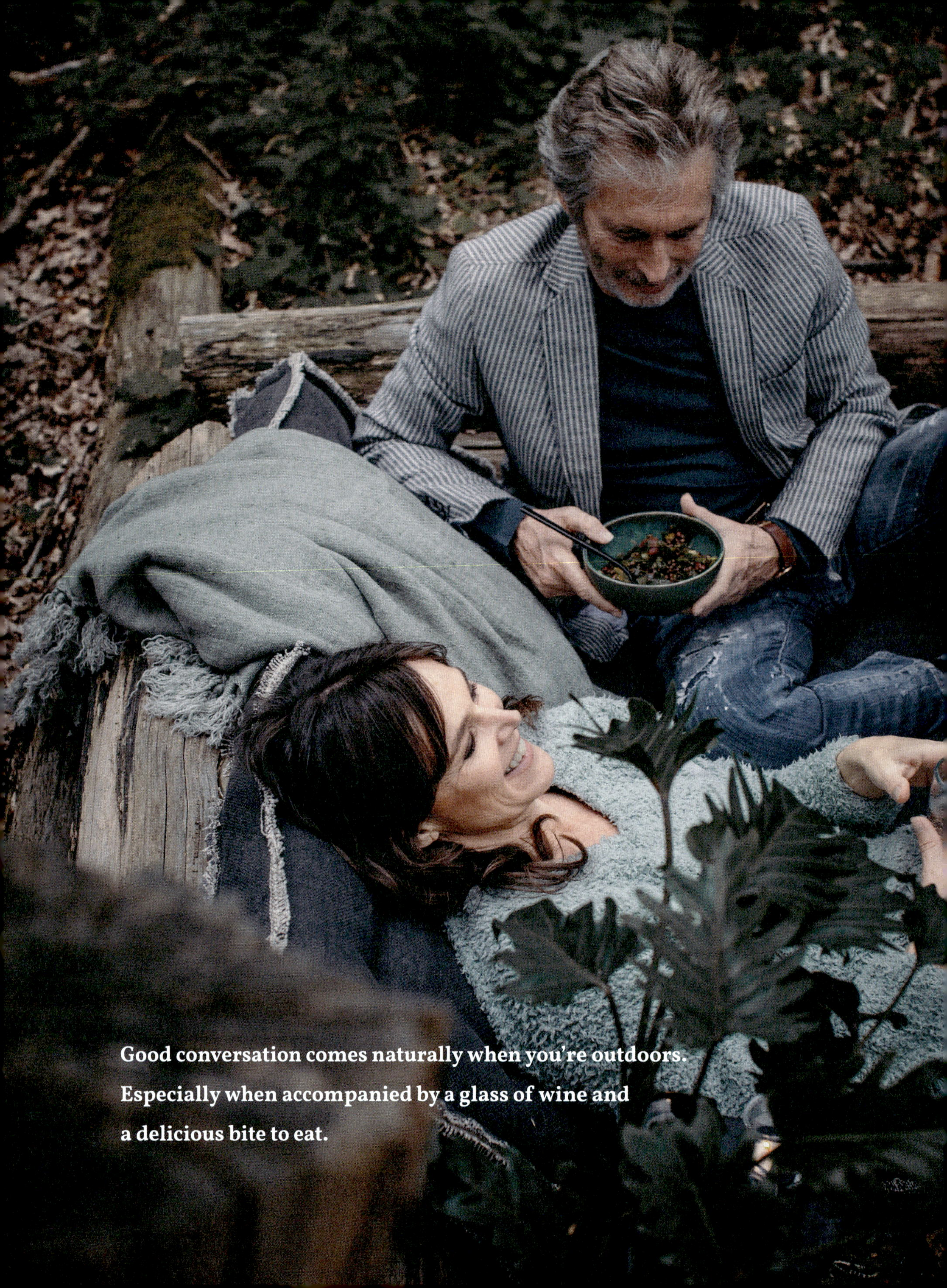

Good conversation comes naturally when you're outdoors. Especially when accompanied by a glass of wine and a delicious bite to eat.

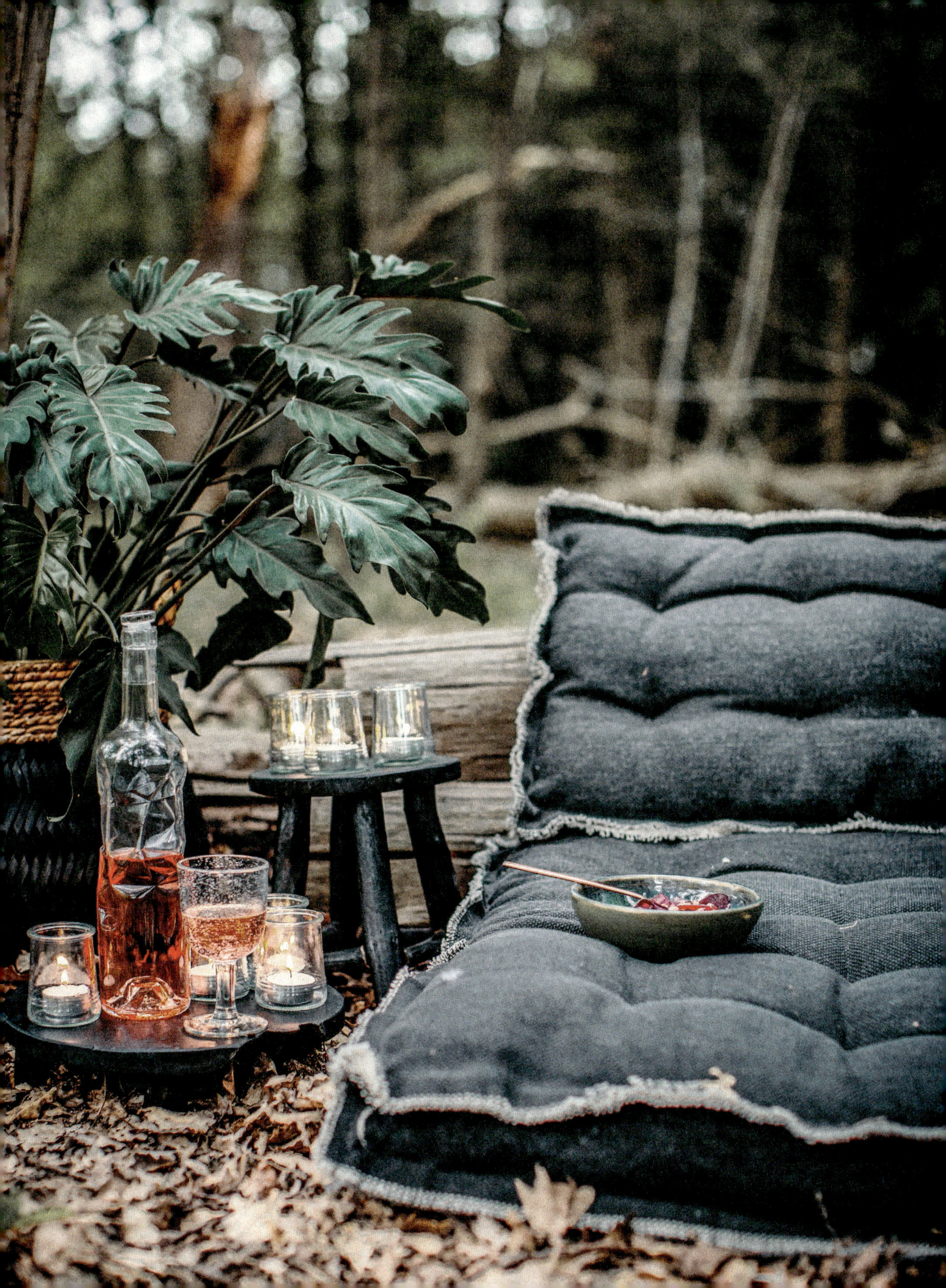

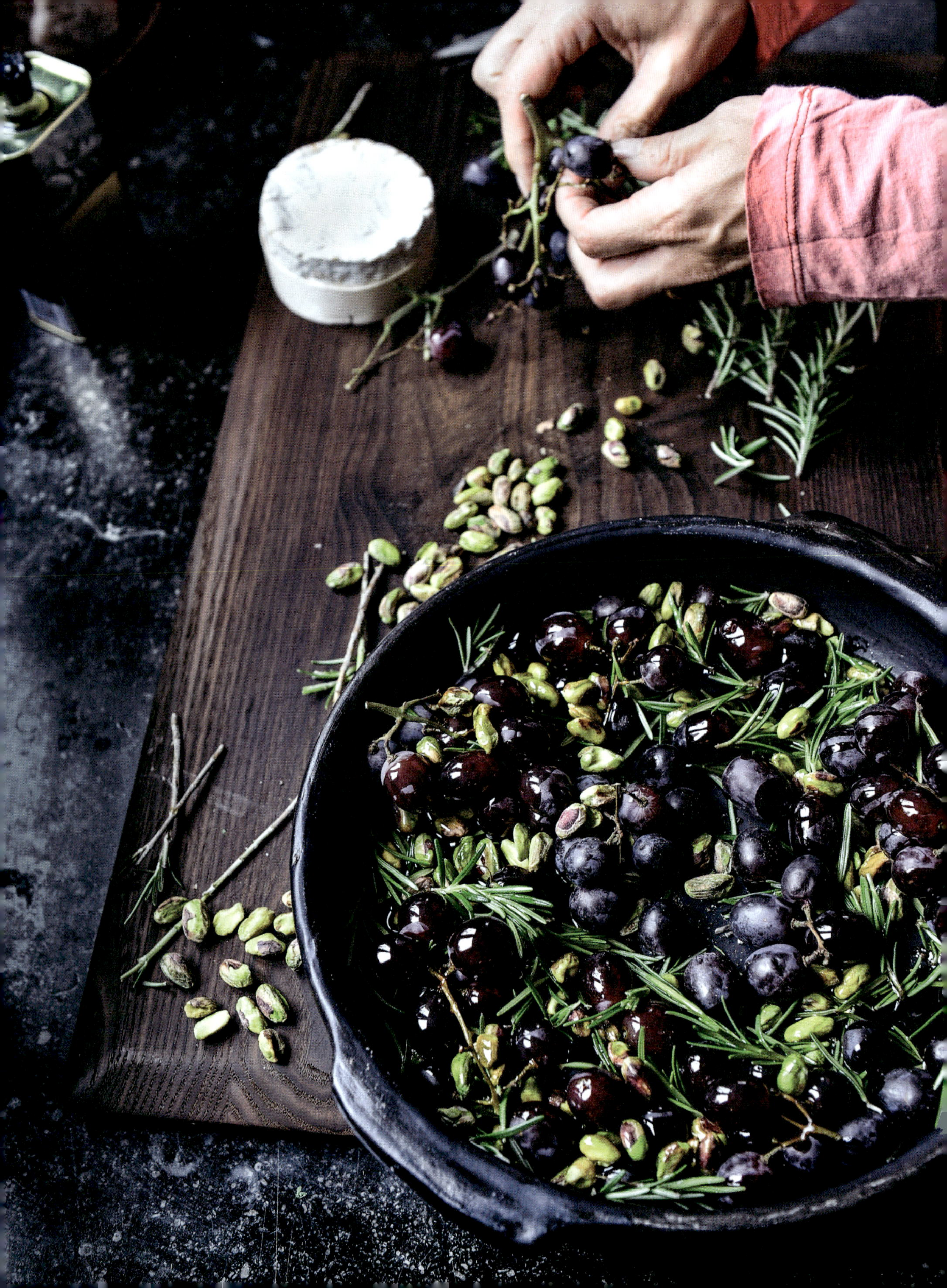

let the oven do the work

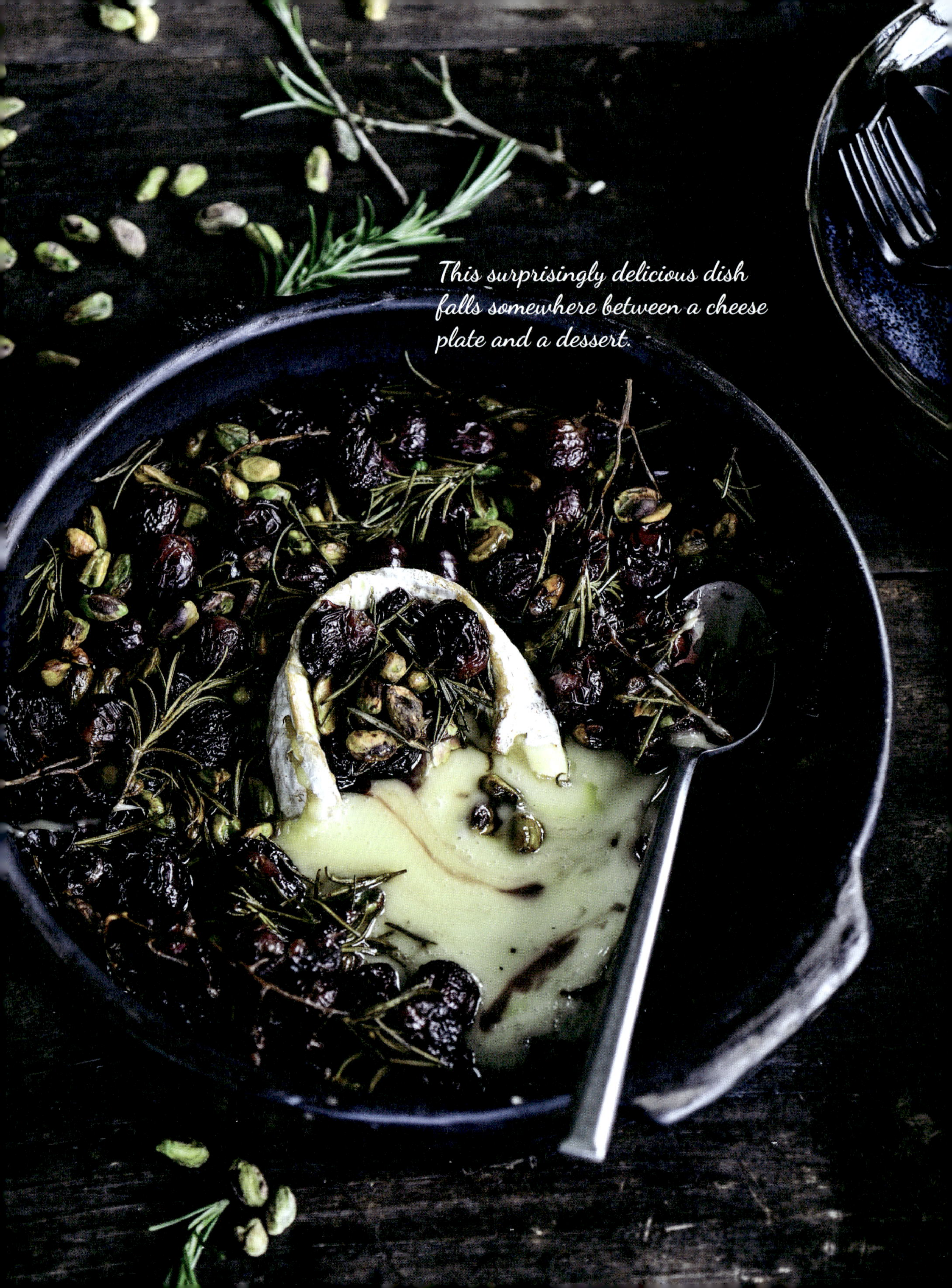
This surprisingly delicious dish
falls somewhere between a cheese
plate and a dessert.

I make this for friends or for when we're not particularly hungry, but still feel like eating something delicious.

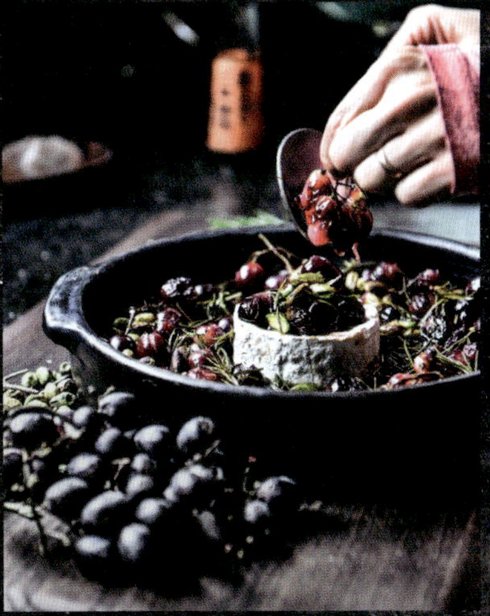

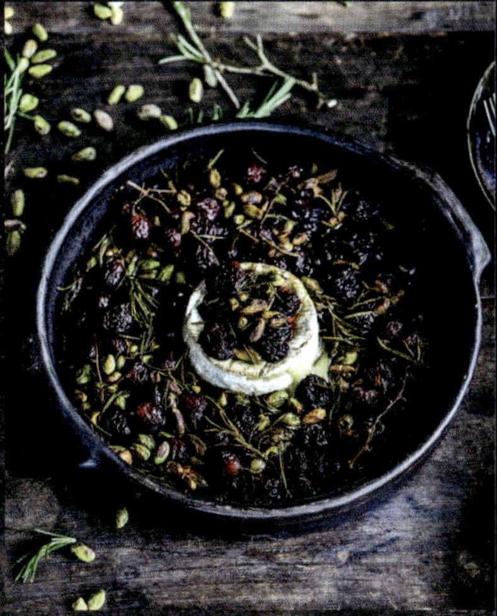

camembert
with grapes and nuts

- **1 large bunch of seedless red grapes**
- **a handful of pistachios**
- **5 sprigs of rosemary**
- **camembert (or brie)**

Preheat the oven to 350 °F (180 °C). Cut the grapes into smaller bunches and place them in a baking dish. Remove the rosemary leaves from the stems and sprinkle them over the grapes. Add the nuts and season generously with black pepper. Drizzle a splash of olive oil over the grapes and bake for 15 to 20 minutes in the oven, or longer if the grapes are large. Score the camembert a couple of times and put the cheese in the oven during the last 10 minutes of cooking. Spoon some of the melted camembert cheese onto a plate and add some grapes and nuts. Delicious!

TIP: GRAPES
Grapes and bananas contain more sugar than other fruits, which is why I see them as nature's candy and only eat them occasionally. Consider this dish more as comfort food, given that it contains too much sugar for a low-carb dish.

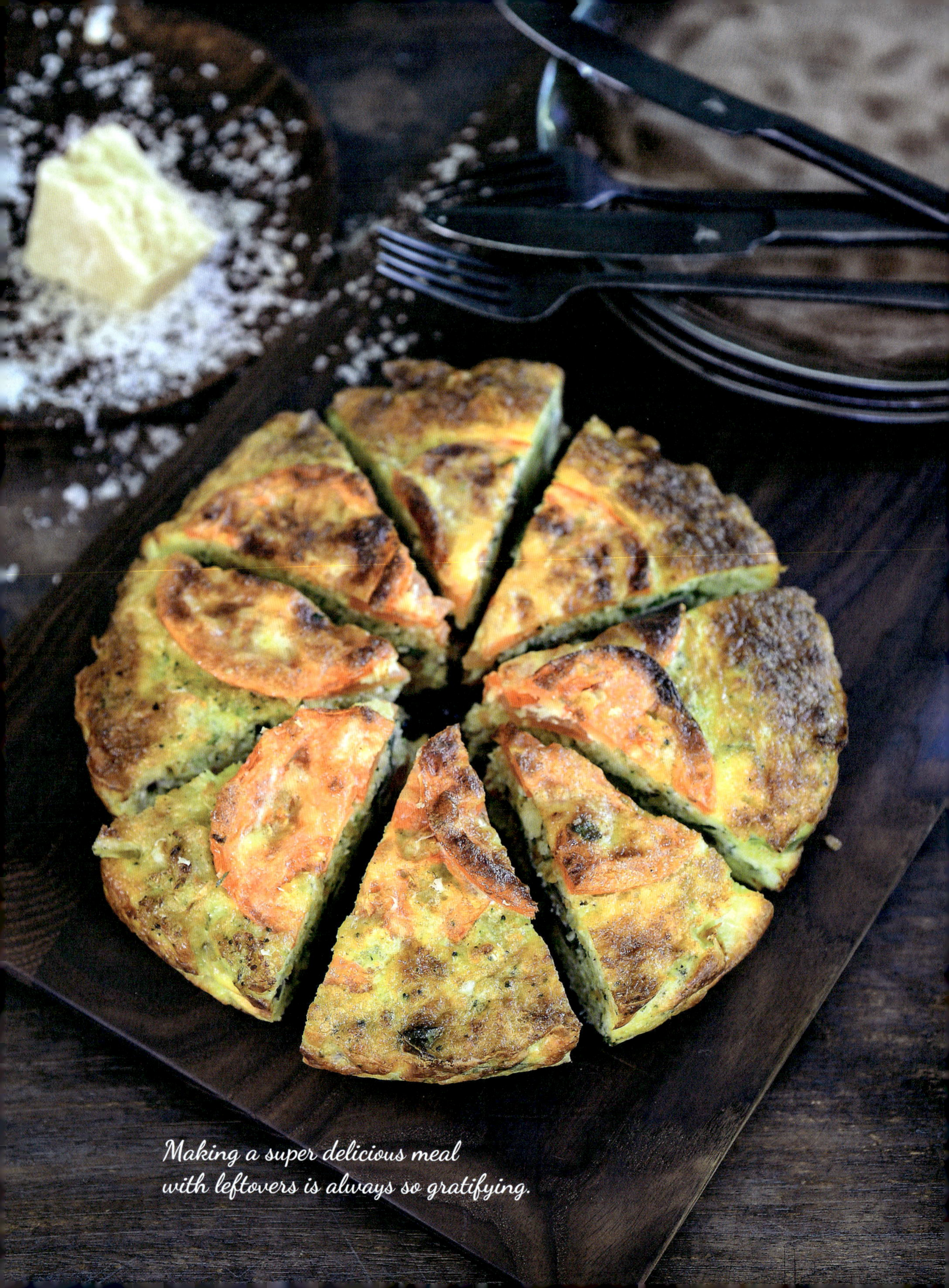

Making a super delicious meal with leftovers is always so gratifying.

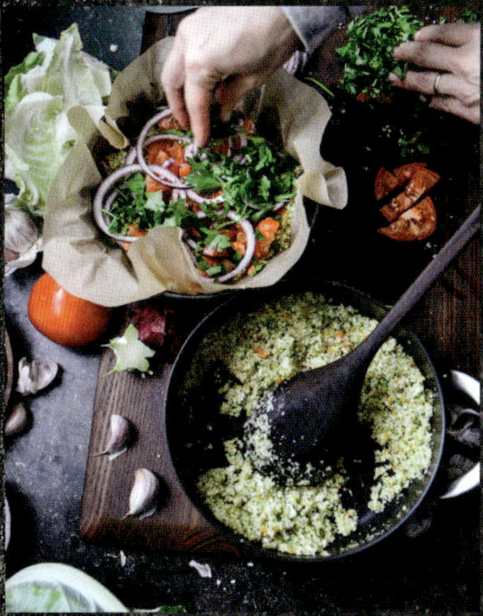

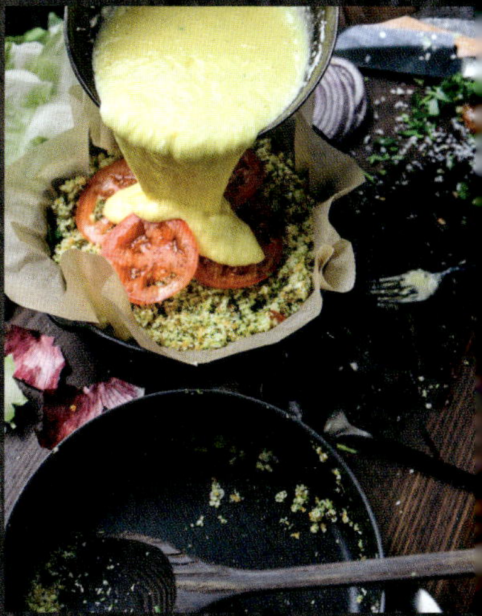

no-waste-recipe

quiche

✓ keto

- **3 eggs (about 1 egg per 5 oz/150 g vegetables)**
- **1 lb (450 g) leftover vegetables and herbs**
- **7 fl oz (200 ml) cream**
- **¾ oz (20 g) Parmesan cheese + ¼ oz (5 g) extra**

extra: parchment paper

Preheat the oven to 350 °F (180 °C). Dice the hard vegetables into smaller pieces, put them in the blender and blend them into fine crumbs with the same texture as cauliflower rice. If you can't blend them all at once, blend each vegetable separately. Sauté the vegetables in plenty of olive oil. Three minutes should be enough to make sure the vegetables will soften enough during cooking. Season with plenty of salt and pepper. Meanwhile, chop the softer vegetables into small pieces: for example, onions into rings, zucchini into cubes, and tomatoes into slices. Finely chop the herbs. Line a baking dish with parchment paper. Spoon all the vegetables and herbs into the dish. I like to finish with a couple of slices of tomato on top. Combine the cream with the eggs and grate the Parmesan cheese into the mixture. Season with salt and pepper. Pour the egg mixture over the vegetables and let it soak in between the vegetables. Garnish with the extra Parmesan cheese. Bake the quiche in the oven for 30 to 45 minutes, or until the eggs are set and a crispy crust forms on top of the quiche.

TIP: NO-WASTE RECIPE
You can make a delicious quiche with any leftover vegetables and herbs you may have in the fridge, anything goes. The fun thing about this recipe is that your quiche will taste different every time, and it feels great not to have to throw anything away. It's also ideal for when you need to eat while on the go.

TIP: VEGETABLES
Hard vegetables: cauliflower, celeriac, broccoli, turnips …
Soft vegetables: tomatoes, zucchini, onions, mushrooms …
Leftover herbs: parsley, chives, fresh garlic …

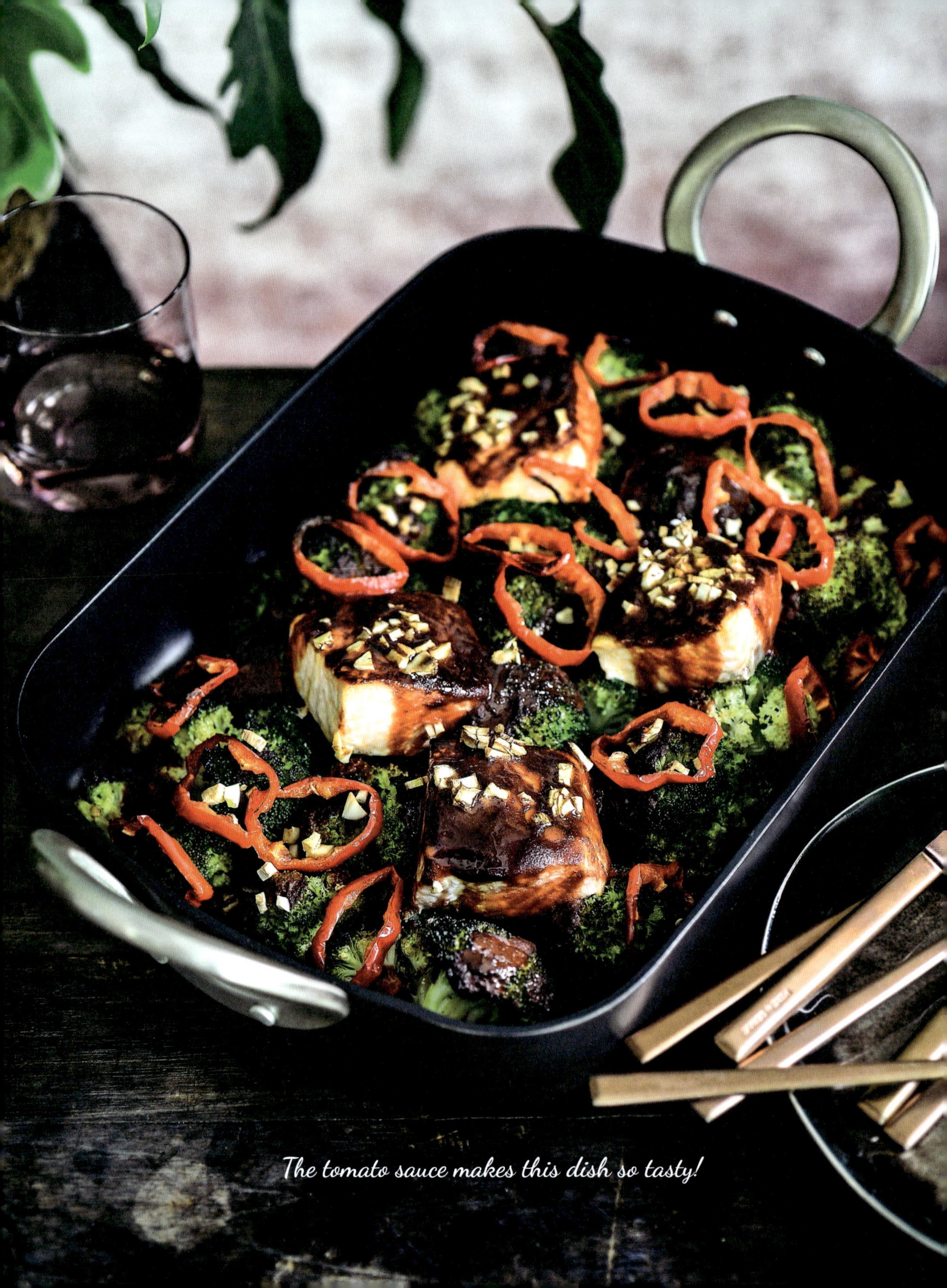

The tomato sauce makes this dish so tasty!

oven-baked salmon ✓keto

with broccoli and delicious tomato sauce

- **10½ oz (300 g) salmon fillet, without skin**
- **1 head of broccoli**
- **7 oz (200 g) strained tomatoes or tomato puree (see tip on page 107)**
- **1 pointed sweet red pepper**

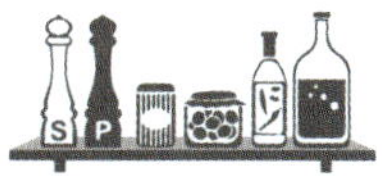

– soy sauce –
– balsamic vinegar –
– fresh garlic –

Preheat the oven to 350 °F (180 °C). Cut the florets from the broccoli and cook them for 3 minutes in water with a splash of olive oil. Put them in a baking dish. Slice the salmon into four pieces and place the fish on top of the broccoli. Season with salt and pepper. Stir 6 tablespoons of soy sauce, 3 tablespoons of balsamic vinegar and 3 tablespoons of water into the strained tomatoes. Spoon the sauce mostly over the salmon and a little bit over the broccoli.

Finely chop 2 cloves of garlic and sprinkle over the salmon. Slice the pointed sweet pepper into rings and distribute them evenly over the salmon and broccoli. Pour a thin drizzle of olive oil over the vegetables and bake the dish in the oven for 20 minutes until the salmon is cooked through.

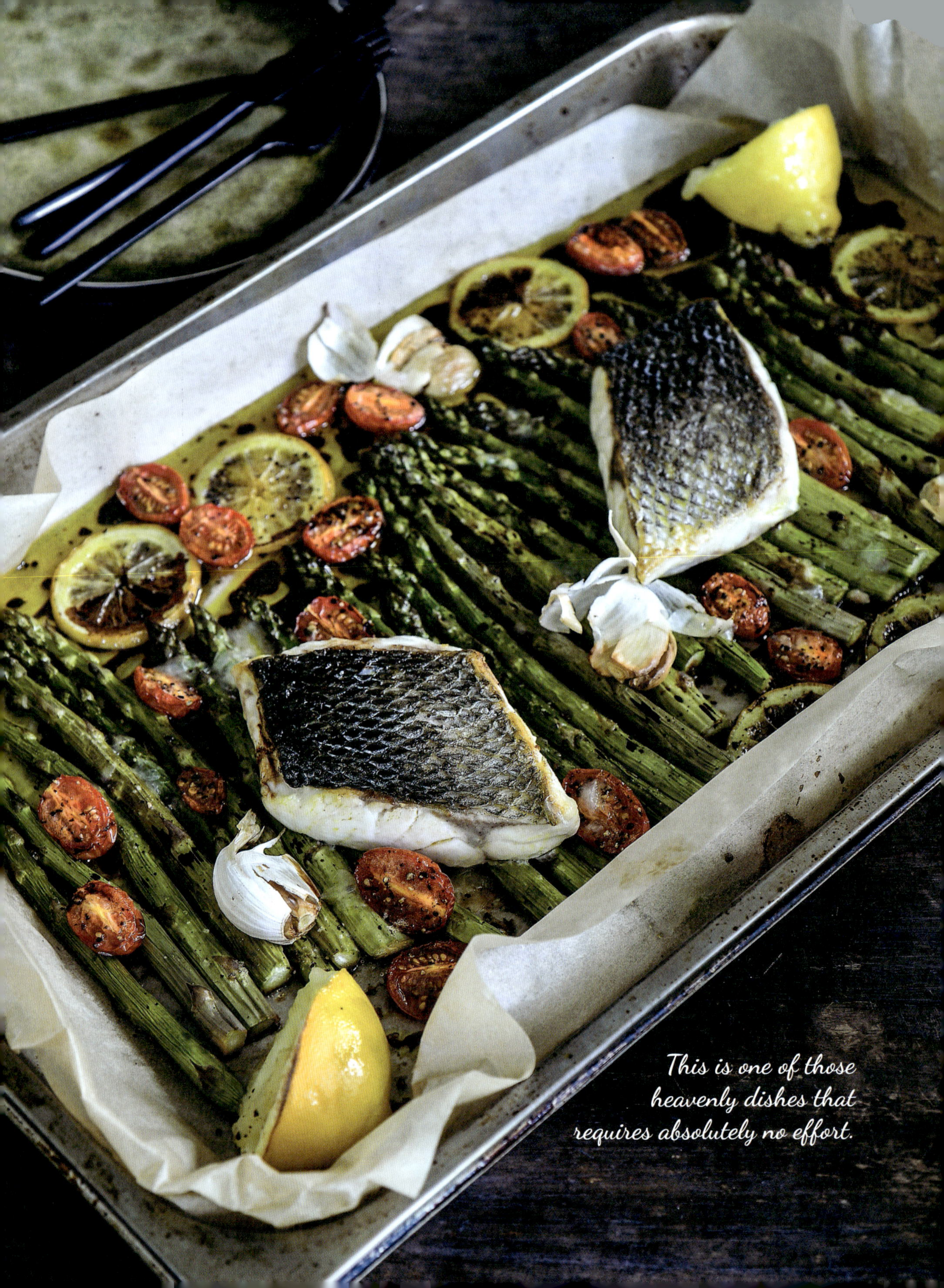

This is one of those heavenly dishes that requires absolutely no effort.

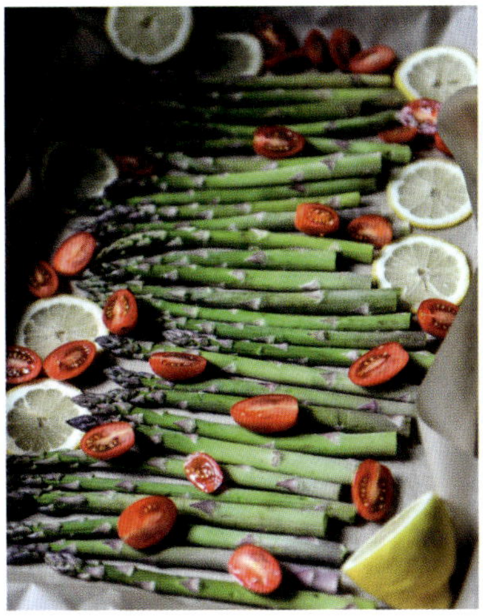

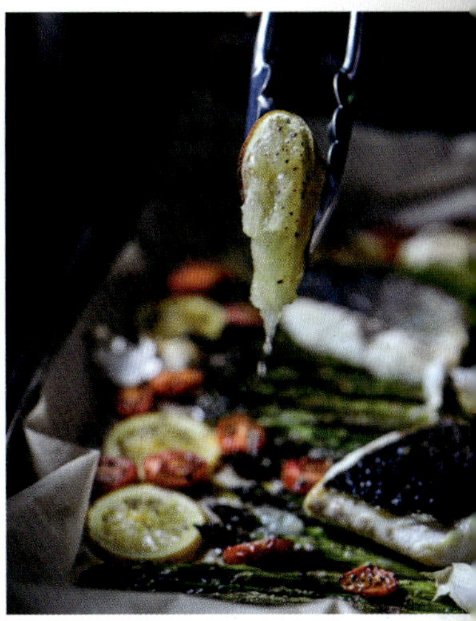

sea bass
keto

with green asparagus

- 2 sea bass fillets, with skin
- 2 bunches of green asparagus
- 15 cherry tomatoes
- 2 lemons

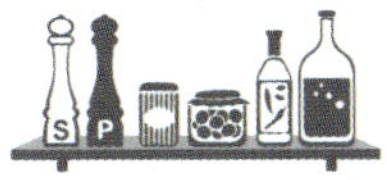

– soy sauce –

extra: parchment paper

Preheat the oven to 350 °F (180 °C). Line a baking dish with parchment paper. Cut off the hard ends and place the asparagus in the baking dish. Cut the cherry tomatoes in half and arrange them among the asparagus. Cut 1 lemon into slices and the other in half. Put the lemon slices with the asparagus. Season with salt and pepper and drizzle some olive oil over the top. Bake in the oven for 25 minutes. Season the fish with salt and pepper and rub the fish with olive oil. Cook the fish with the vegetables in the oven during the final 10 minutes of cooking. Remove the dish from the oven once the fish is tender. Squeeze the lemon halves out over the asparagus and pour a small amount of soy sauce over the dish. Arrange the fish and vegetables on the plates.

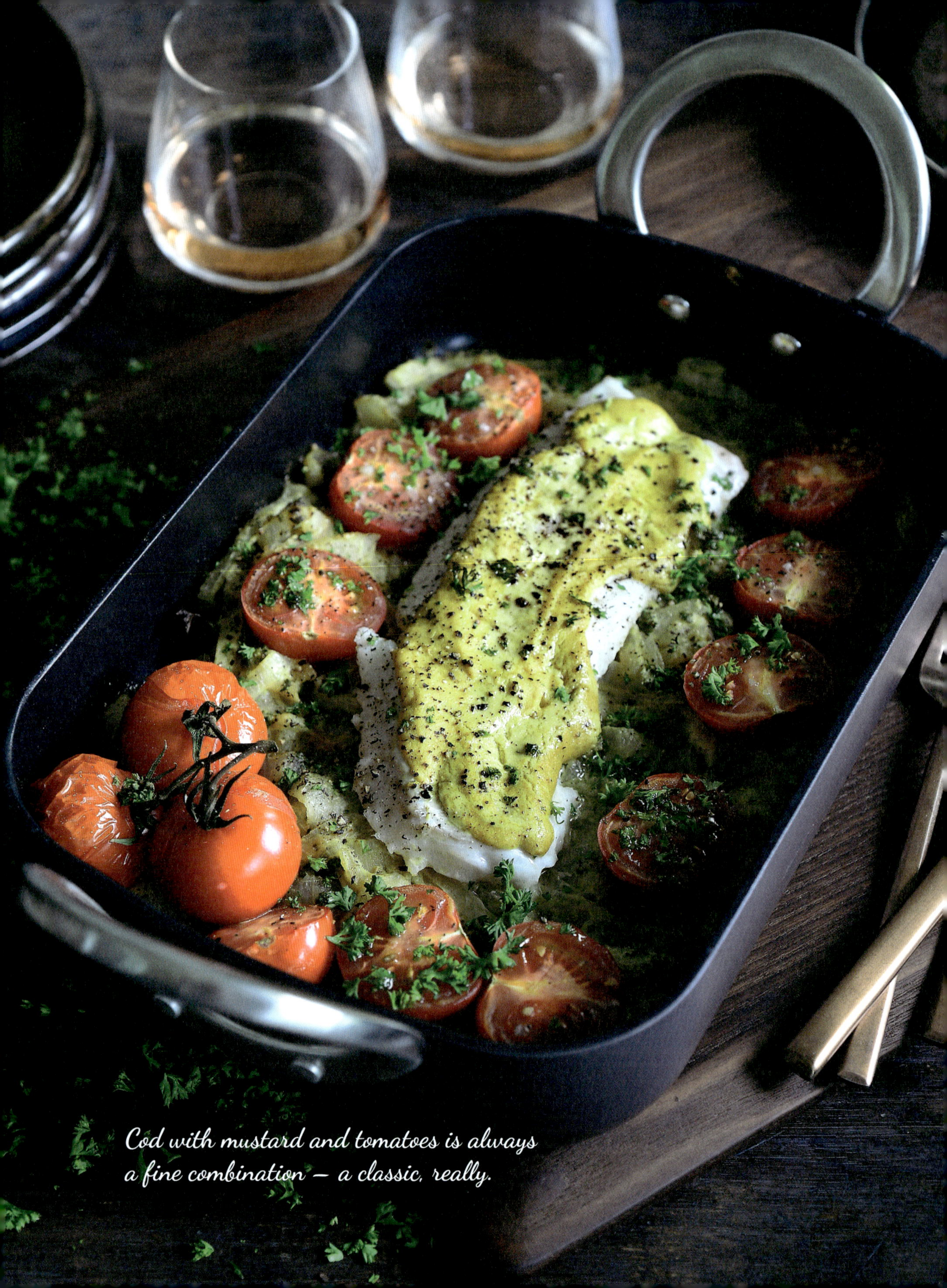

Cod with mustard and tomatoes is always a fine combination – a classic, really.

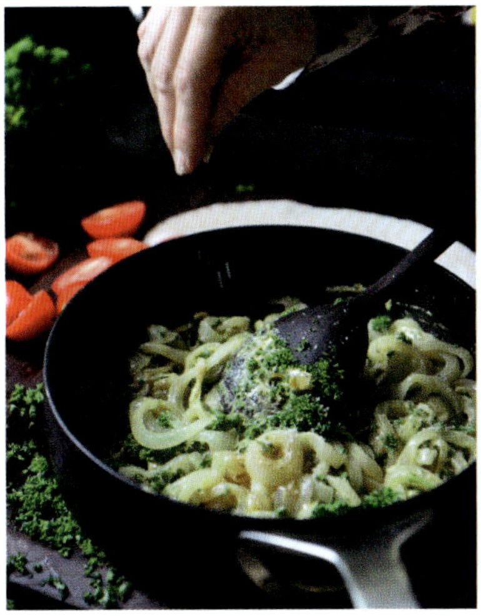

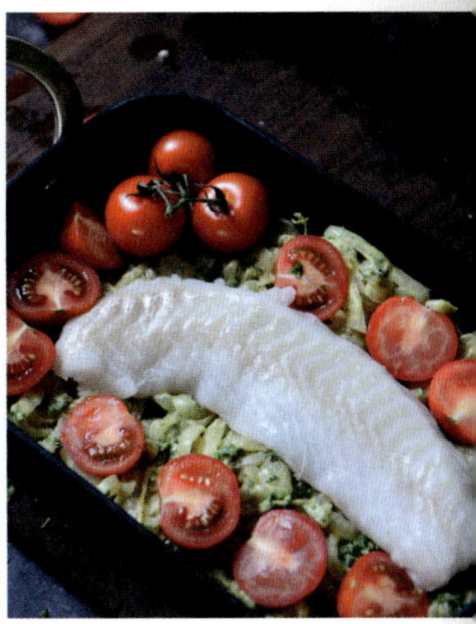

cod
✓ keto

with mustard

- **3 or 4 large yellow onions**
- **10 medium-sized tomatoes**
- **2 cod fillets**
- **a handful of curly-leaf parsley**

Slice the onions and sauté them, covered, for 4 minutes in plenty of olive oil. Stir occasionally but not too often, giving the onions time to brown. Cut the tomatoes in half and finely chop the parsley. Preheat the oven to 350 °F (180 °C). Remove the pan from the heat and season the onions with salt and pepper. Add 2 to 3 tablespoons of mustard and half the parsley.
Stir everything thoroughly and spoon the onions into a baking dish. Flatten them slightly with the back of a spoon. Arrange the tomatoes with the cut side up on top and place the fish in the middle. Combine 1 tablespoon of mustard with 1 tablespoon of olive oil and coat the fish with the mixture. Season the tomatoes with salt and pepper, drizzle some olive oil over the top and bake in the oven for 10 minutes. Serve in the baking dish.

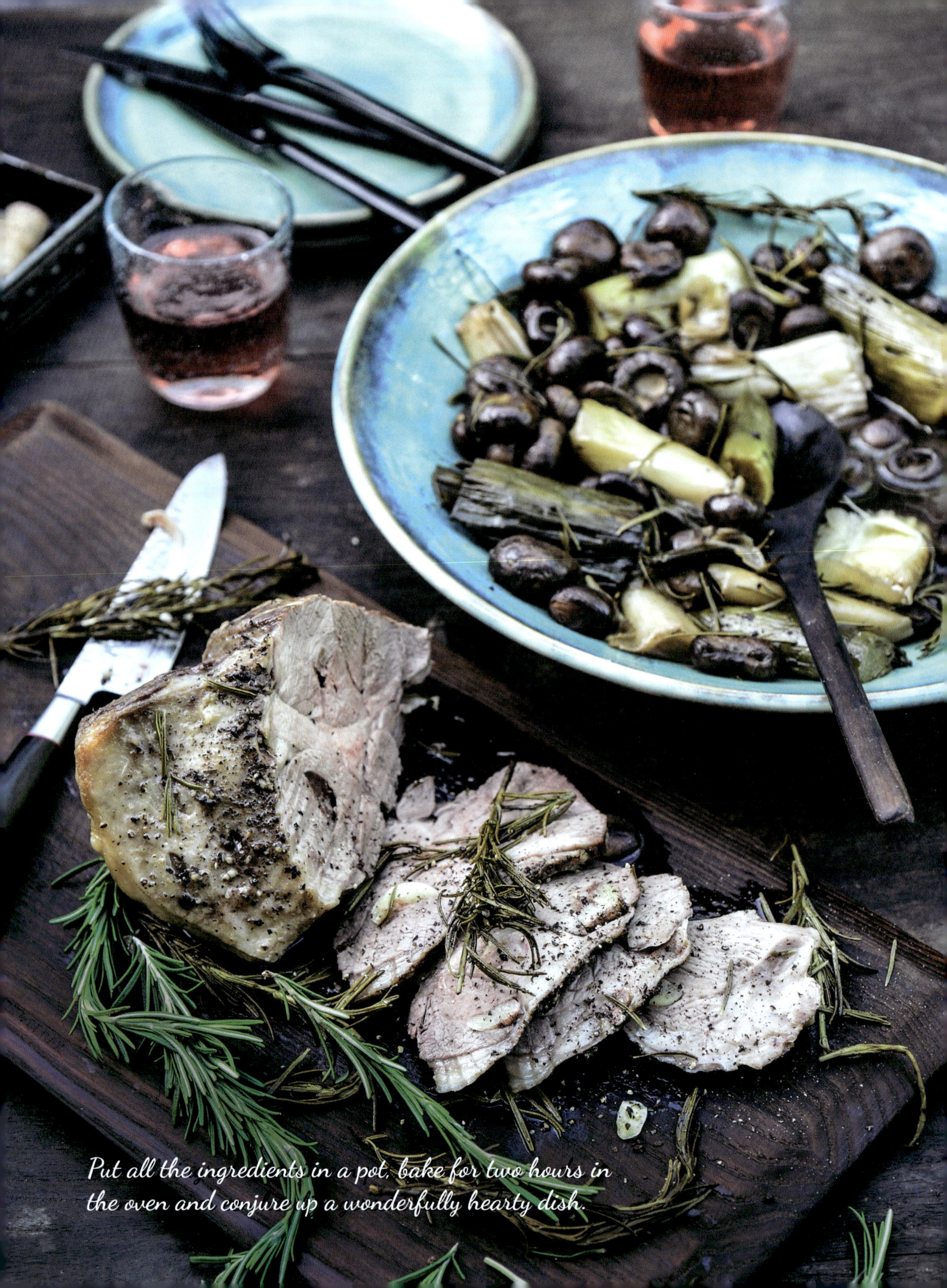

Put all the ingredients in a pot, bake for two hours in the oven and conjure up a wonderfully hearty dish.

If you are having guests over who enjoy a fine piece of meat, look no further! Simple, surprising and scrumptious.

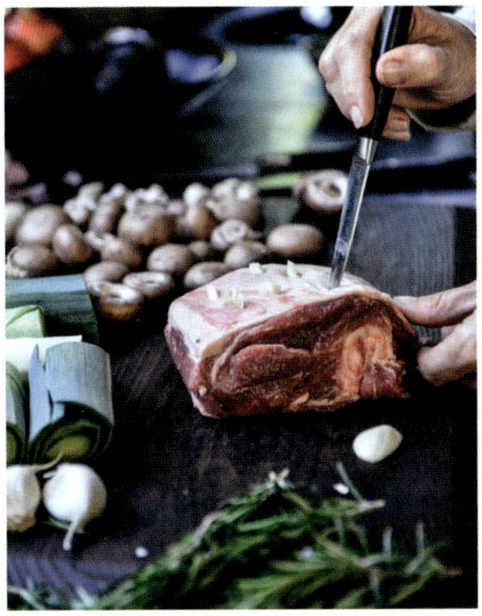

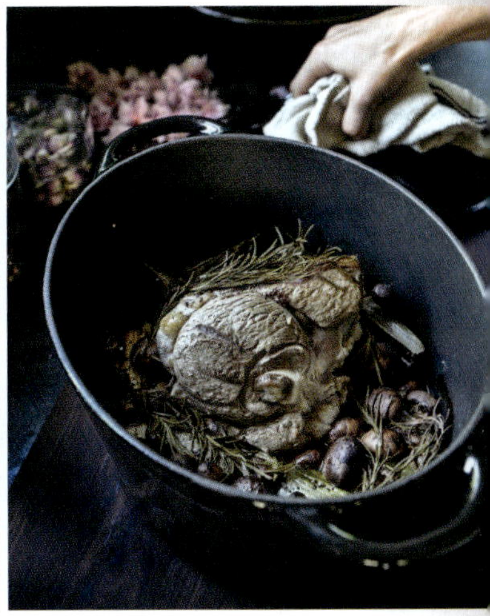

leg of lamb

keto

with leeks, mushrooms and rosemary

- **leg of lamb for 2 people**
- **3 leeks**
- **a little over 1 lb (500 g) brown mushrooms**
- **2 bunches of rosemary**

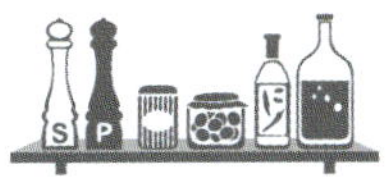

- fresh garlic -

Preheat the oven to 350 °F (180 °C). With a knife, score ten cuts measuring ¾ inches (2 cm) deep in the leg of lamb and fill the cuts with halved cloves of garlic. Use a large, sturdy ovenproof pot with a lid. Slice the leeks into 2-inch (5 cm) pieces and put them in the pot. Remove the stems from the mushrooms and place them on top of the leeks. Put one bunch of rosemary on top of the vegetables. Season with salt and pepper and pour plenty of olive oil over the top. Put the leg of lamb on top of the vegetables, season with salt and pepper and distribute the second bunch of rosemary evenly over the top. Drizzle some olive oil over the meat. Cover the pot and bake for 2 hours in the oven. I like to serve this on an attractive dish.

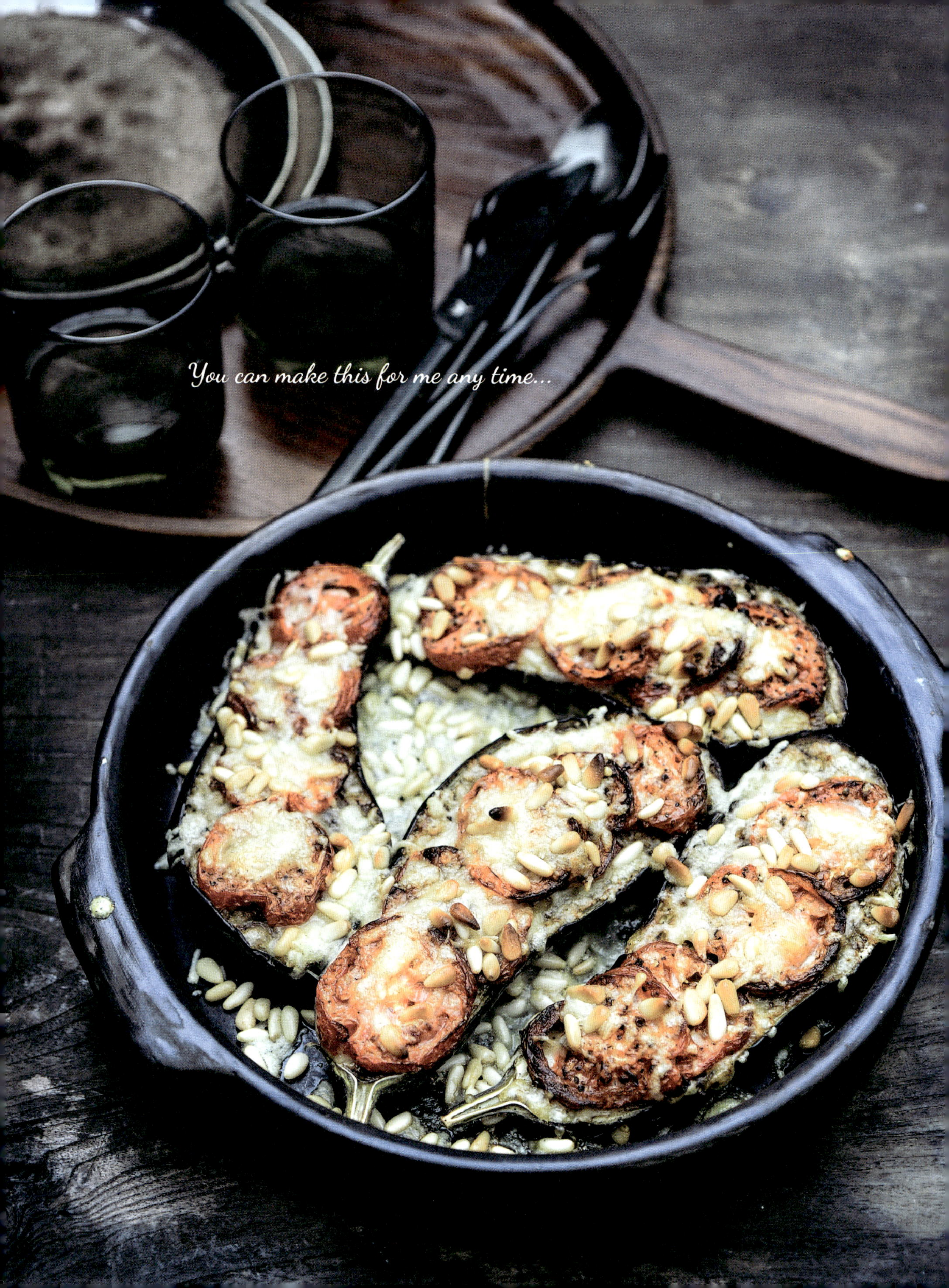
You can make this for me any time...

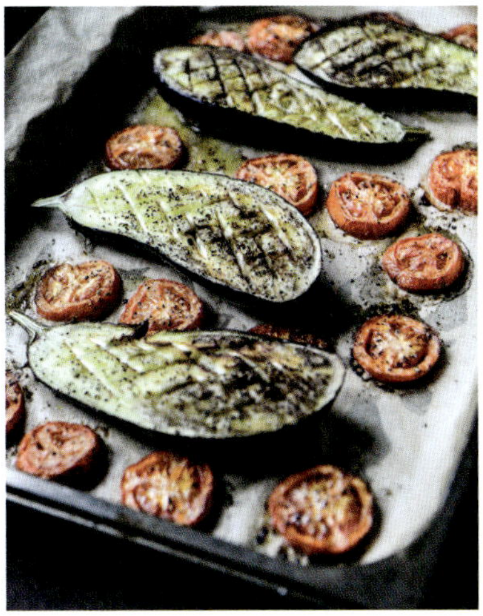

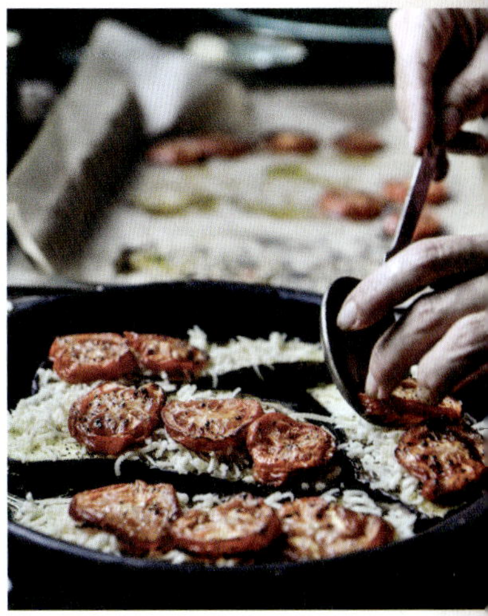

✓ keto

eggplant
and tomato gratin

- **2 eggplants**
- **4 tomatoes**
- **3½ oz (100 g) Gruyère cheese**
- **a handful of pine nuts**

extra: parchment paper

Preheat the oven to 350 °F (180 °C). Slice the eggplants in half. With a knife, score the flesh in a crisscross pattern and drizzle some olive oil over the top. Season with salt and pepper and place the eggplants cut side up on a baking tray lined with parchment paper.
Slice the tomatoes into thick slices and place them between the eggplant halves. Season with salt and pepper and pour a splash of olive oil over the top. Bake the vegetables in the oven for 30 minutes.
Remove the vegetables from the oven and transfer the eggplant to a baking dish. Scatter half the Gruyère over the eggplants, place the cooked tomato slices on top and top off with the remaining cheese. Garnish with the pine nuts and bake in the oven for another 5 to 10 minutes until the cheese has melted.

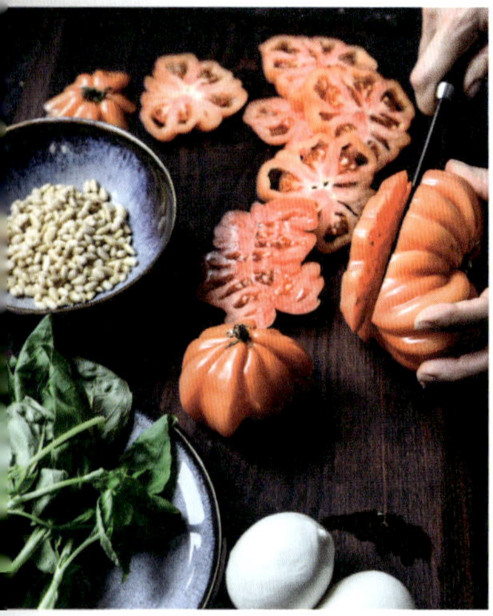
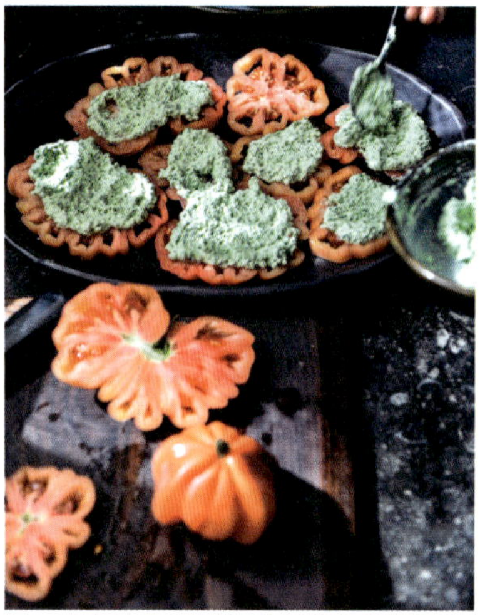

tomato with burrata ✓keto

- **2 balls burrata cheese (see tip)**
- **3 to 4 tomatoes (see tip)**
- **2 bunches of basil (1½ oz/40 g)**
- **a handful of pine nuts**

Preheat the oven to 350 °F (180 °C). Put the burrata together with three quarters of the pine nuts and three quarters of the basil in a blender, season with salt and pepper and blend to form a pesto. Slice the tomatoes, put them in a baking dish, distribute the cheesy pesto over the tomatoes and scatter the remaining pine nuts on top. Bake in the oven for about 20 minutes.
Serve the tomatoes in the baking dish and garnish with the remaining basil.

TIP: BURRATA
Burrata is a fresh Italian cheese made from mozzarella and cream. This makes the cheese creamier and more flavorful than mozzarella.

TIP: TOMATOES
When they're in season, I like to use beefsteak tomatoes because of their lovely shape.

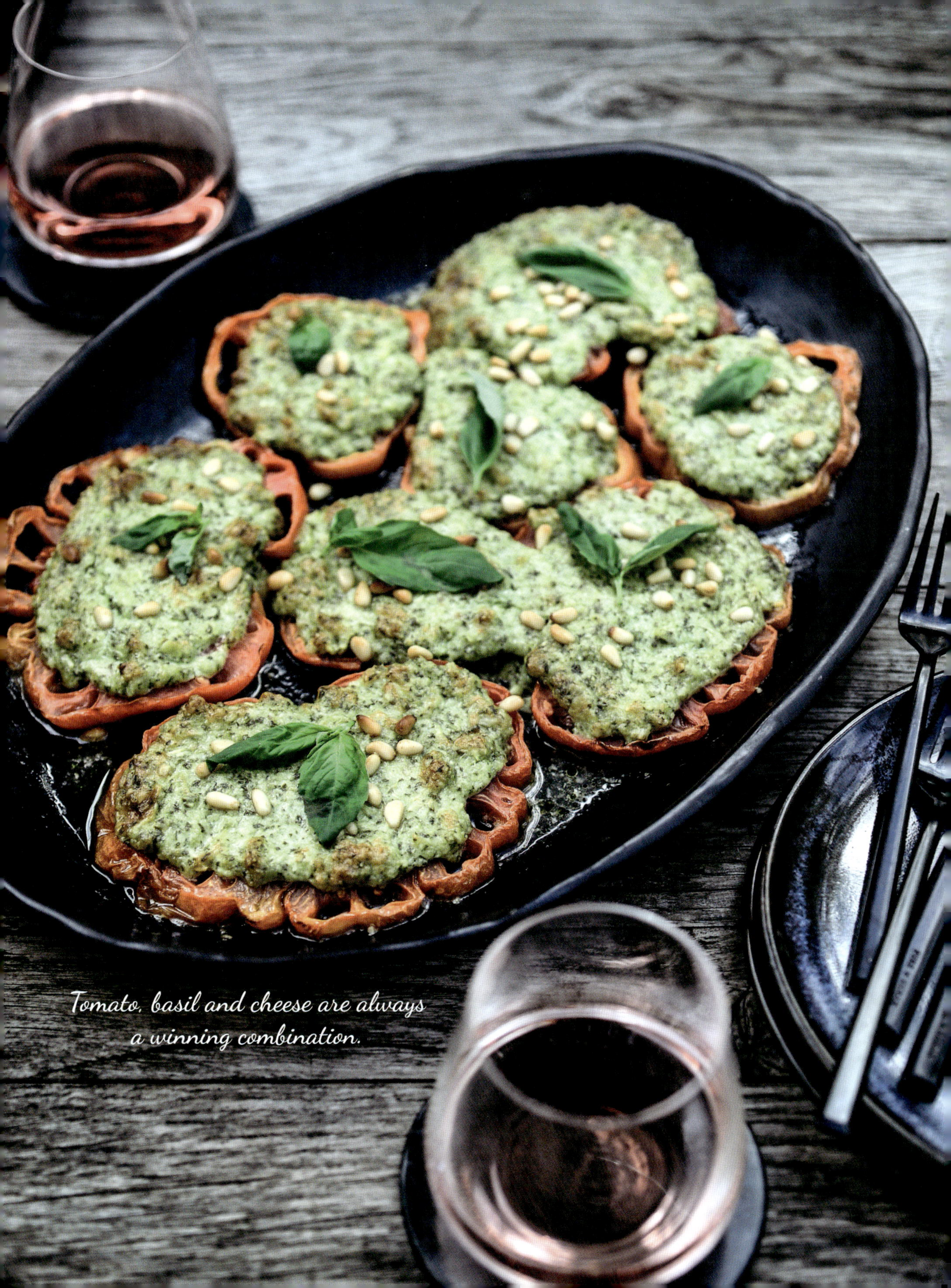

Tomato, basil and cheese are always a winning combination.

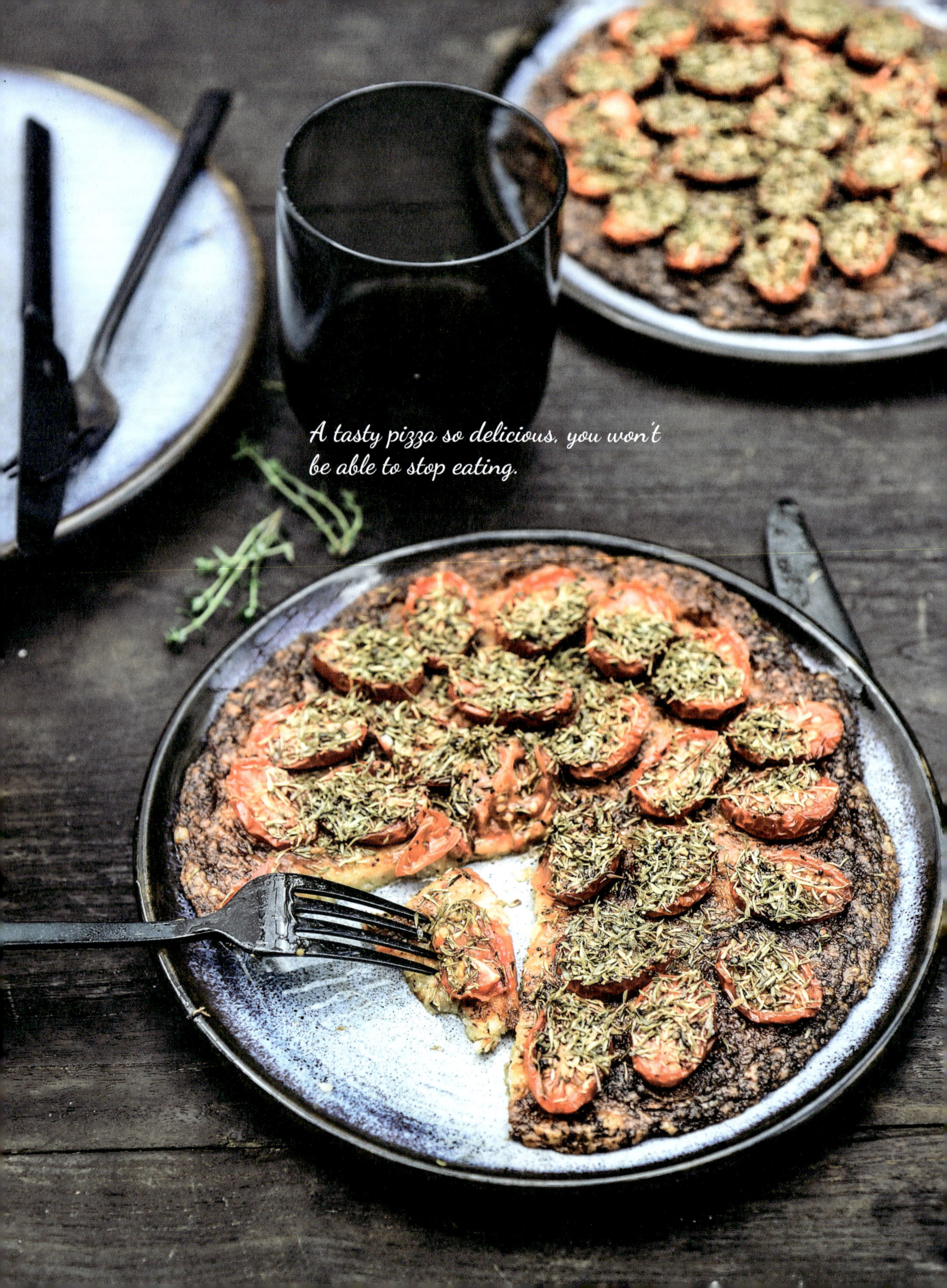
A tasty pizza so delicious, you won't
be able to stop eating.

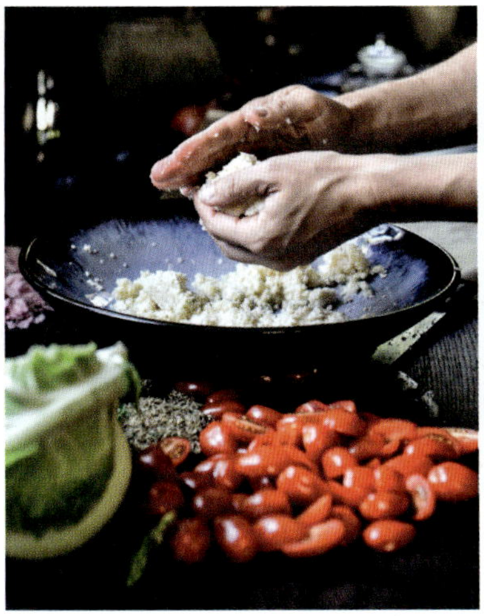
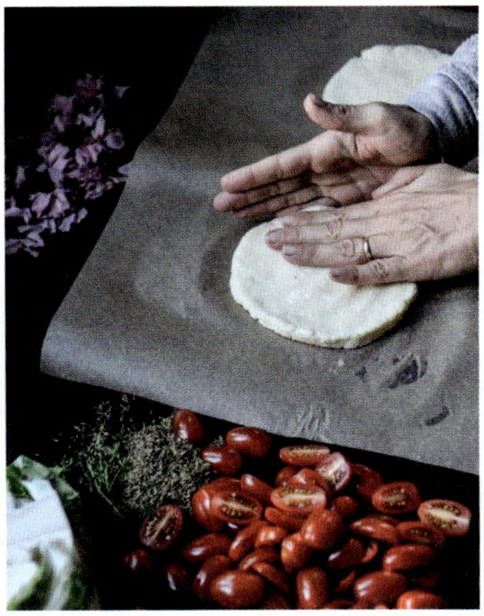
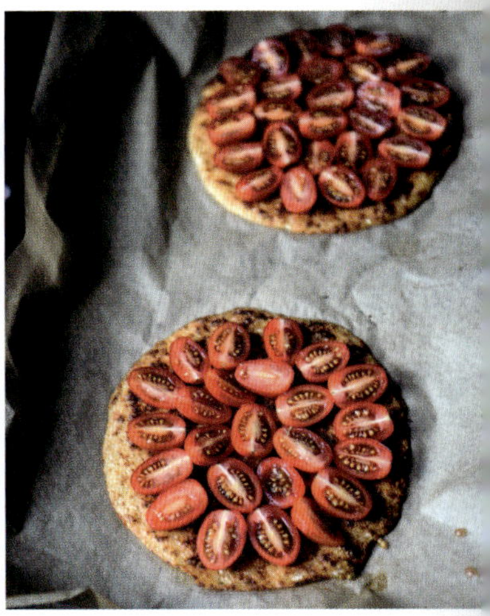

pizza with tomatoes ✓ keto

and a cheesy cauliflower base

- **¼ cauliflower (about 7 oz/200 g)**
- **7 oz (200 g) Gruyère**
- **7 oz (200 g) cherry tomatoes**
- **dried thyme**

extra: parchment paper

Preheat the oven to 350 °F (180 °C). Finely chop the cauliflower and combine with the Gruyère in a blender to form a sort of dough. Shape the dough into two balls and flatten them to a thickness of about ¼ inch (0.5 cm) on a baking sheet lined with parchment paper.

Bake the pizza bases for 20 to 30 minutes in the oven until they are light brown.

Meanwhile, slice the tomatoes in half. Remove the pizza bases from the oven and arrange the tomatoes on top, putting them close to each other. Scatter plenty of dried thyme over the pizzas, season with salt and pepper, drizzle a generous splash of olive oil over the top and bake in the oven for another 20 minutes.

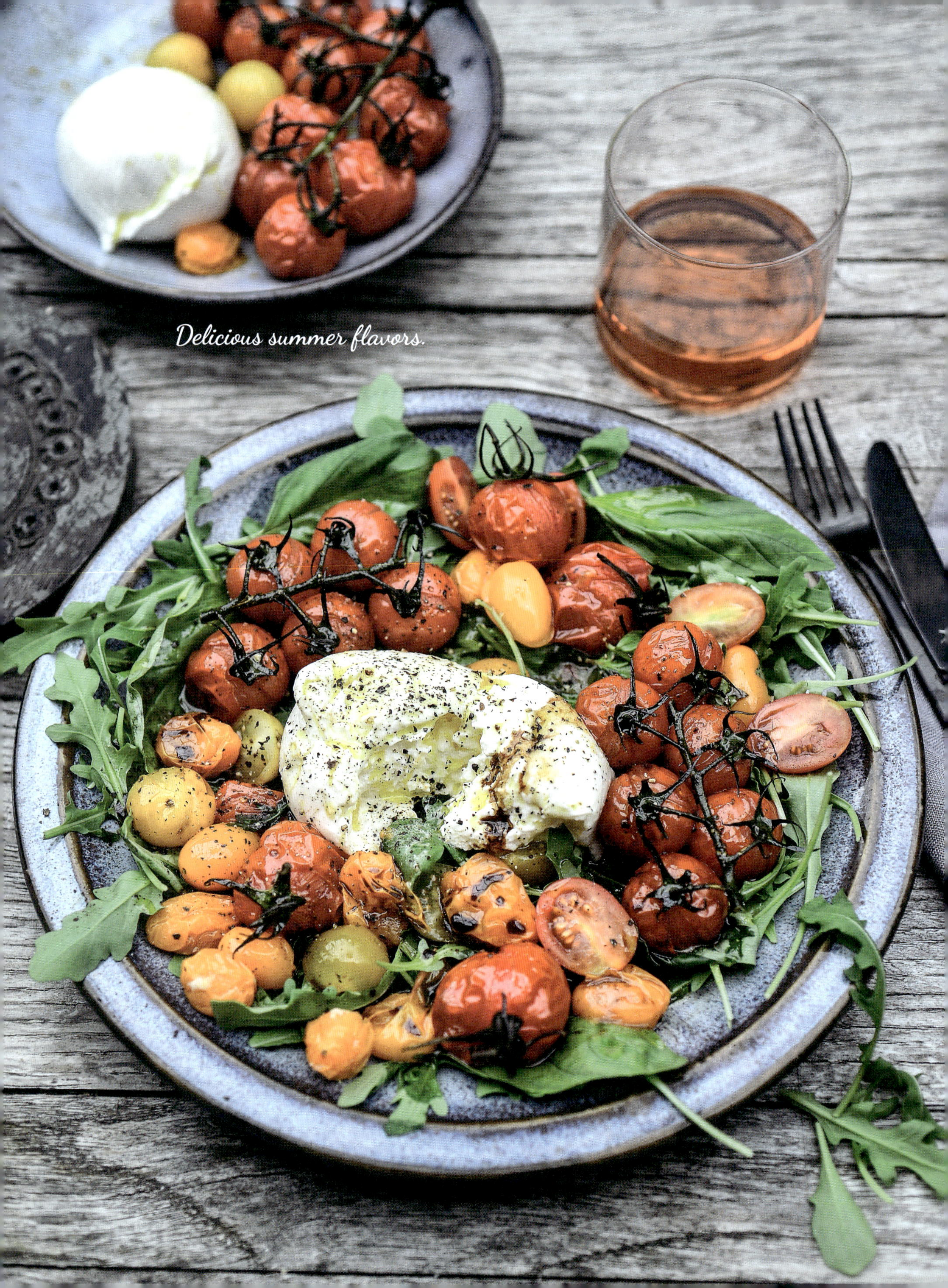

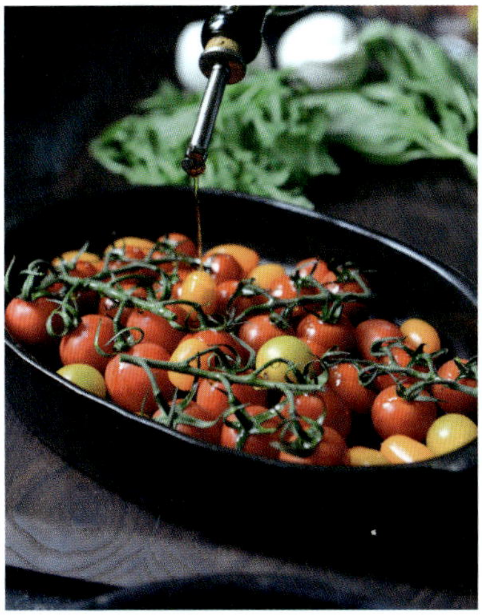

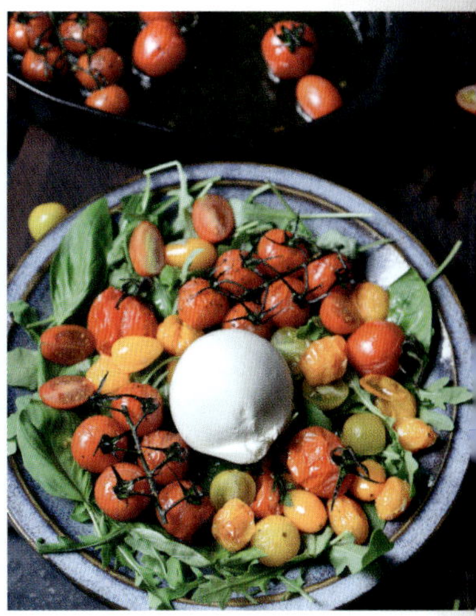

burrata
with baked cherry tomatoes

- **2 balls burrata cheese**
- **a little over 1 lb (500 g) cherry tomatoes, in different colors**
- **1 bunch of basil**
- **3½ oz (100 g) arugula**

– balsamic vinegar –

Preheat the oven to 350 °F (180 °C). Put three quarters of the tomatoes in a baking dish and bake for 20 minutes in the oven. Slice the remaining tomatoes in half. Distribute the arugula and the basil over two plates. Place the cooked and raw tomatoes on top and place a ball of burrata in the middle. Season with salt and pepper and pour plenty of olive oil and a bit of balsamic vinegar over the arugula, tomatoes and burrata.

TIP: KETO AND BALSAMIC VINEGAR

Balsamic vinegar is made from grape must and therefore generally contains quite a lot of carbs. Some of the cheaper balsamic vinegars even have added sugar. If you would like to make this recipe keto-friendly, use apple cider vinegar instead of balsamic vinegar.

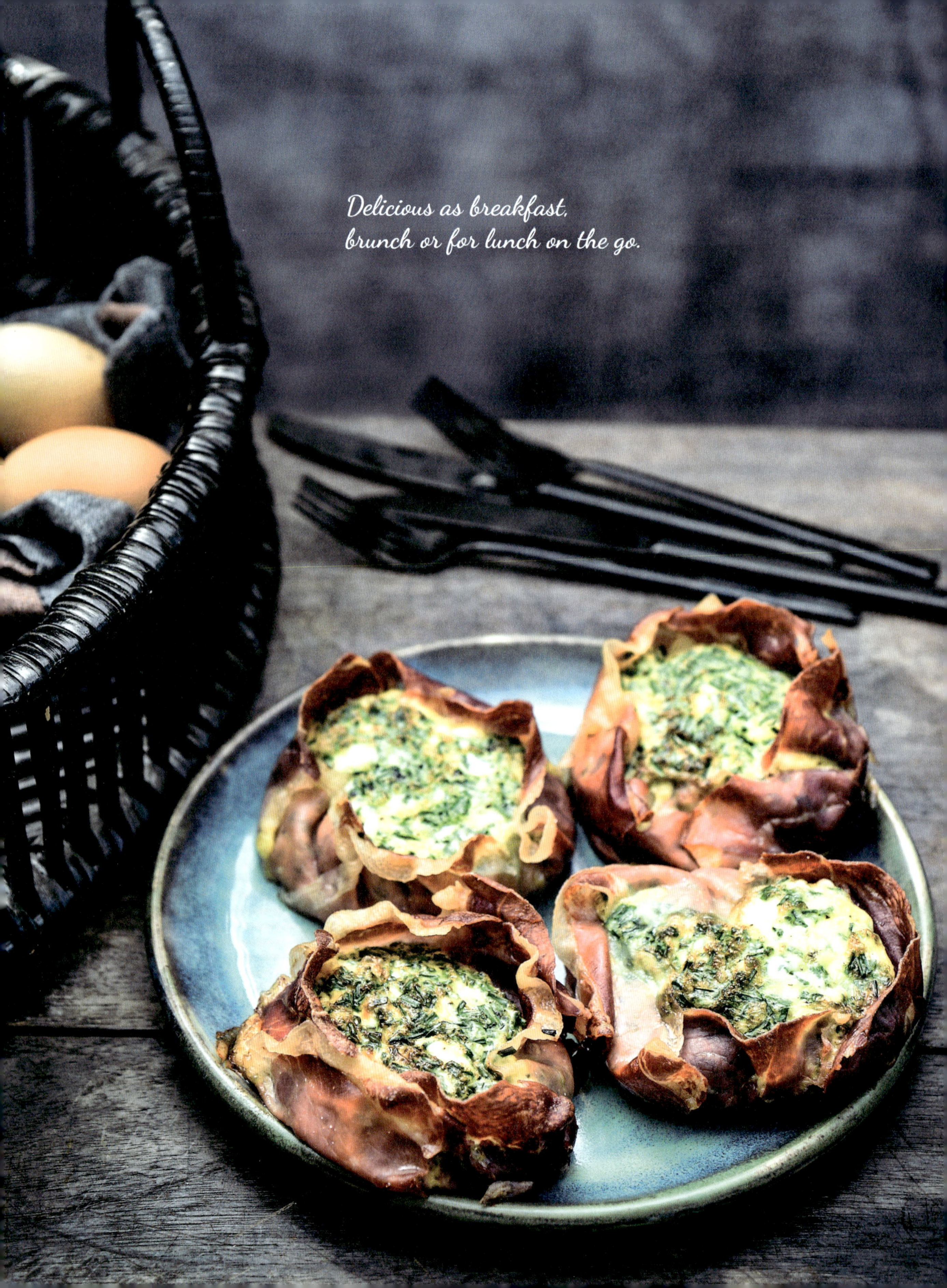

*Delicious as breakfast,
brunch or for lunch on the go.*

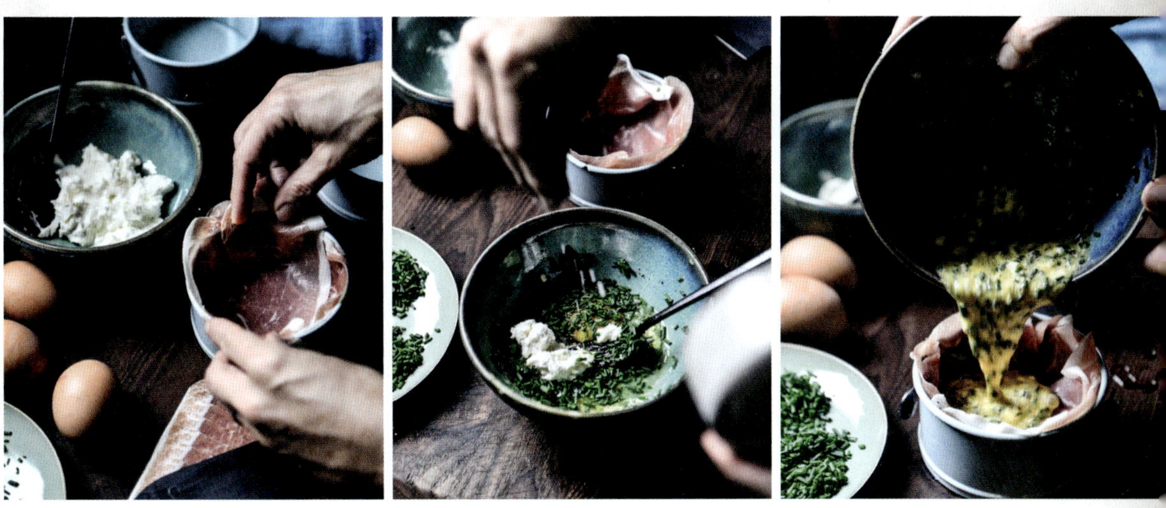

Mini quiche with ham ✓ keto

- 12 slices dry-cured ham (prosciutto)
- 4 eggs
- 4 tablespoons mascarpone
- ¾ oz (20 g) chives

extra: molds (ramekins or muffin tins)

Preheat the oven to 212 °F (100 °C). Place three slices of ham in each mold, making sure to cover the sides and bottom of the mold. Finely chop the chives. Briefly place the mascarpone in the oven to soften it. Raise the oven temperature to 350 °F (180 °C). Beat each egg separately with 1 tablespoon of mascarpone, some chives, pepper and a little bit of salt. The mixture doesn't have to be completely smooth. If it contains some mascarpone lumps, that's fine. Pour the egg mixture into the molds and bake for 15 minutes in the oven. Serve slightly warm.

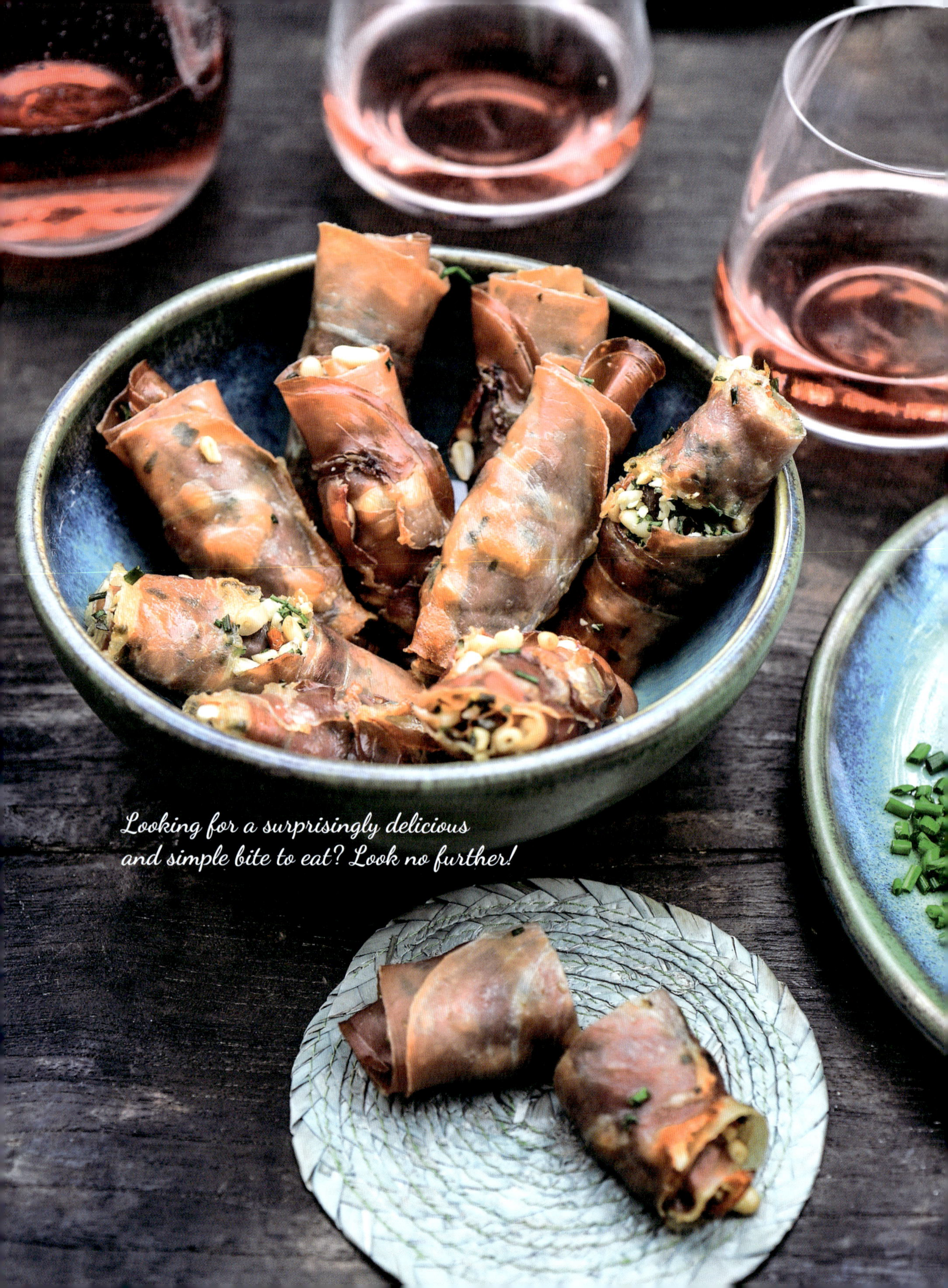
Looking for a surprisingly delicious
and simple bite to eat? Look no further!

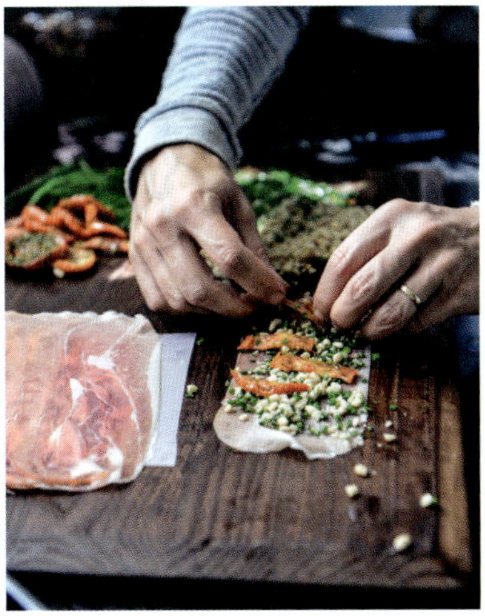

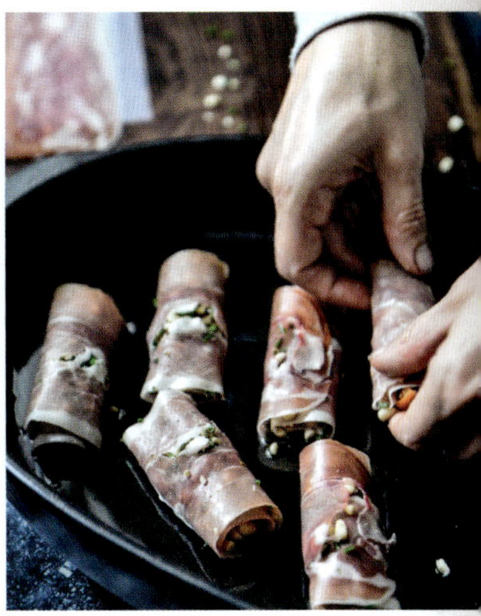

ham rolls

keto

with pine nuts and sundried tomatoes

Ingredients for 10 rolls:

- **10 slices of firm dry-cured ham (see tip)**
- **a handful of pine nuts (about 3 oz/90 g)**
- **10 sundried tomatoes**
- **¾ oz (20 g) chives**

Preheat the oven to 350 °F (180 °C). Coarsely chop the pine nuts. Finely chop the chives and dice the sundried tomatoes. Put the ham slices on a work surface and distribute the pine nuts, tomatoes and chives over the slices. Season with black pepper and roll them up. It doesn't matter if they're not rolled up tightly, as they will shrink and firm up during cooking. Place the ham rolls in a baking dish and bake them for 15 minutes in the oven.

TIP: HAM

Choose thicker and firmer dry-cured ham slices, as these are easier to roll up. You can also use thin slices of ham, but it will be harder to roll them up properly.

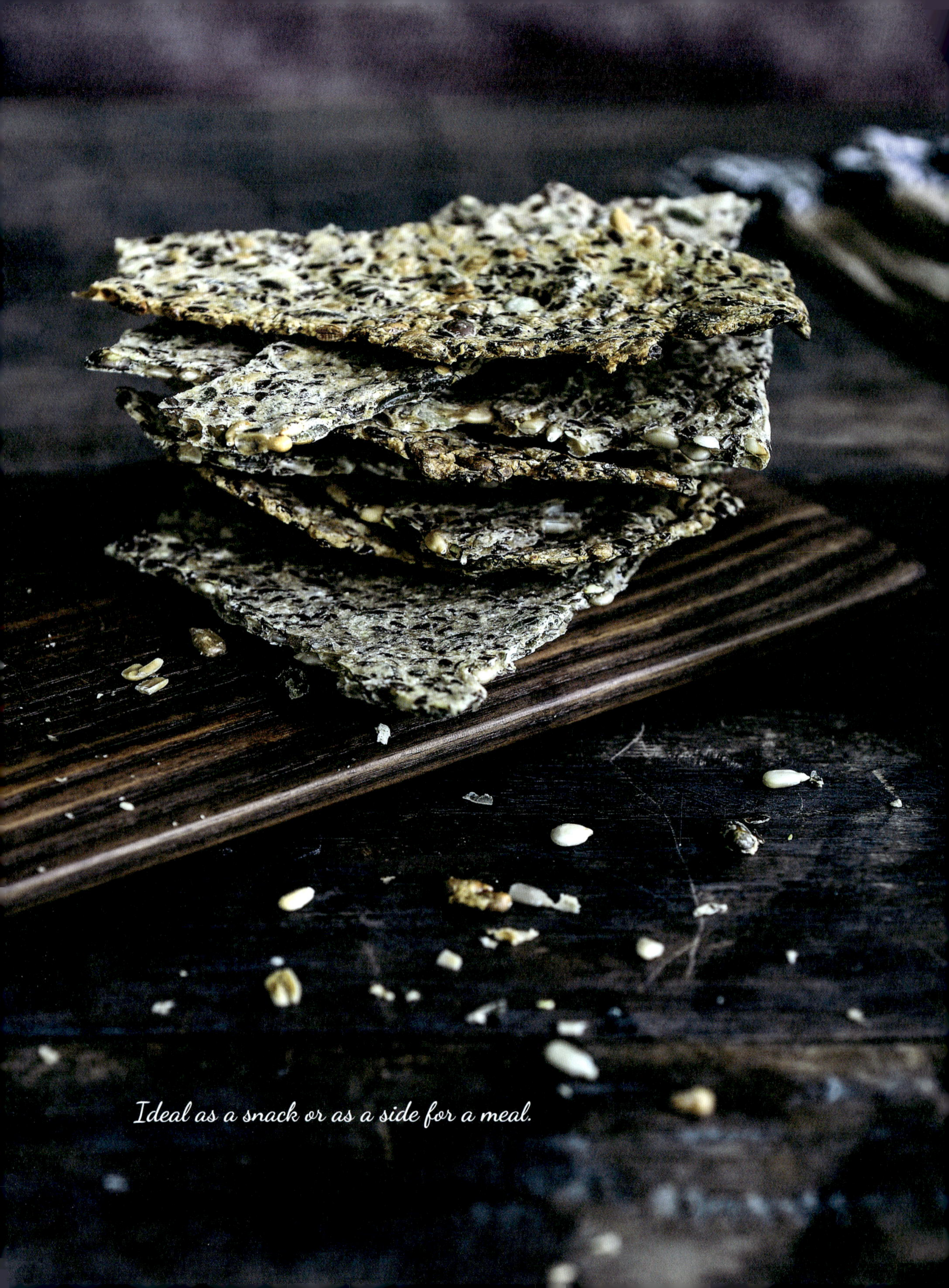

Ideal as a snack or as a side for a meal.

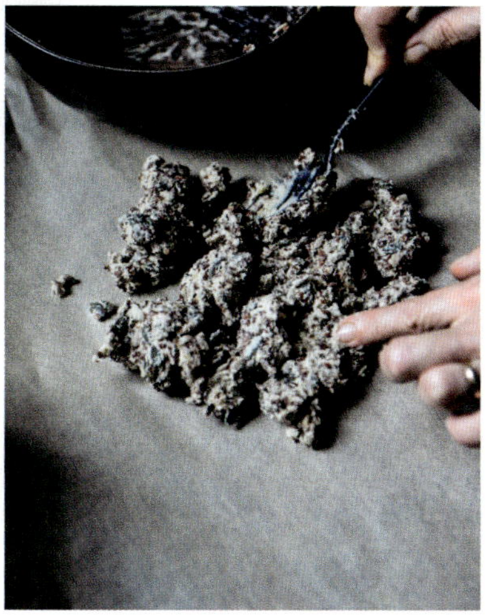
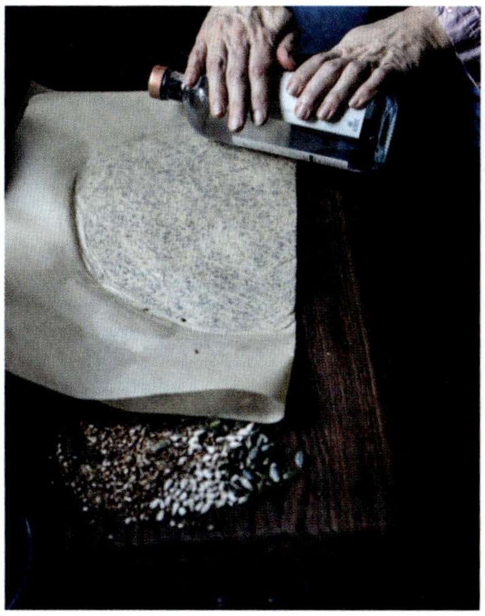
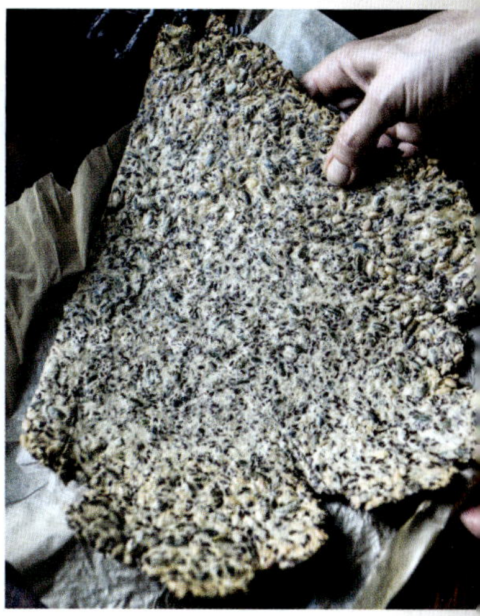

seed crackers ✓ keto

- **4 tablespoons sunflower seeds**
- **4 tablespoons flaxseeds**
- **4 tablespoons pumpkin seeds**
- **2 oz (50 g) oatmeal**

extra: parchment paper

Preheat the oven to 350 °F (180 °C). Combine the seeds with the oatmeal and season with salt and pepper. Bring ½ cup (125 ml) water to a boil and add it to the seed mixture and mix to form a firm dough. Take a large sheet of parchment paper and spoon the dough onto one half of the sheet. Fold the other half of the sheet over the dough and roll the dough out between the parchment paper to a thickness of about ⅛ inch (3 mm) (see tip). Remove the top layer of the parchment paper. Bake in the oven for 20 minutes but turn the cracker over after 13 minutes. If the cracker doesn't come off the parchment paper easily, wait a little longer.
Once the cracker is dry, let it cool and then break it into pieces.

TIP: SEEDS
You can use leftover seeds in nut cake, the recipe for which you will find on page 160, or add them to your breakfast fruit, together with some coconut milk or full-fat yogurt.

TIP: ROLLING PIN
If you don't have a rolling pin, a bottle or something else works fine for rolling out the dough.
It doesn't matter what you use, as long as you can roll out the dough with it.

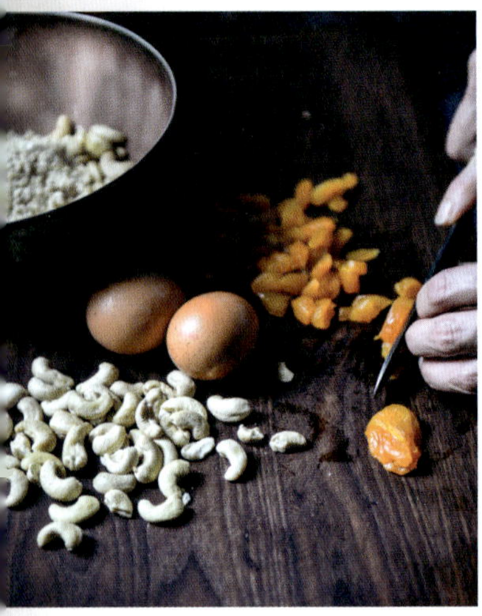 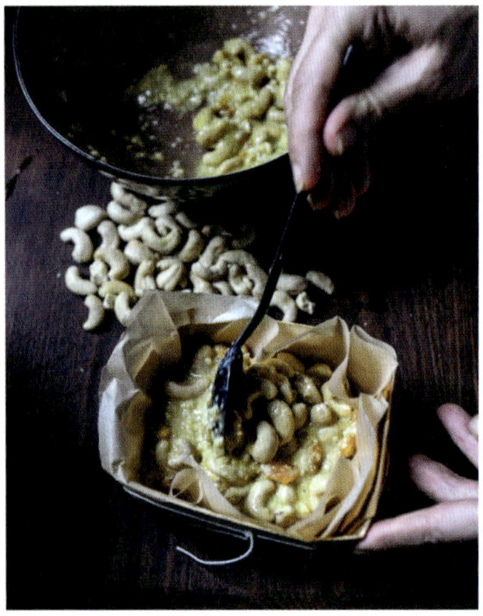

cashew cake

- **7 oz (200 g) cashews (see tip)**
- **3½ oz (100 g) dried apricots (see tip)**
- **2 eggs**
- **4 tablespoons coconut milk**

extra: parchment paper

Preheat the oven to 350 °F (180 °C). Grind a third of the nuts to form a coarse flour. Dice the apricots into small pieces. Combine the whole and ground nuts and the apricots, mixing well. Add the eggs and the coconut milk. Line a baking dish with parchment paper and spoon the batter into the dish. Bake in the oven for 20 minutes or until the dough is completely dry.

TIP: NUTS AND APRICOTS
Cashews are soft, making them ideal for quick and easy cakes.
You can also use other nuts, but these are often harder; in that case, bake your cake longer in the oven. Let the cake cool completely before slicing it, if you can wait that long. I like to use soft apricots that are not completely dry, otherwise the cake becomes too dry.

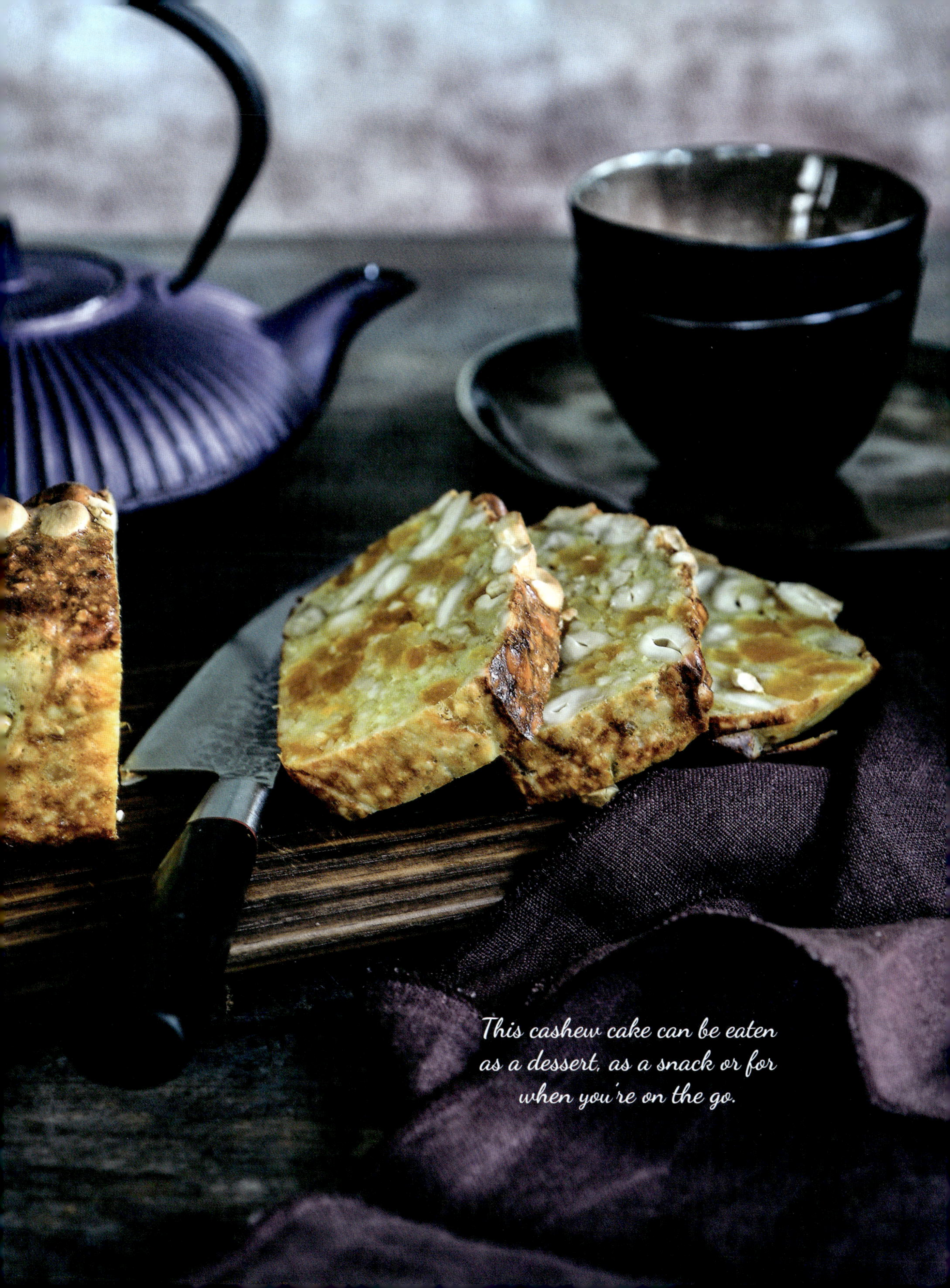

This cashew cake can be eaten as a dessert, as a snack or for when you're on the go.

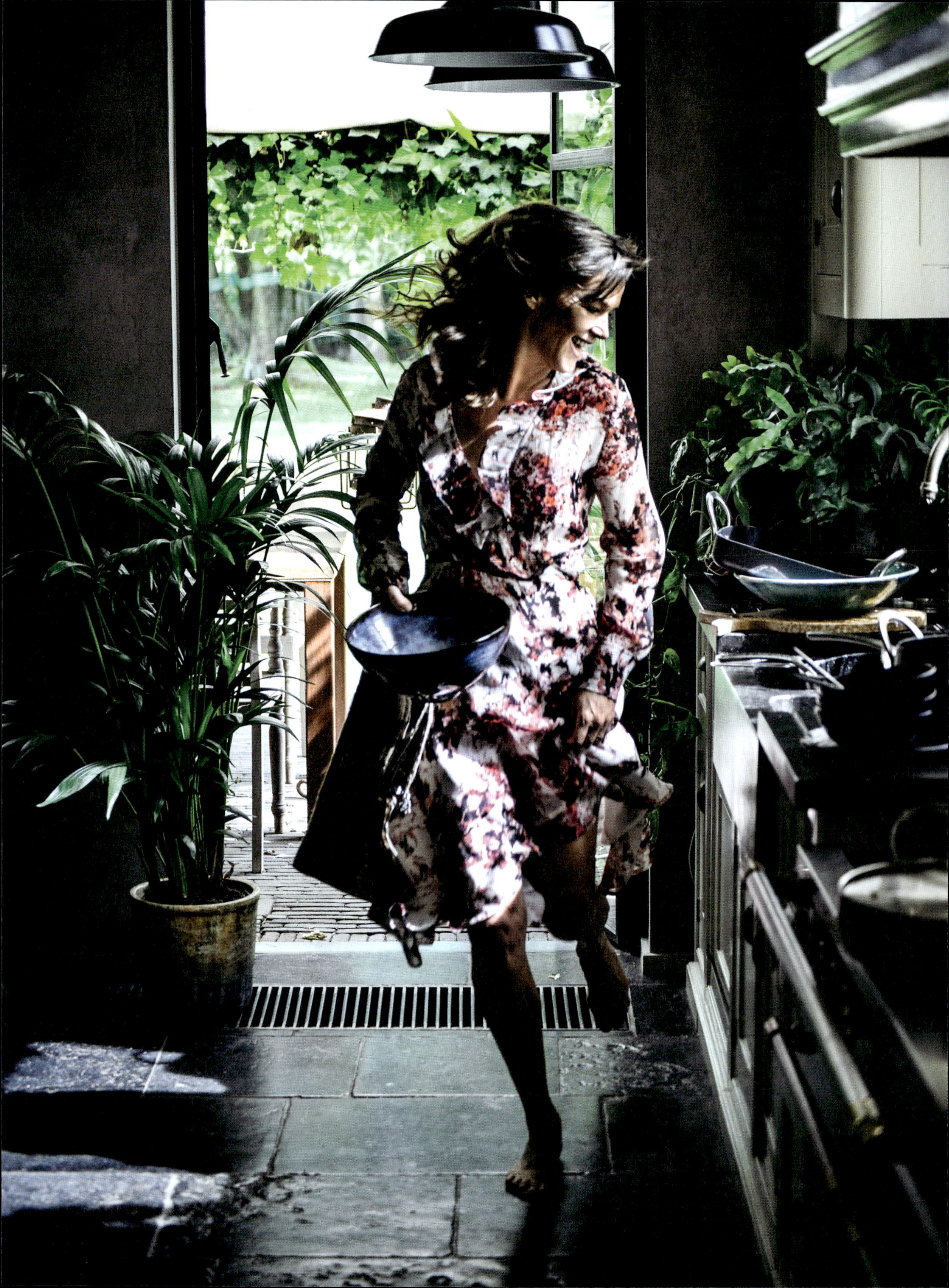

Rituals...

I am a huge fan of rituals. They add a different dimension to everyday things such as preparing food. Instead of letting cooking become part of the daily drudgery, you can turn it into an inspiring moment. Rituals give you structure and mental space, as well as making normal chores valuable and fun. During a ritual, you are not looking for any reward or recognition. Instead, you are enjoying the small things in life. Your food will also taste better, as you appreciate your own personal engagement in creating it.

Create your own rituals

I have to get dinner ready again! No, we shouldn't have to do anything. We should want to do it ☺. And it's all in our own hands: we can either turn it into something boring, or something beautiful, just the way we want it. Find enjoyment in your work, be creative and spontaneous. Prepare your food with undivided attention, use your favorite ingredients, keep it simple and manageable, and keep it healthy for you and your loved ones. We tend to place a lot of importance on eating and dining, but we forget to focus on how we prepare food. Why should that be any less important? Embrace the Ayurvedic concept that the preparation of food has something spiritual to it. Turn your kitchen into an inspiring workplace, your workspace. Use beautiful, high-quality products and surround yourself with attractive, fun things that make you happy. Don't be afraid to get your hands dirty. For instance, this year I painted the entire kitchen myself. By doing that, I feel like I'm a part of my kitchen and, now more than ever, it's become my own creative space.

Scientific research

For some it's no surprise that the French, known for their love of food, have many culinary rituals. Perhaps that's also the reason why French children will eat almost anything.
French schools devote ample attention to fresh, healthy food, and children are even served a first course, main course and dessert at lunchtime. Scientific research shows that, when eating is preceded by ritual, the food tastes better. In one experiment, two different groups of people were given chocolate. One group ate the chocolate as usual, while the other group had to break up the chocolate in a special way before eating it. The second group found that they had more fun eating the chocolate. Researchers agree: rituals often improve quality of life and increase enjoyment.

What is a ritual?

The dictionary definition of a ritual is an act or a series of acts as part of a ceremony, acts that symbolize something. Others describe a ritual as a symbolic activity, usually involving repeated and unusual behavior, occurring in set ways and set sequences. Rituals are also found in the animal kingdom. Rituals can be anything that's out of the ordinary: behaviors, words, sounds, dance, singing, actions ... It's completely up to you.

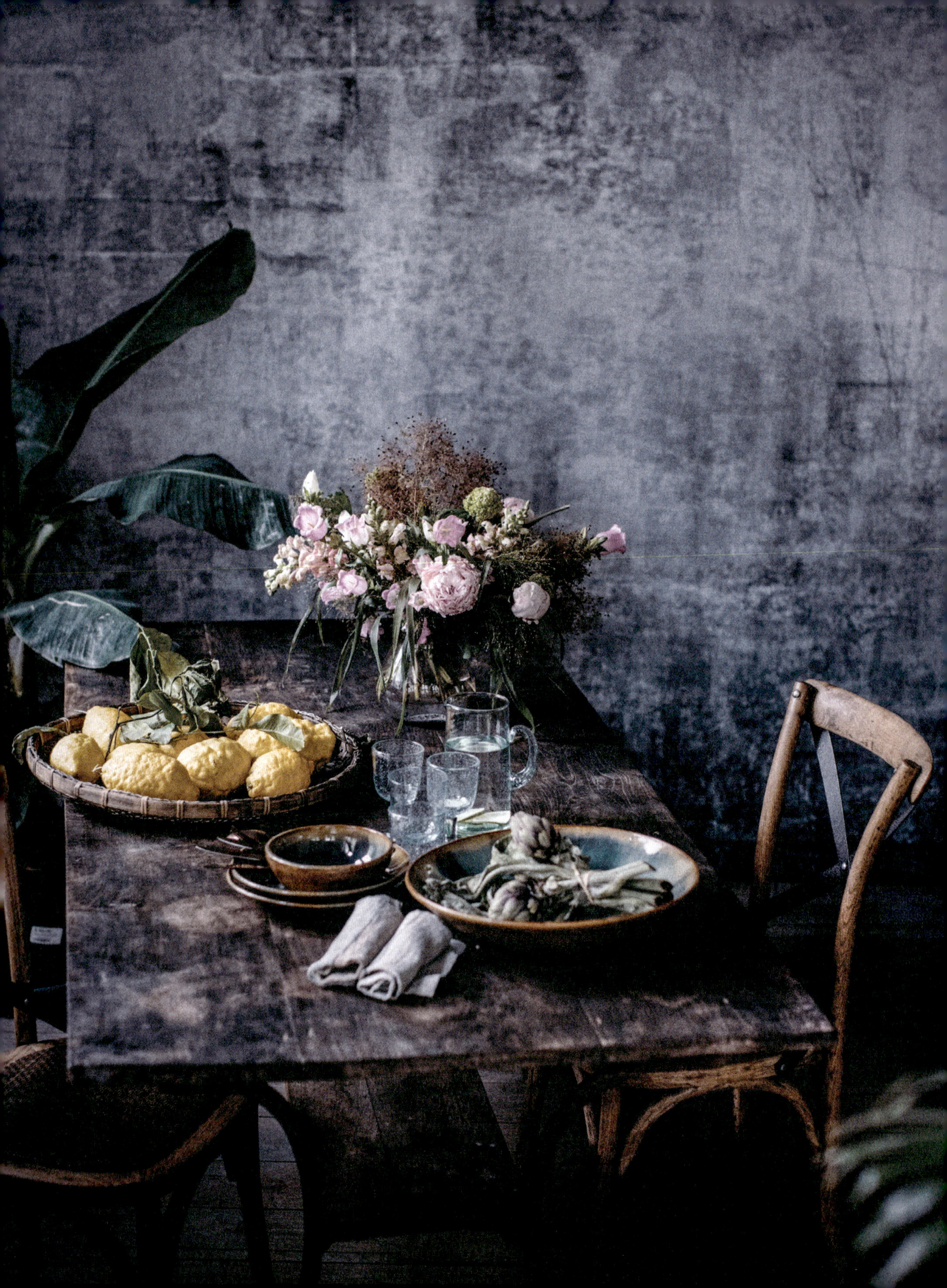

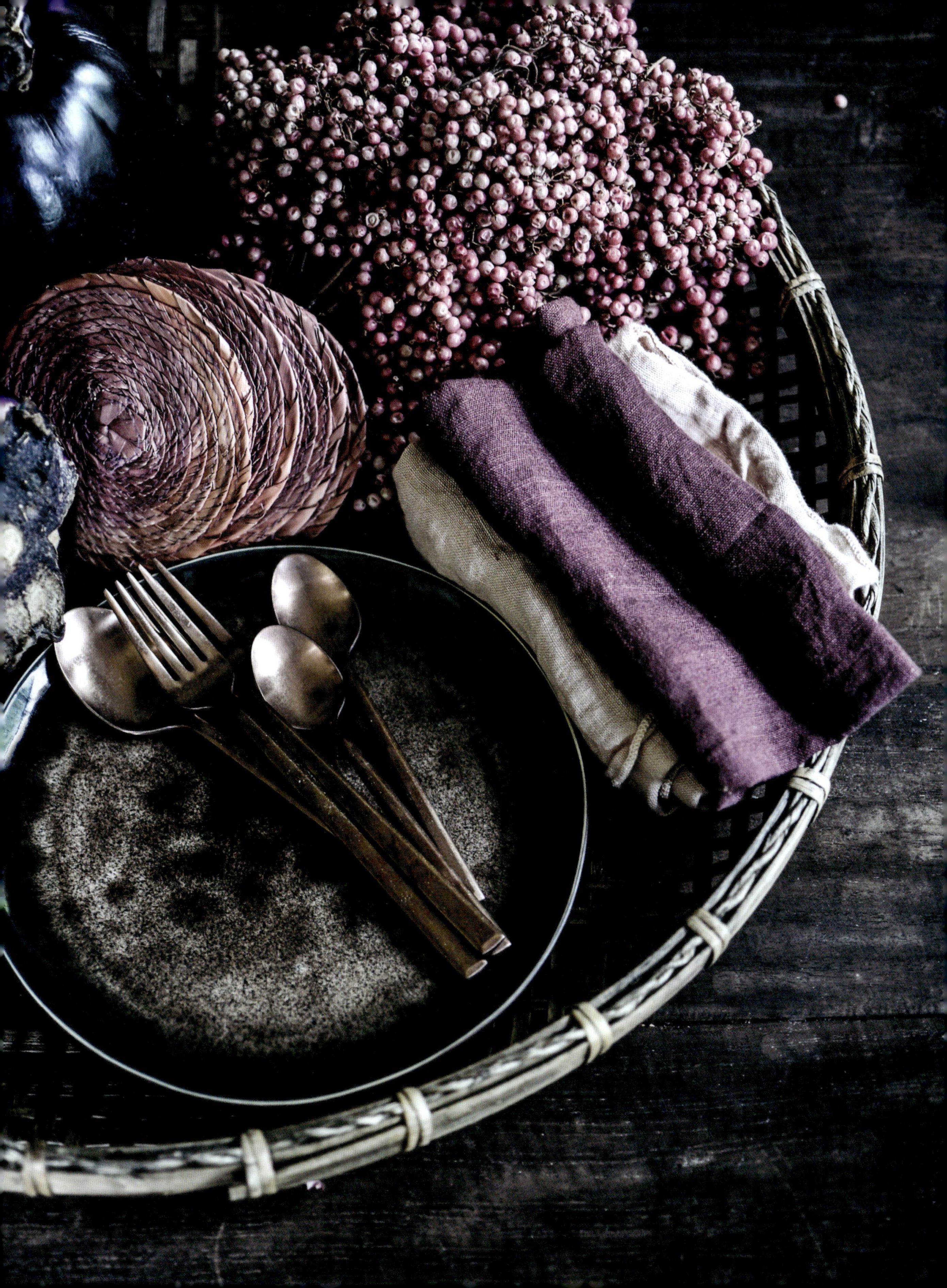

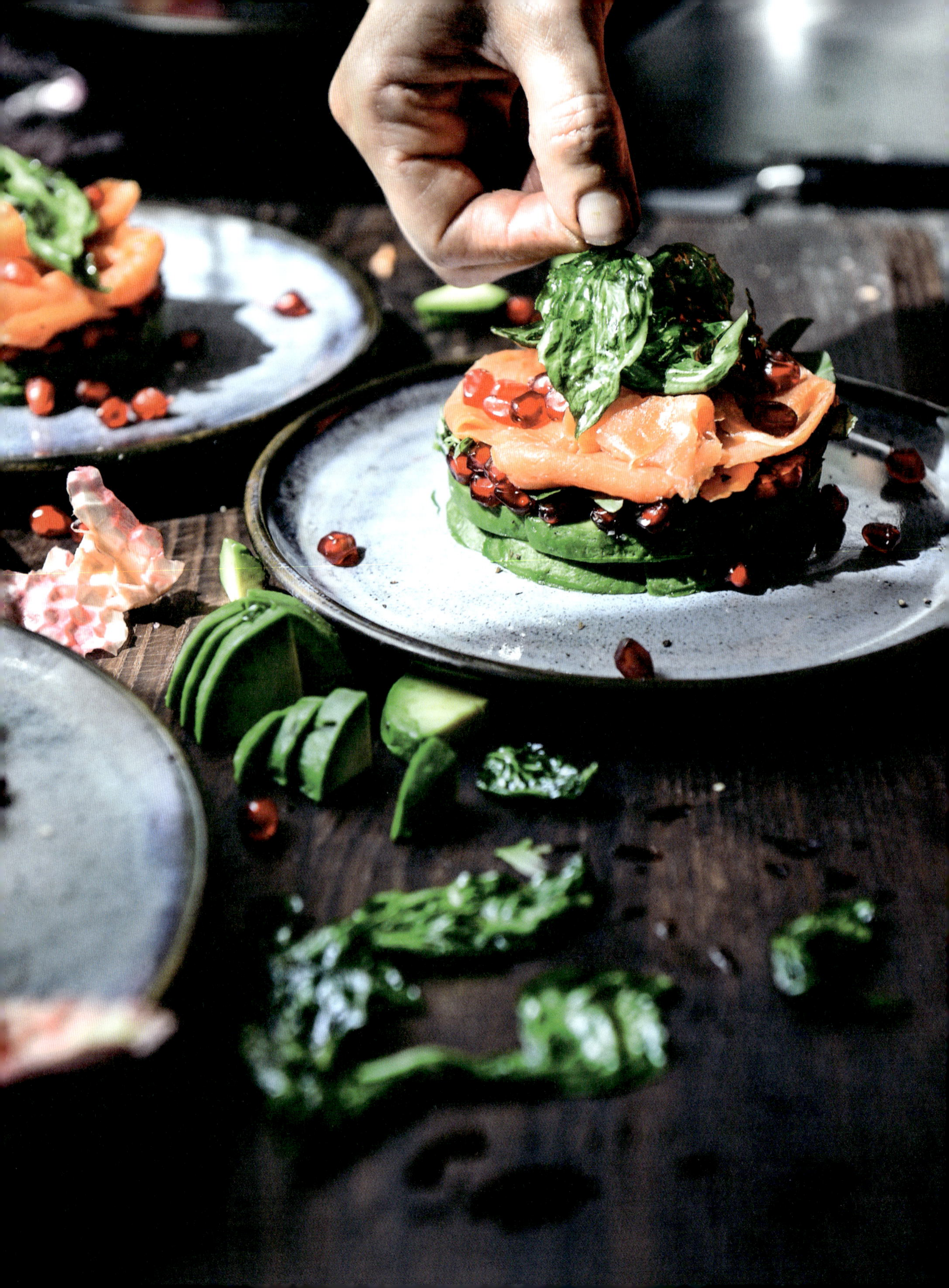

chic

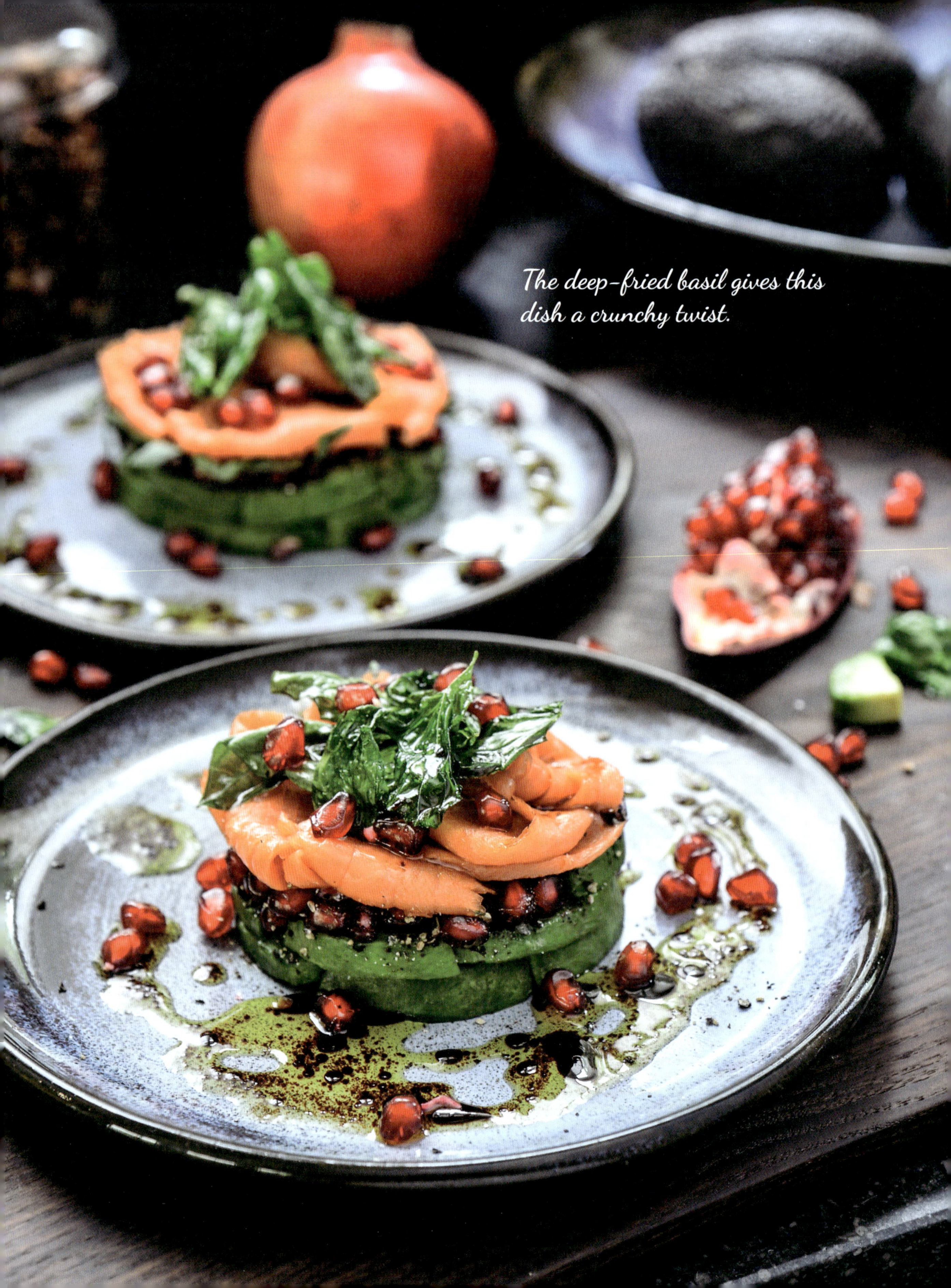
The deep-fried basil gives this
dish a crunchy twist.

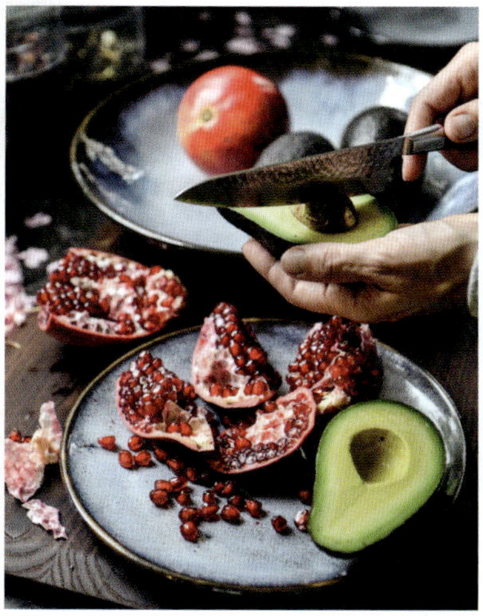
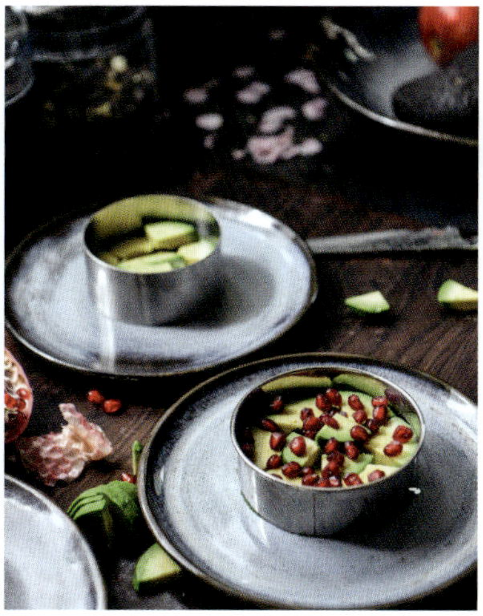
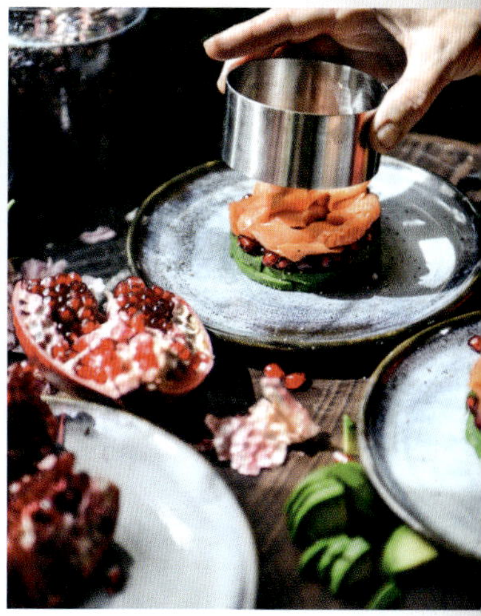

smoked salmon

with avocado, pomegranate and basil

- **3½ to 5 oz (100 to 150 g) smoked salmon**
- **the seeds from ¼ pomegranate**
- **1 avocado**
- **1 bunch of basil (¾ oz/20 g)**

– balsamic vinegar –

extra: cooking rings

Cut the avocado in half and remove the seed and skin. Slice the flesh into ¼-inch (0.5 cm) slices and divide them evenly between the two cooking rings. Remove the best-looking leaves from the basil. Finely chop the remaining leaves and scatter over the avocado. Season with pepper and a little bit of salt. Sprinkle some pomegranate seeds over the avocado and place pieces of smoked salmon on top. Pour some olive oil or coconut oil in a small pan and deep-fry the remaining basil leaves in the oil. Make sure not to get burnt, as the oil might spatter a bit. I throw in about four leaves or so and then immediately cover the pan. After about five seconds, I remove the leaves from the oil and drain them on a paper towel.
Place the deep-fried leaves on top of the salmon, remove the cooking ring and garnish with some pomegranate seeds, olive oil and balsamic vinegar.

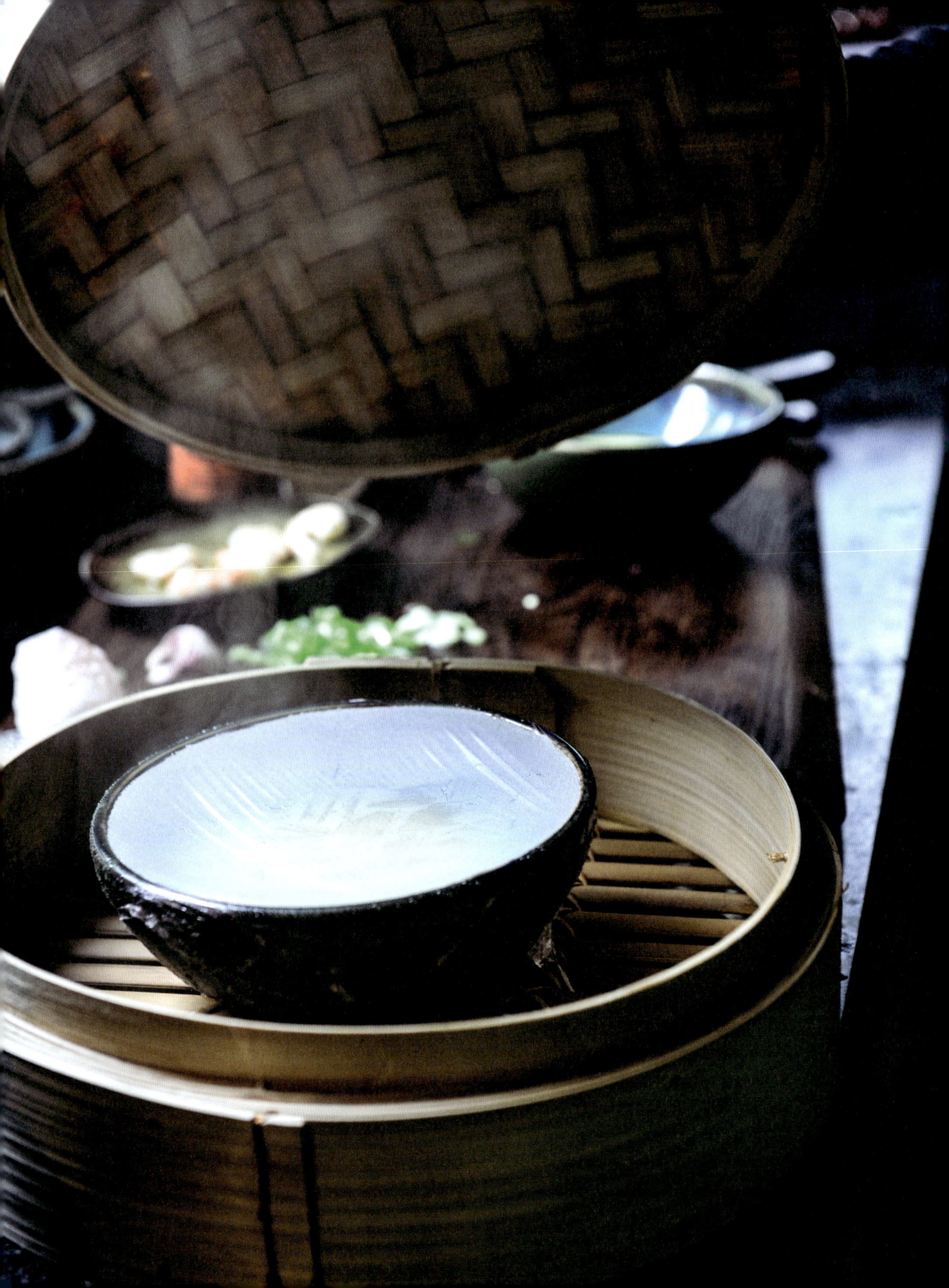

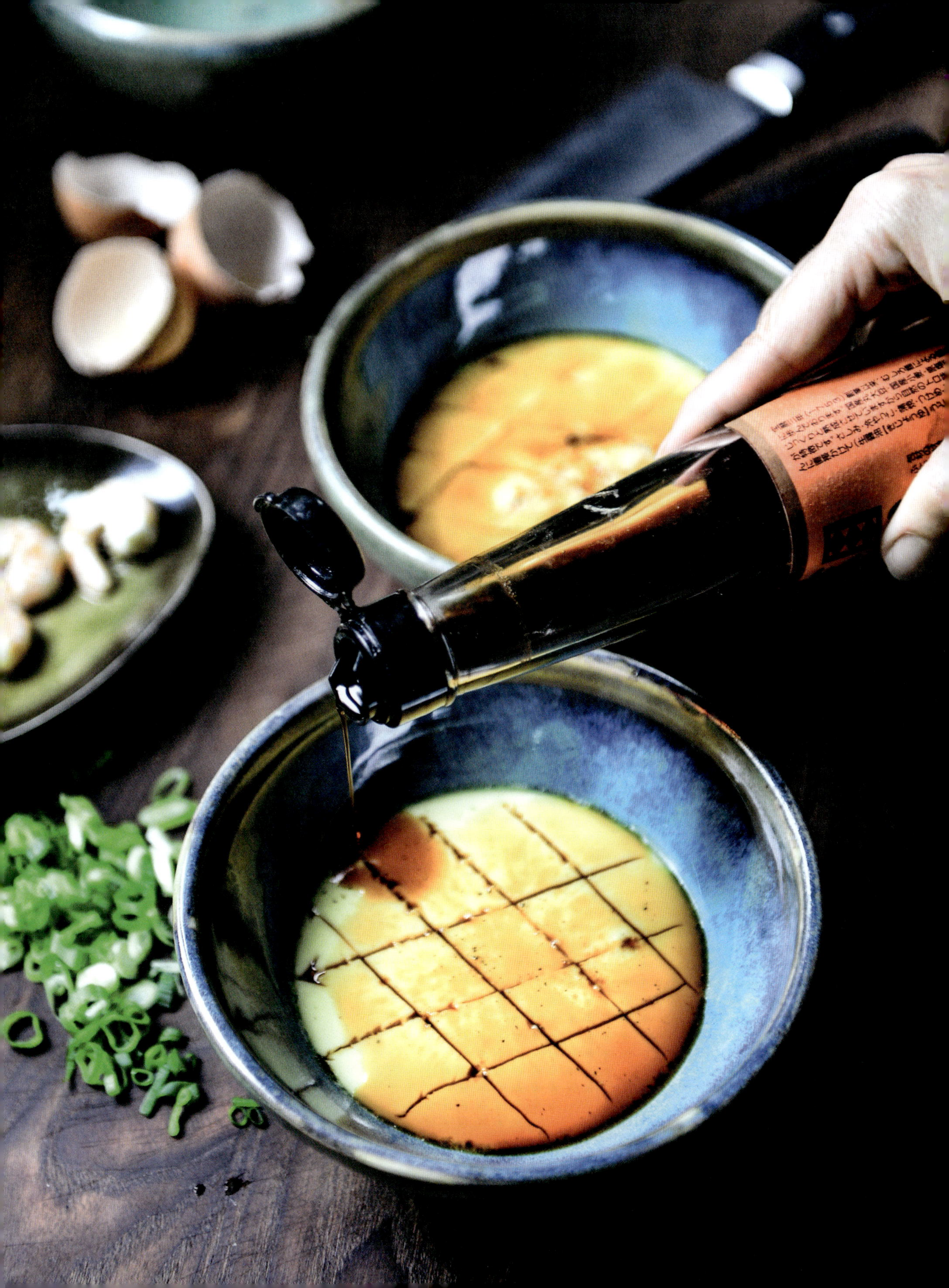

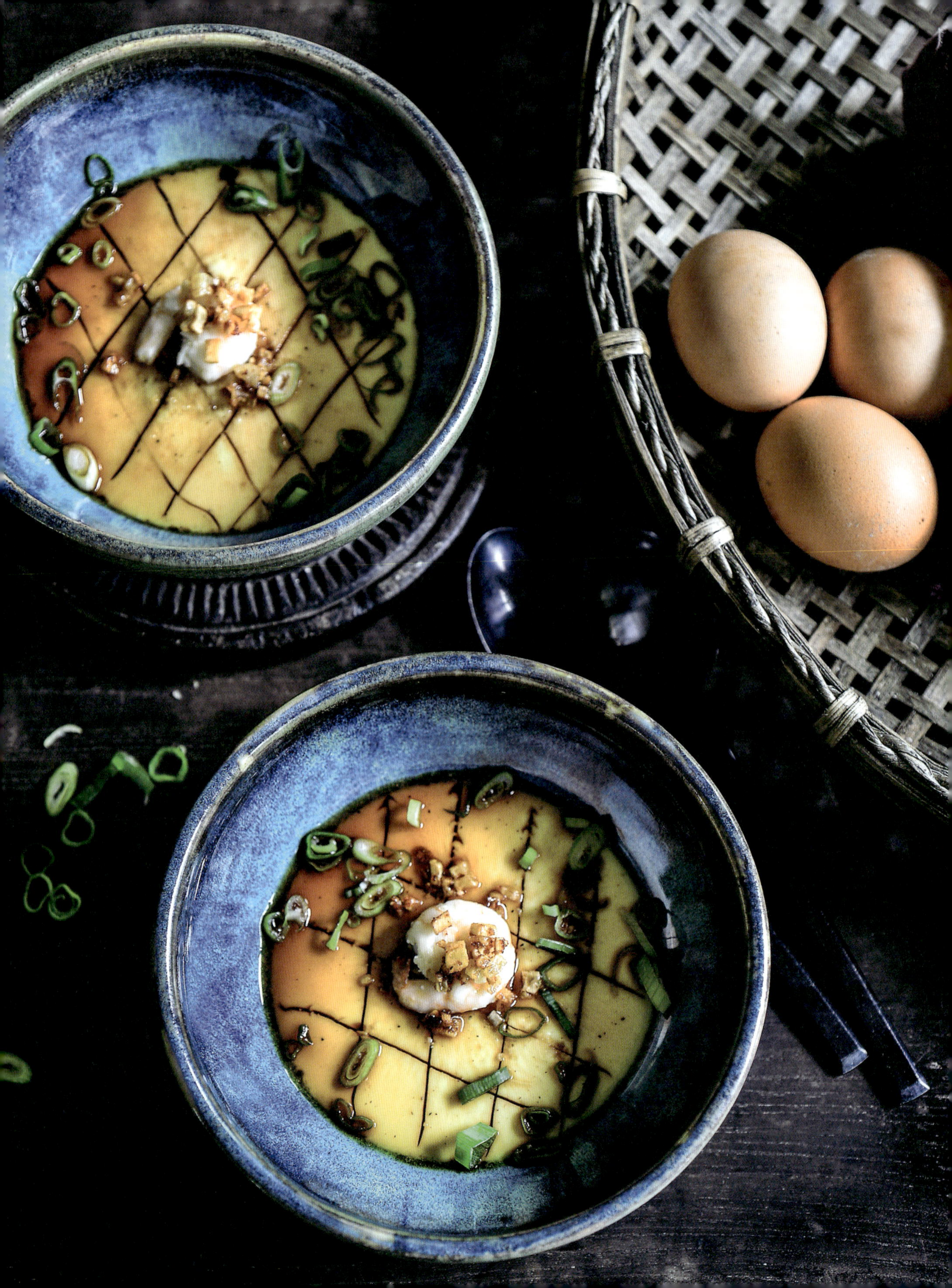

Chinese-style steamed eggs

✓ keto

This dish is an omelet, but with a very different texture. The combination with the soy sauce makes this a particularly unique dish. I usually serve this as a (filling) first course.

- **2 eggs**
- **1 spring onion**
- **2 large shrimp, peeled**

– soy sauce –
– fresh garlic –

Break the eggs in a bowl. Take half an egg shell, fill it eight times with water and add the water to the eggs (see tip). Add some white pepper and salt and beat the eggs together. Distribute the eggs evenly over two bowls but pour the eggs through a sieve to remove the air bubbles and make sure that the surface is nice and smooth. Cover the bowls with plastic film and place a bowl on top to prevent water drops from falling into the egg mixture whilst steaming. Put the bowls in a steamer basket and steam for 10 minutes (see tip).

Finely chop a clove of garlic and sauté in olive oil. Add the shrimp. Finely chop the spring onion. Remove the bowls from the steamer basket. Score a crisscross pattern into the eggs. Pour 1 tablespoon of soy sauce into each bowl and garnish with the shrimp, the garlic and the spring onion.

TIP: WATER

If you use too much water, the eggs will be watery. If it looks too much like a normal omelet, then you've not used enough water.

TIP: STEAMING

You can also place the bowls in a microwave oven for 1 minute instead of steaming the eggs.

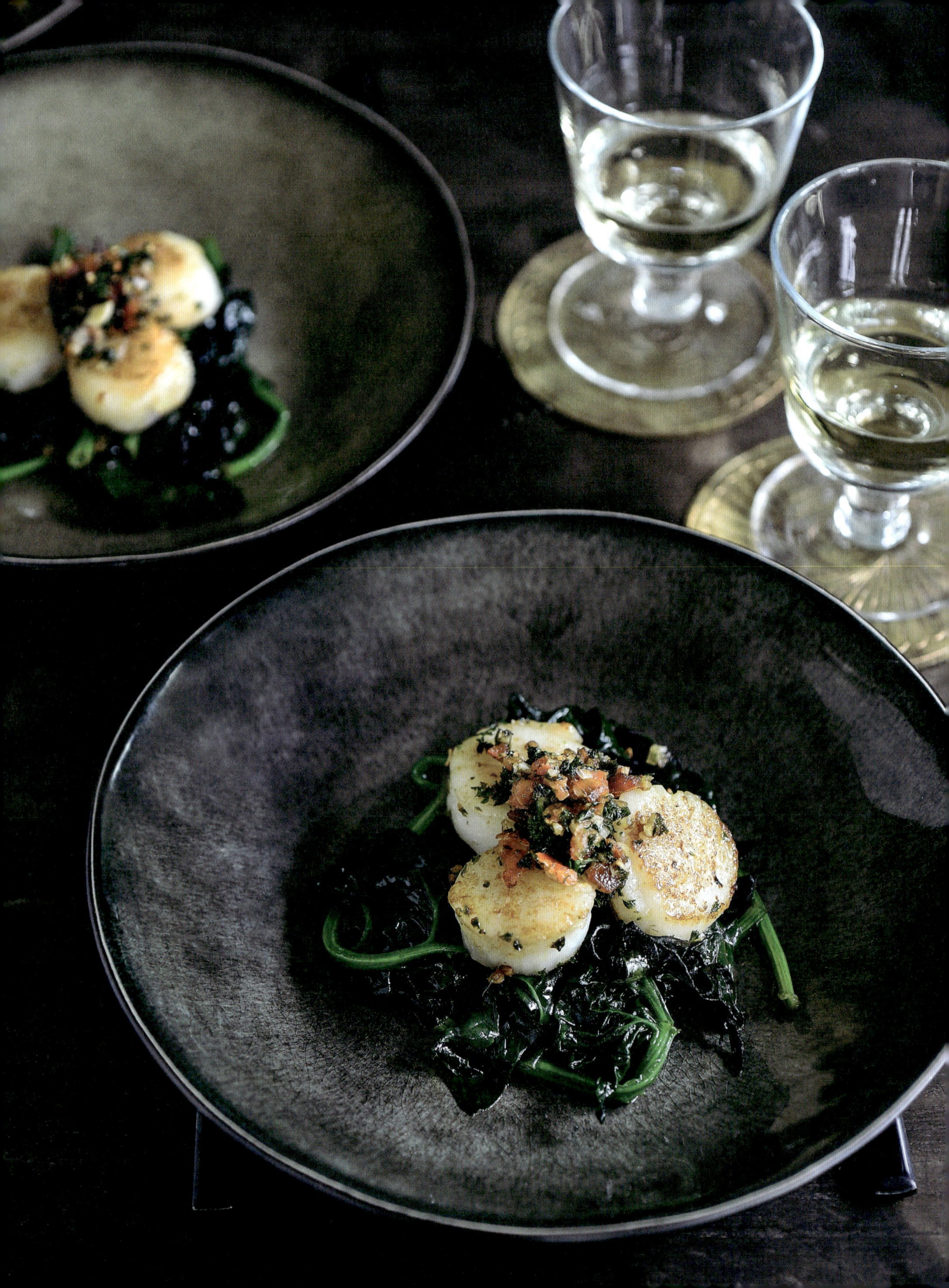

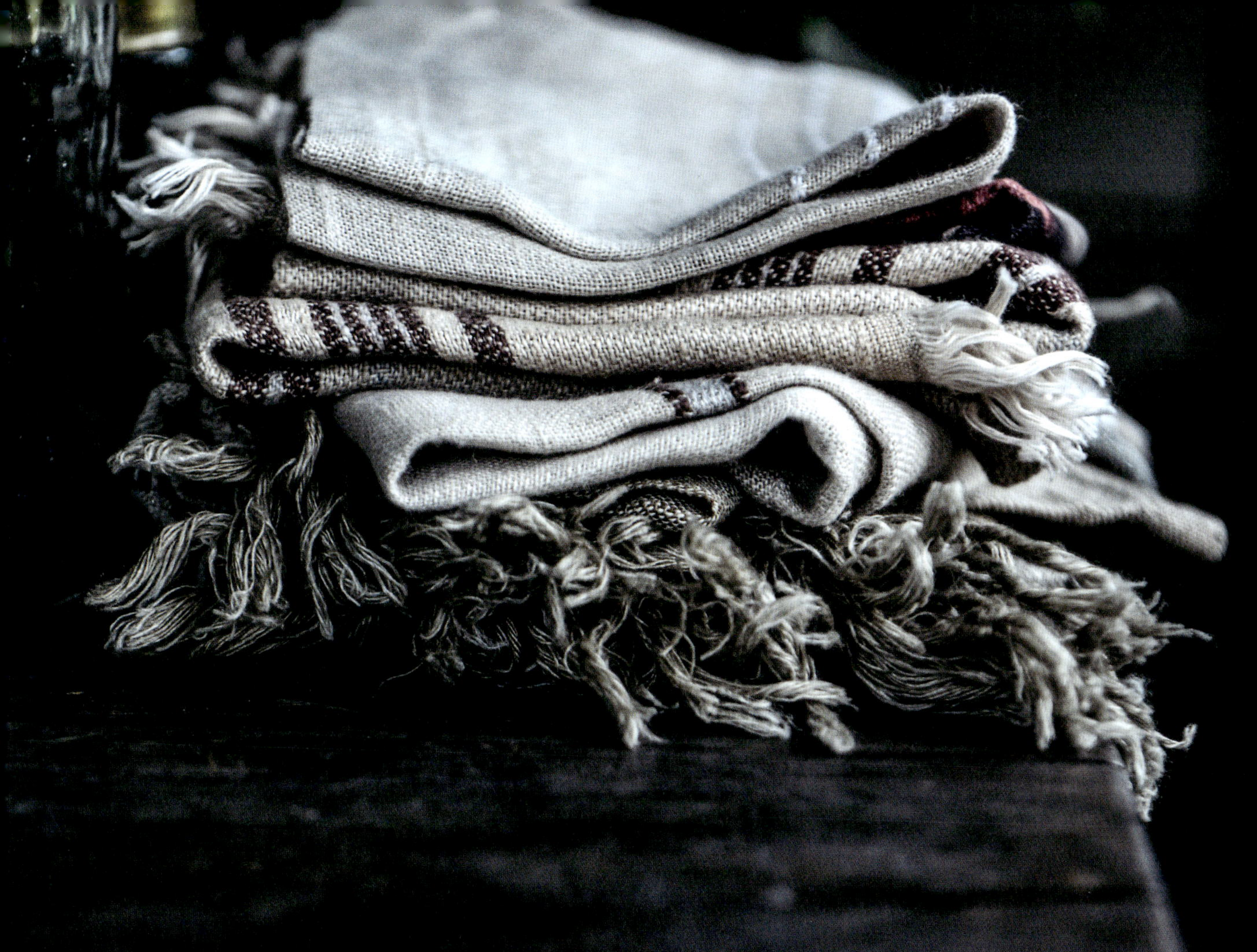

scallops ✓keto

with spinach and herbs

- 6 scallops
- 5 oz (150 g) organic spinach
- 6 sundried tomatoes
- a handful of curly-leaf parsley

- fresh garlic -

Sauté the spinach in plenty of olive oil and season with salt and pepper. Finely chop the sundried tomatoes, 2 cloves of garlic and the curly-leaf parsley and sauté in a pan with some olive oil. After 2 minutes, add the scallops and cook them for 1 to 2 minutes on each side. Season with salt and pepper. Spoon the spinach onto the plates and place the scallops and herbs on top.

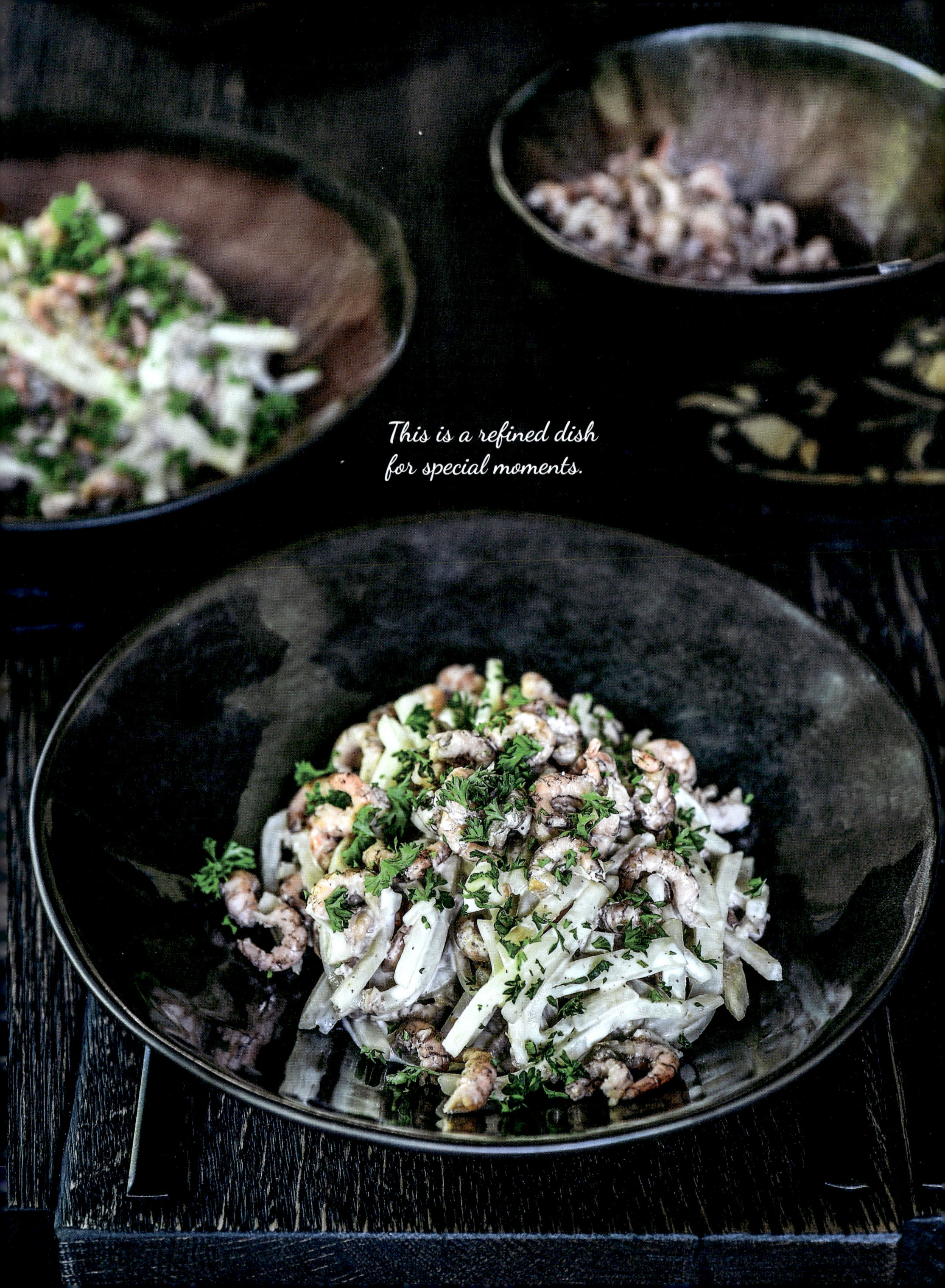

This is a refined dish for special moments.

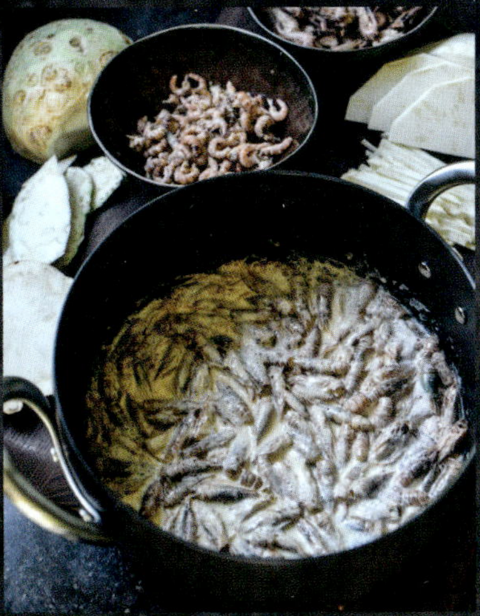

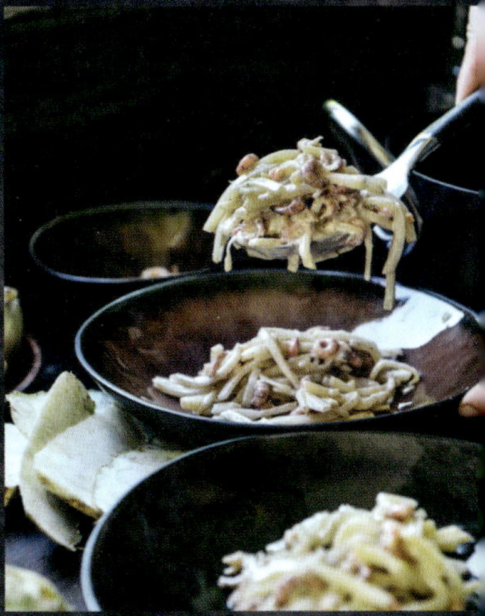

celeriac ✓keto

with brown shrimp

- **14 oz (400 g) celeriac**
- **7 oz (200 g) unpeeled and 3½ oz (100 g) peeled brown shrimp (see tip)**
- **8 fl oz (225 ml) cream**
- **¾ oz (20 g) parsley, finely chopped**

Peel the shrimp and set the heads aside. Put the shrimp heads in a pan, add the cream, and bring to the boil. Let the cream simmer for about 3 minutes. Remove from the heat and let the liquid rest. Peel and slice the celeriac into thin slices. Slice them once more into matchsticks. Cook the celeriac for about 3 minutes in salted water with a generous splash of olive oil. Drain off the water and add another splash of olive oil to the celeriac. Return to the heat and stir occasionally to make sure that the water has completely evaporated. Strain the cream with a sieve into a bowl. Press the last drops of cream out of the shrimp heads. Season with black pepper and a little bit of salt.
Remove the celeriac from the heat, add the cream and stir in the brown shrimp.
Garnish with finely chopped parsley.

TIP: SHRIMP
I buy at least 7 oz (200 g) of unpeeled shrimp (you need them to make the sauce) and an additional 3½ oz (100 g) of peeled shrimp. This helps me save on time. But when I do have time, I buy 14 oz (400 g) of unpeeled shrimp. They are without a doubt tastier!

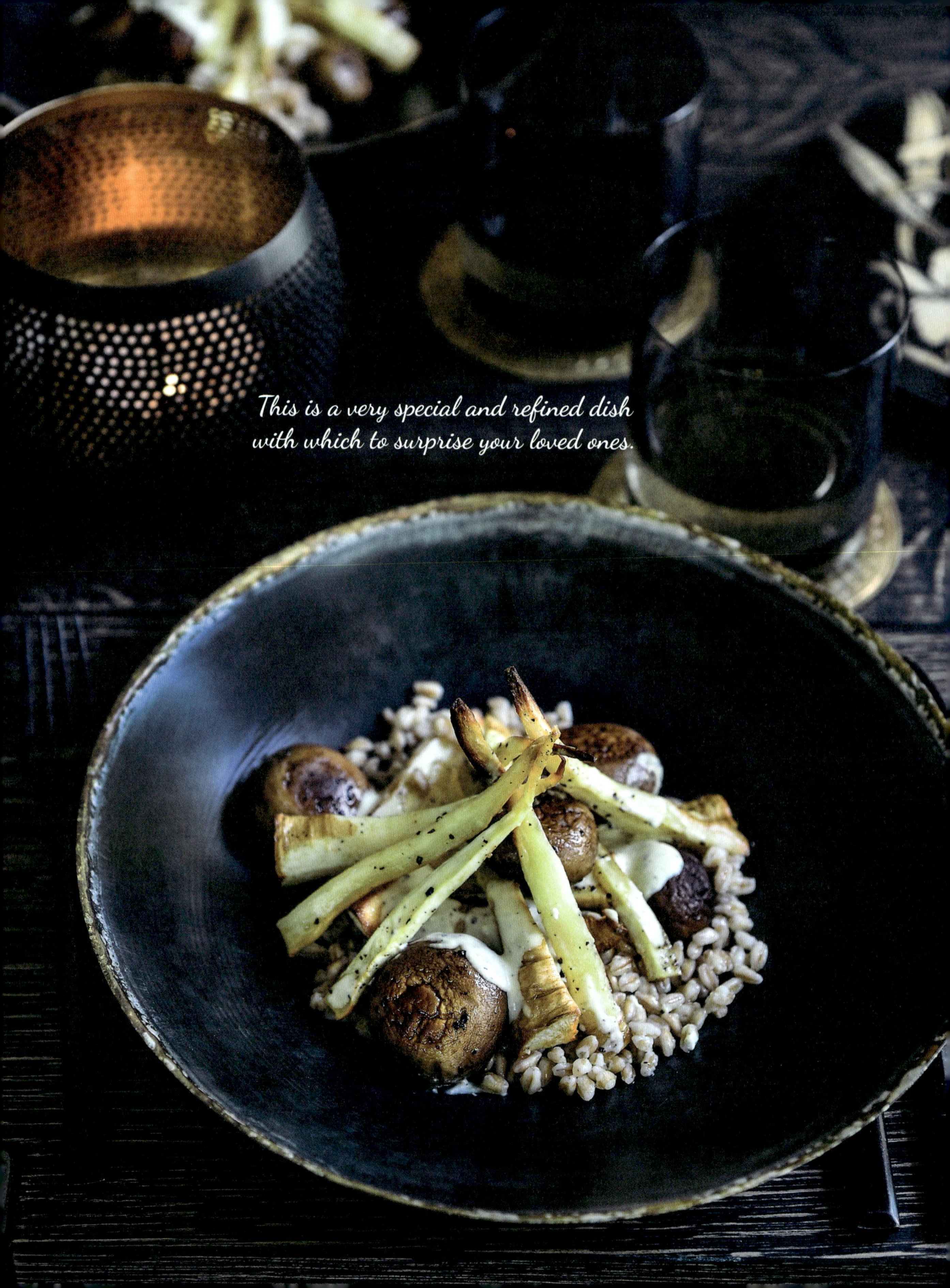

This is a very special and refined dish with which to surprise your loved ones.

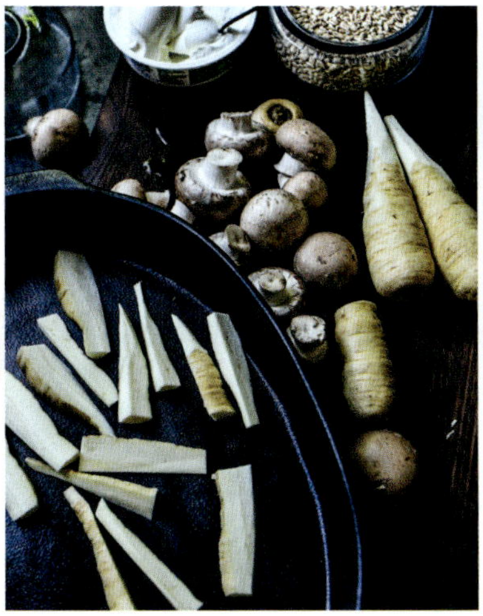
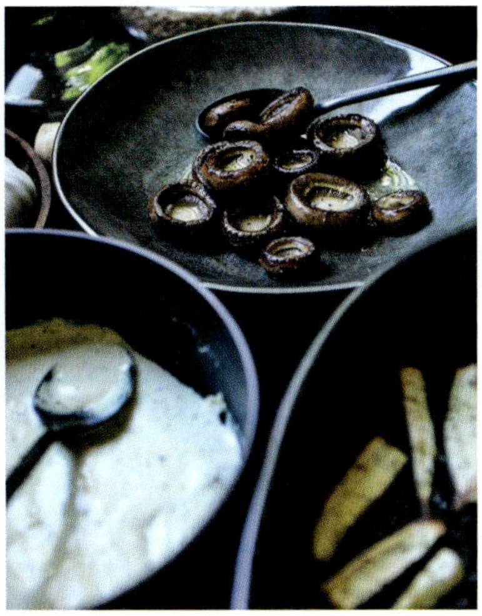
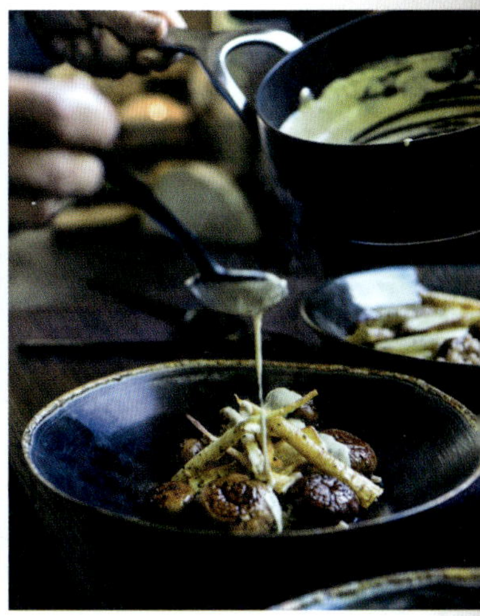

spelt
with parsnip and mushrooms

- **5 oz (150 g) spelt (see tip)**
- **2 parsnips**
- **9 oz (250 g) mushrooms**
- **4 tablespoons mascarpone (about 3½ oz/100 g)**

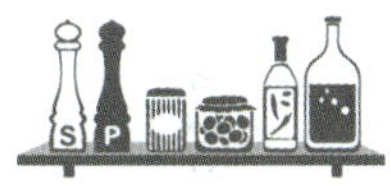

- mild mustard -

Preheat the oven to 350 °F (180 °C). Cut the parsnips in half and slice into long strips. Put the parsnips in a baking dish, season with salt and pepper and drizzle a splash of olive oil over the top. Bake in the oven for 20 minutes. Cook the spelt in salted water with a generous splash of olive oil until tender according to the instructions on the packet (see tip). Remove the mushroom stems and sauté the whole mushroom caps in plenty of olive oil. Season with salt and pepper. Combine the mascarpone with 1 tablespoon of mild mustard and heat the mixture. Add 3 to 4 tablespoons of water until you have a thin sauce. Season with pepper and a little bit of salt. Distribute the spelt evenly onto the plates and place the mushrooms on top. Arrange the parsnip strips next to the mushrooms and finish with the sauce.

TIP: SPELT

I'm talking about the whole grain variety. I often buy precooked spelt, which you only have to cook for 10 minutes. You can only enjoy the health benefits from grains if you use the whole grain instead of the (processed) flour. Whole grains release their sugars more slowly, so you automatically eat less of them. Please note, spelt contains gluten!

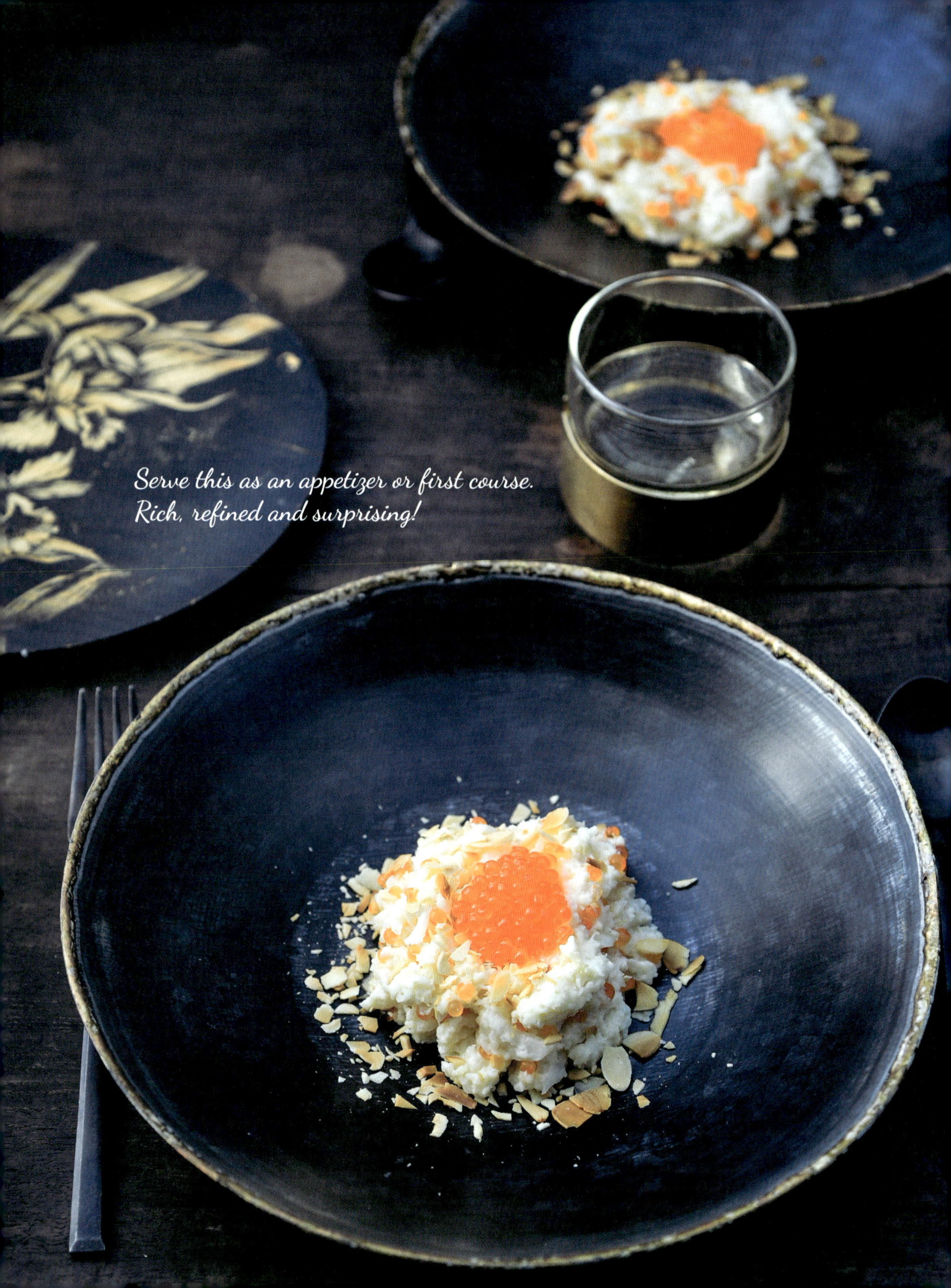

Serve this as an appetizer or first course.
Rich, refined and surprising!

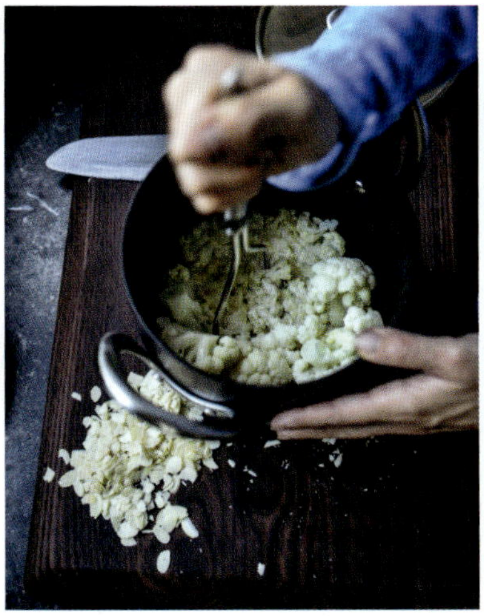 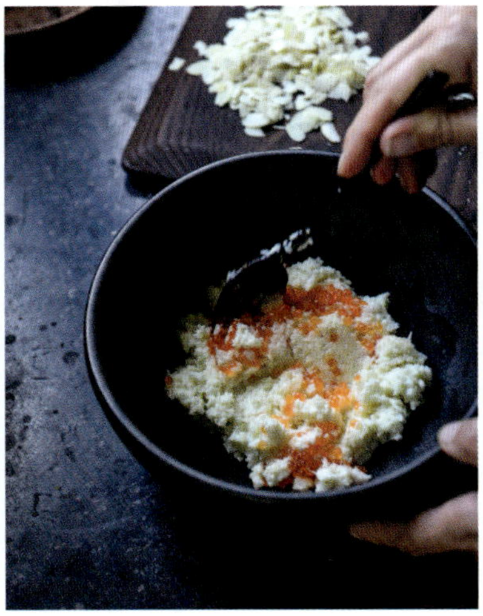 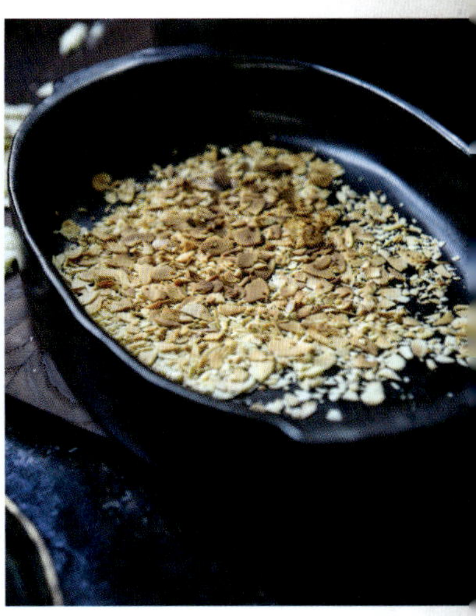

cauliflower puree ✓ keto

with trout roe and sliced almonds

- **¼ cauliflower**
- **1 jar trout roe**
- **3½ fl oz (100 ml) cream**
- **a handful of sliced almonds**

Cook the cauliflower florets until tender in water seasoned with some salt and pepper and a generous splash of olive oil. Coarsely chop the sliced almonds and roast them in the oven or in a pan.
Drain the cauliflower, add the cream and blend the mixture to a puree. Let the puree cool until it is lukewarm before adding the trout roe, otherwise the roe will cook in the puree and turn hard.
Add three quarters of the trout roe and stir into the puree.
Spoon the puree into bowls, scatter some sliced almonds over the top and garnish with the remaining trout roe.

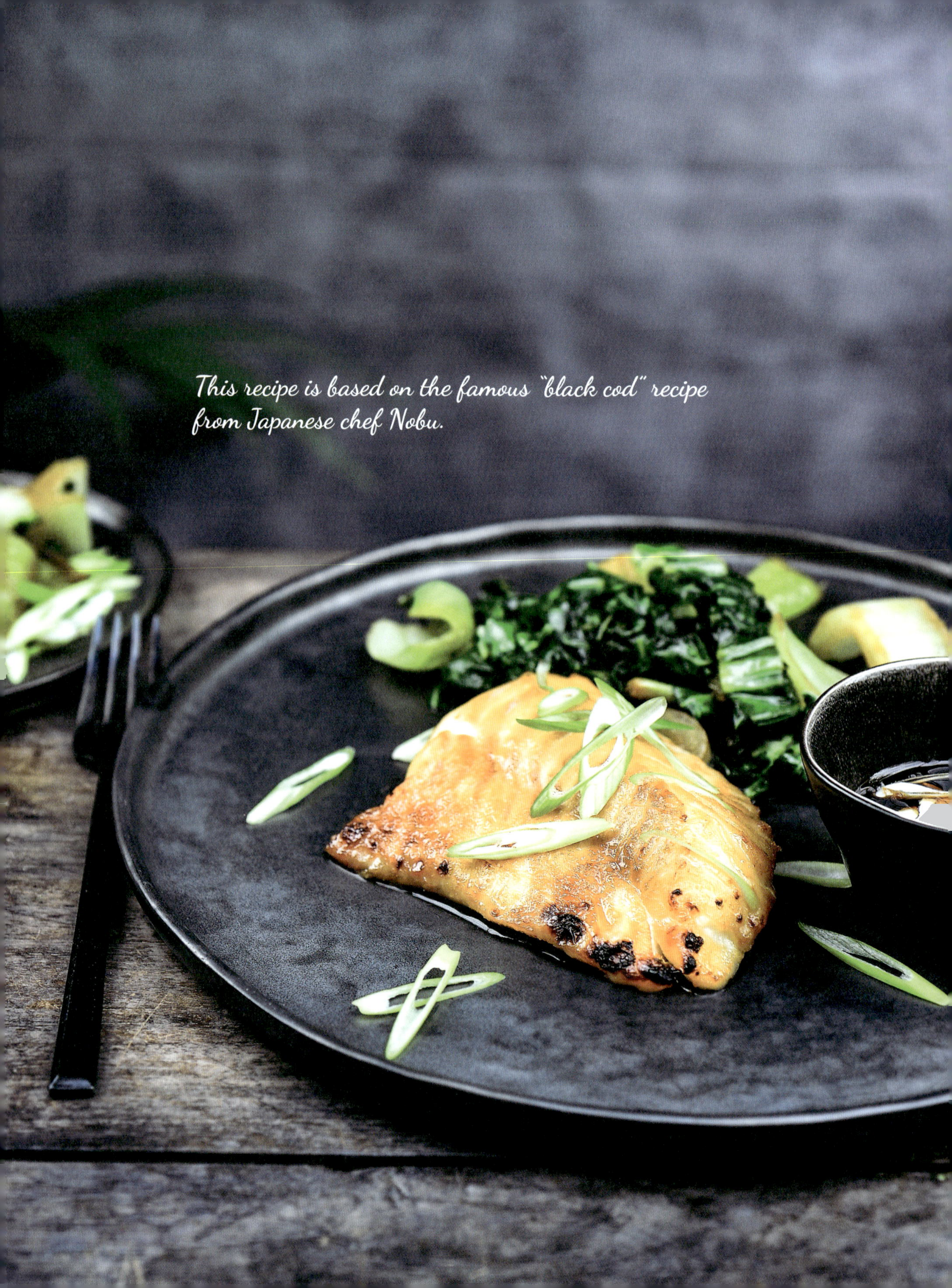

This recipe is based on the famous "black cod" recipe from Japanese chef Nobu.

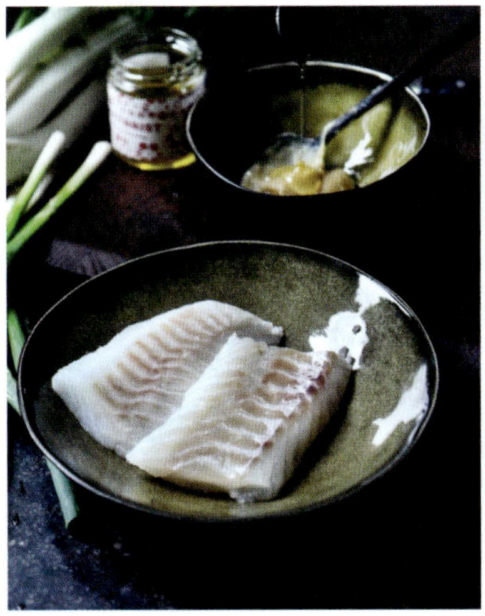

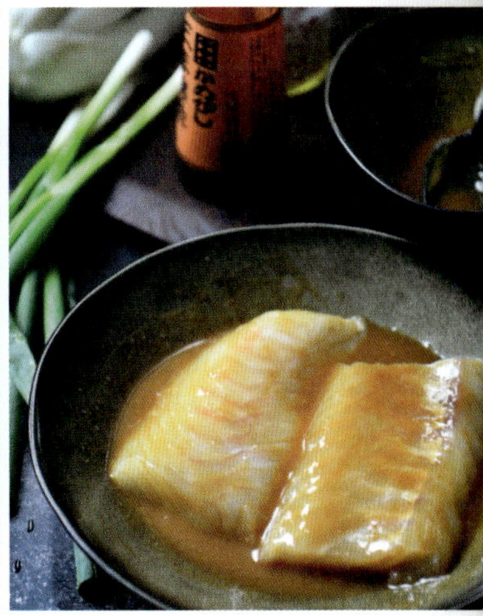

cod ✓ keto
with miso and bok choy

- **2 cod fillets**
- **shiro miso**
- **a little over 1 lb (500 g) bok choy (see tip)**
- **2 spring onions, finely chopped**

– soy sauce –
– honey –

Preheat the oven to 400 °F (200 °C). Combine one large tablespoon of shiro miso with 2 tablespoons of soy sauce and 2 teaspoons of honey. Mix well and rub the mixture over the cod fillets. If you have time, you can leave the fish to marinate in the fridge (see tip). Slice the white part of the bok choy into strips and stir-fry for about 3 minutes in plenty of olive oil. Add 2 tablespoons of soy sauce and continue to stir-fry.

Slice the green part of the bok choy into strips and add to the pan. Bake the fish in the oven for about 10 minutes. Place the cod fillets on the plates and arrange the vegetables next to the fish. Serve with a mixture of soy sauce and olive oil and garnish with the finely chopped spring onions.

TIP: MARINATING

Nobu is one of my favorite chefs. His dishes are of the highest quality, yet simple. I've made a simplified, Western version of his "black cod" dish. Marinate the fish for as long as you can. Nobu marinates the fish for no fewer than four days. A couple of hours should be enough for my version of this dish, but if I'm short on time, I skip the marinating part. Even without marinating, this fish tastes delicious.

TIP: KETO AND SHIRO MISO

One spoonful of shiro miso is about 10 grams and contains 1/10 of an ounce (2.8 g) of carbohydrates. This recipe also works well in a keto diet because you use so little of the miso paste.

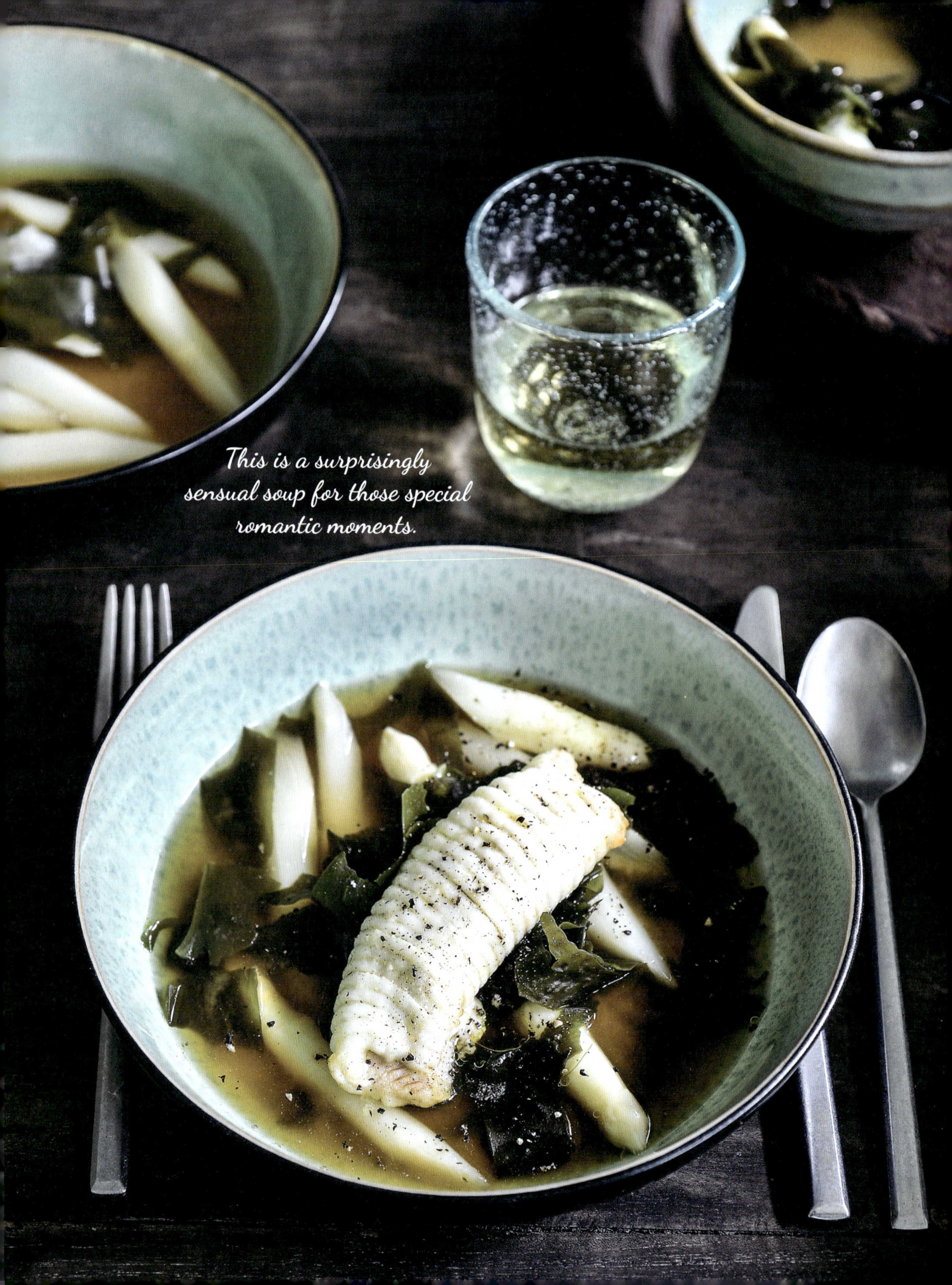
This is a surprisingly
sensual soup for those special
romantic moments.

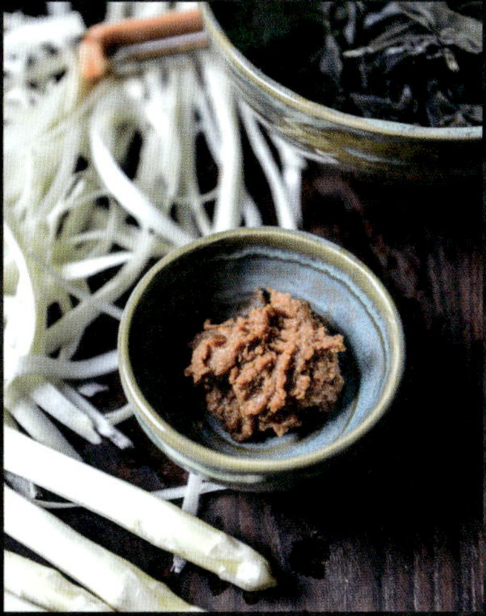
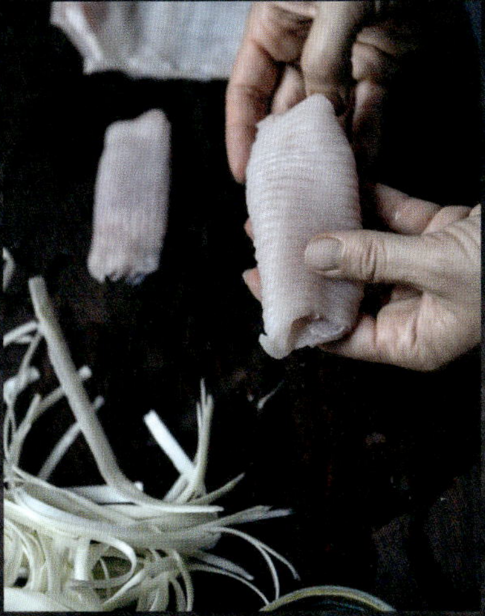
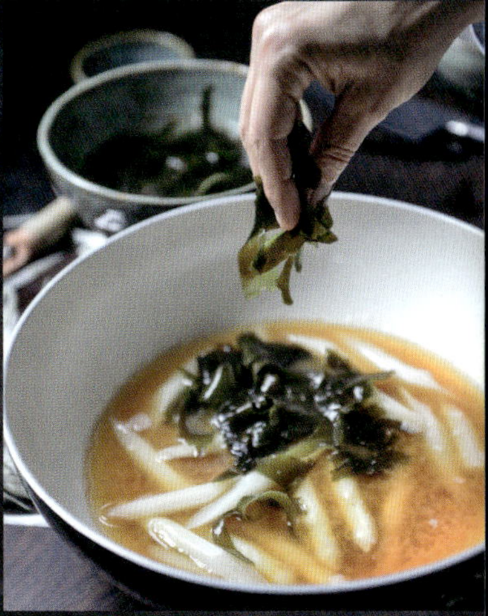

ray with asparagus ✓keto

in a miso soup

- **2 ray fillets (see tip)**
- **1 bunch of white asparagus**
- **6 to 8 dried wakame sheets**
- **2 tablespoons brown miso (barley miso)**

Add lukewarm water to the wakame sheets and leave them to soak for 10 minutes. Preheat the oven to 350 °F (180 °C). Peel the asparagus with a vegetable peeler and cut off the hard ends. Pour 3 cups (750 ml) of water into a pan and cook the asparagus until tender. Roll up the ray fillets with the inside facing outwards so you can see those gorgeous ridges. Put them in a baking dish and bake for about 15 minutes in the oven.
Dissolve the miso in a bit of lukewarm water. Remove the pan from the heat once the asparagus is tender and strain the dissolved miso through a sieve into the pan with the water and asparagus. Throw away the hard bits of miso left in the sieve. Remove the soaked wakame from the water and add to the miso soup. Serve the asparagus and the miso soup in two deep dishes and place a piece of ray on top of the soup.

TIP: RAY
Take the straight, middle part of the ray wing and have it boned or bone it yourself, which is quite easy to do. Scrape a knife along the bone, starting from the thick part of the wing.

TIP: WAKAME AND MISO
It's better not to let the wakame cook, as it becomes rubbery. The same goes for miso: don't cook the miso, that way it retains its full flavor.

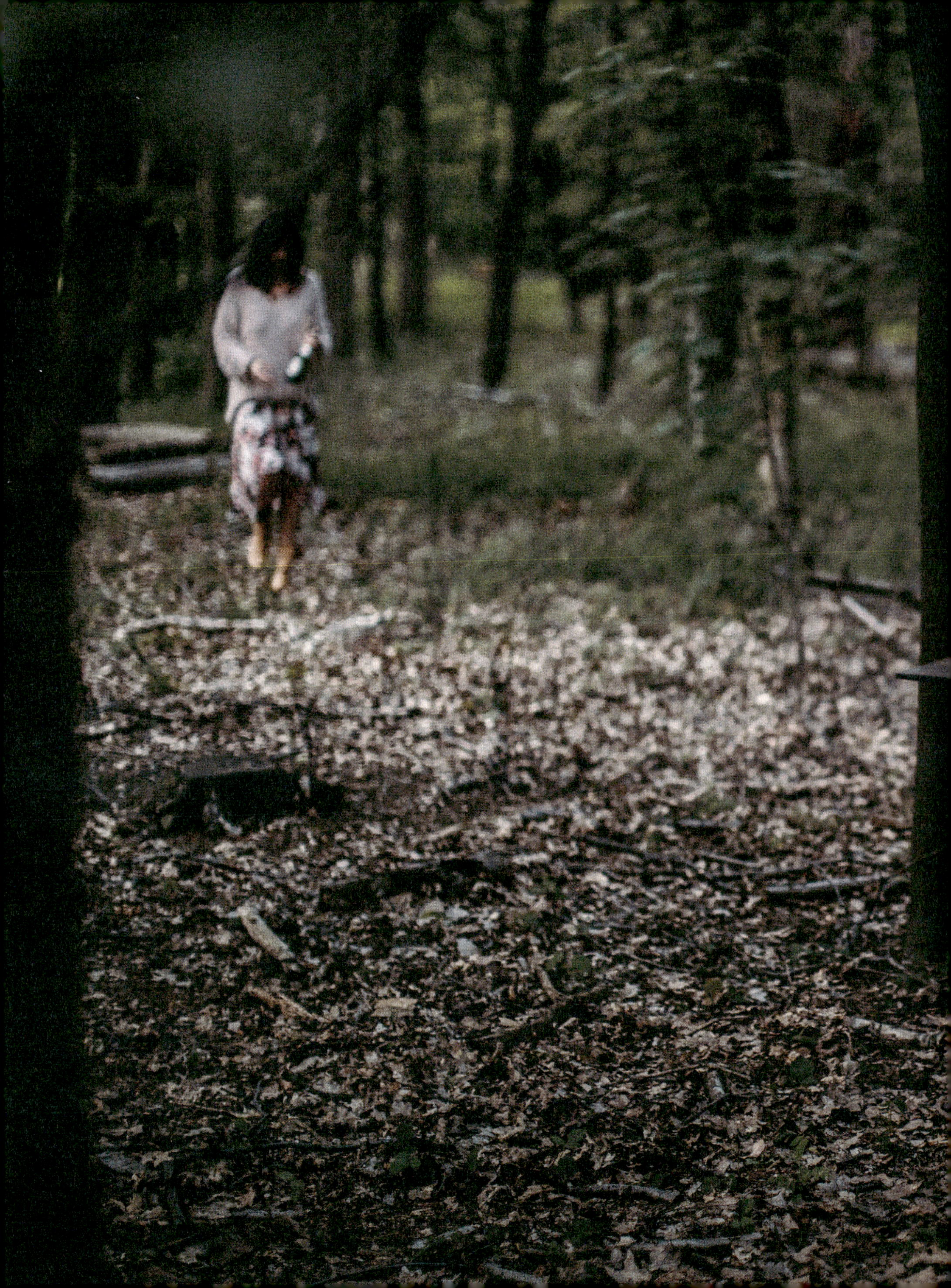

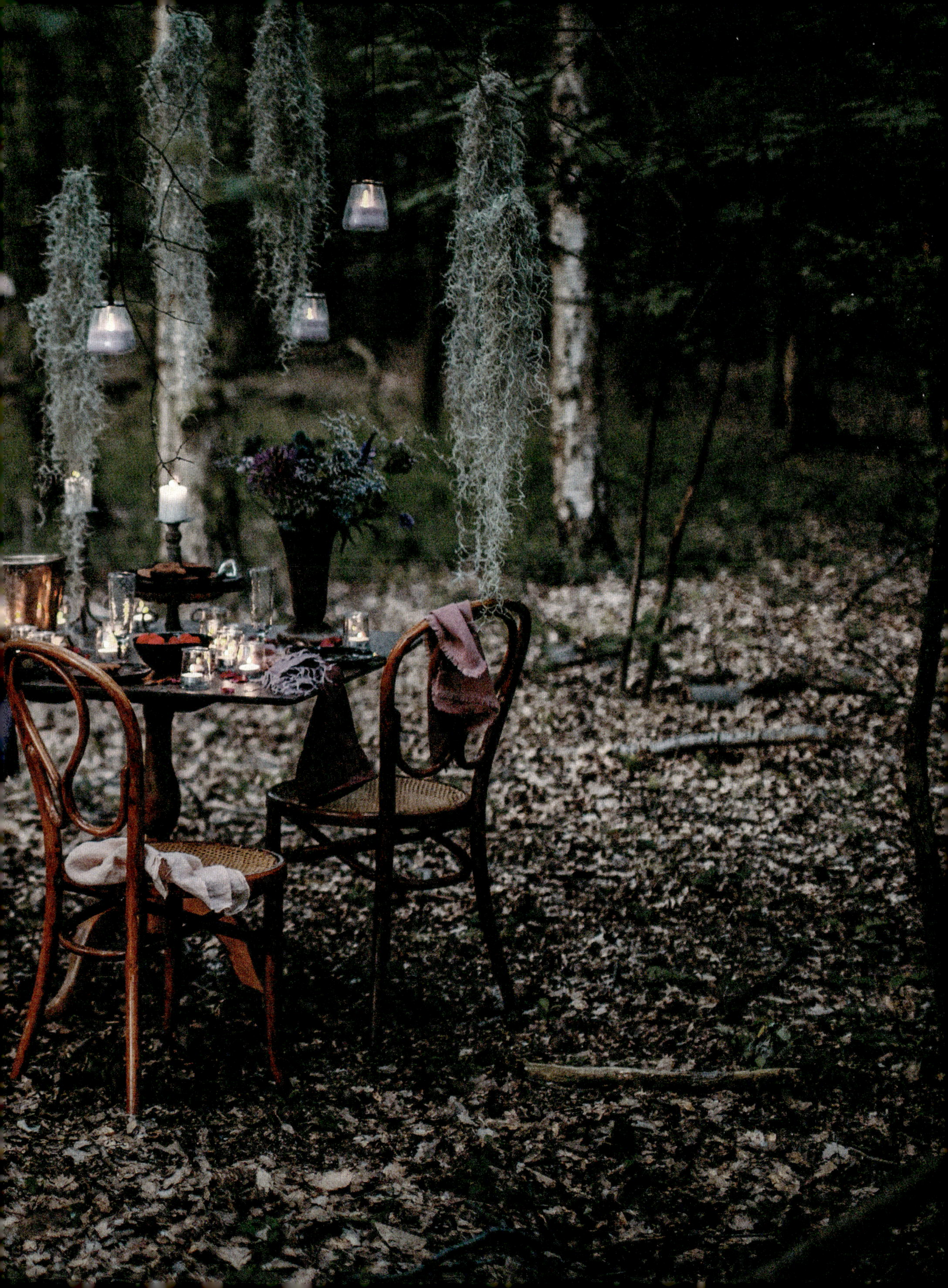

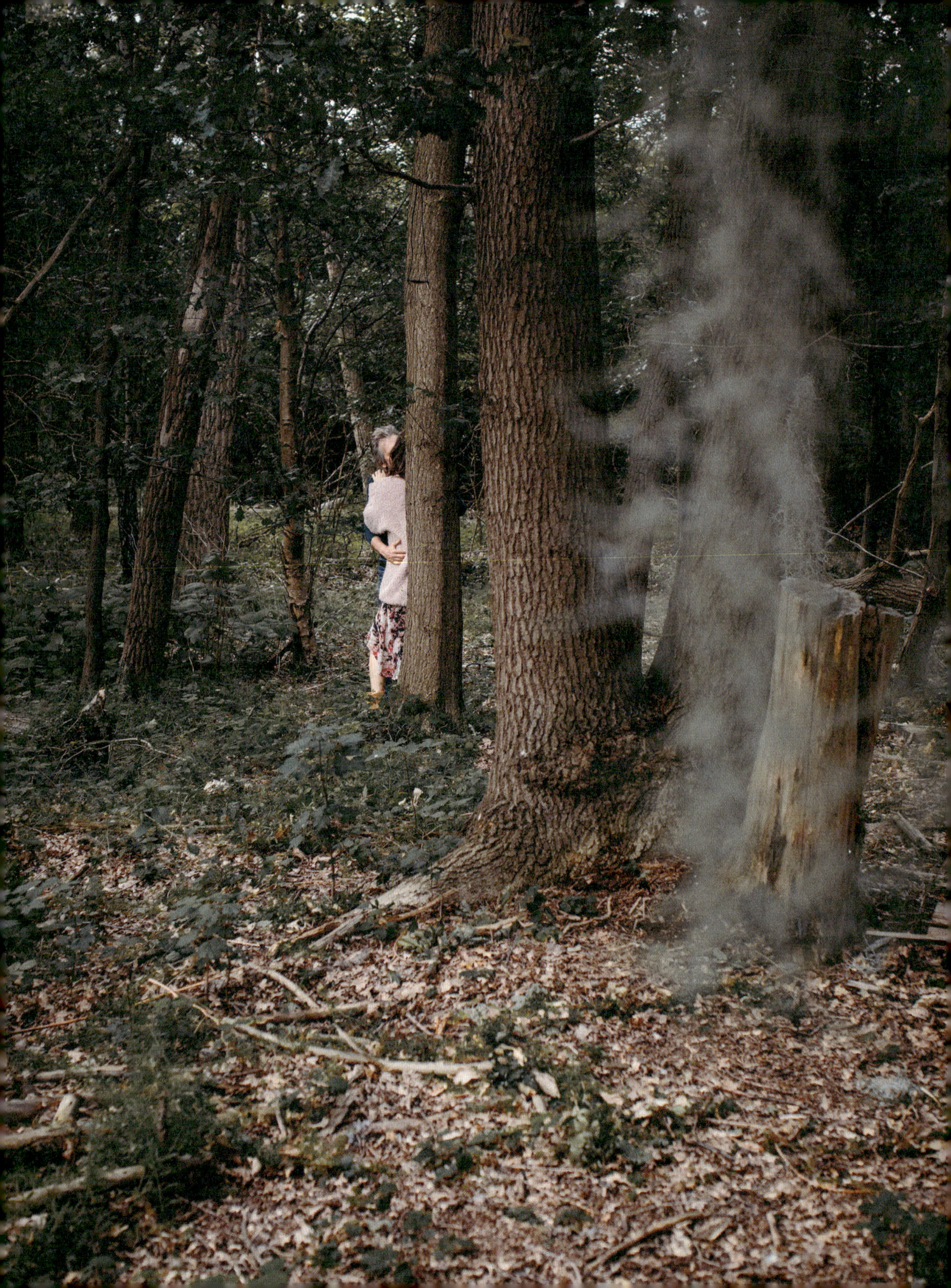

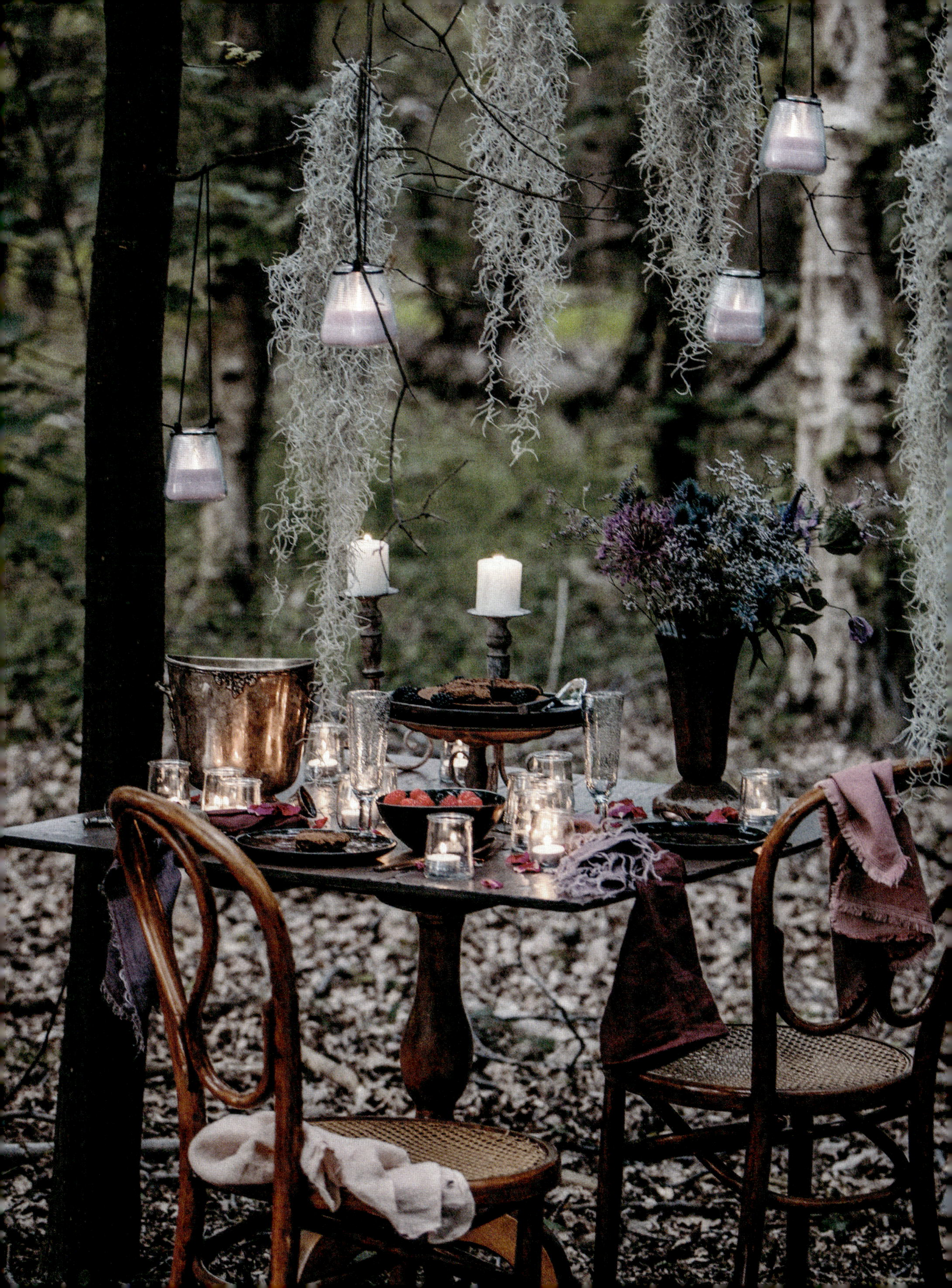

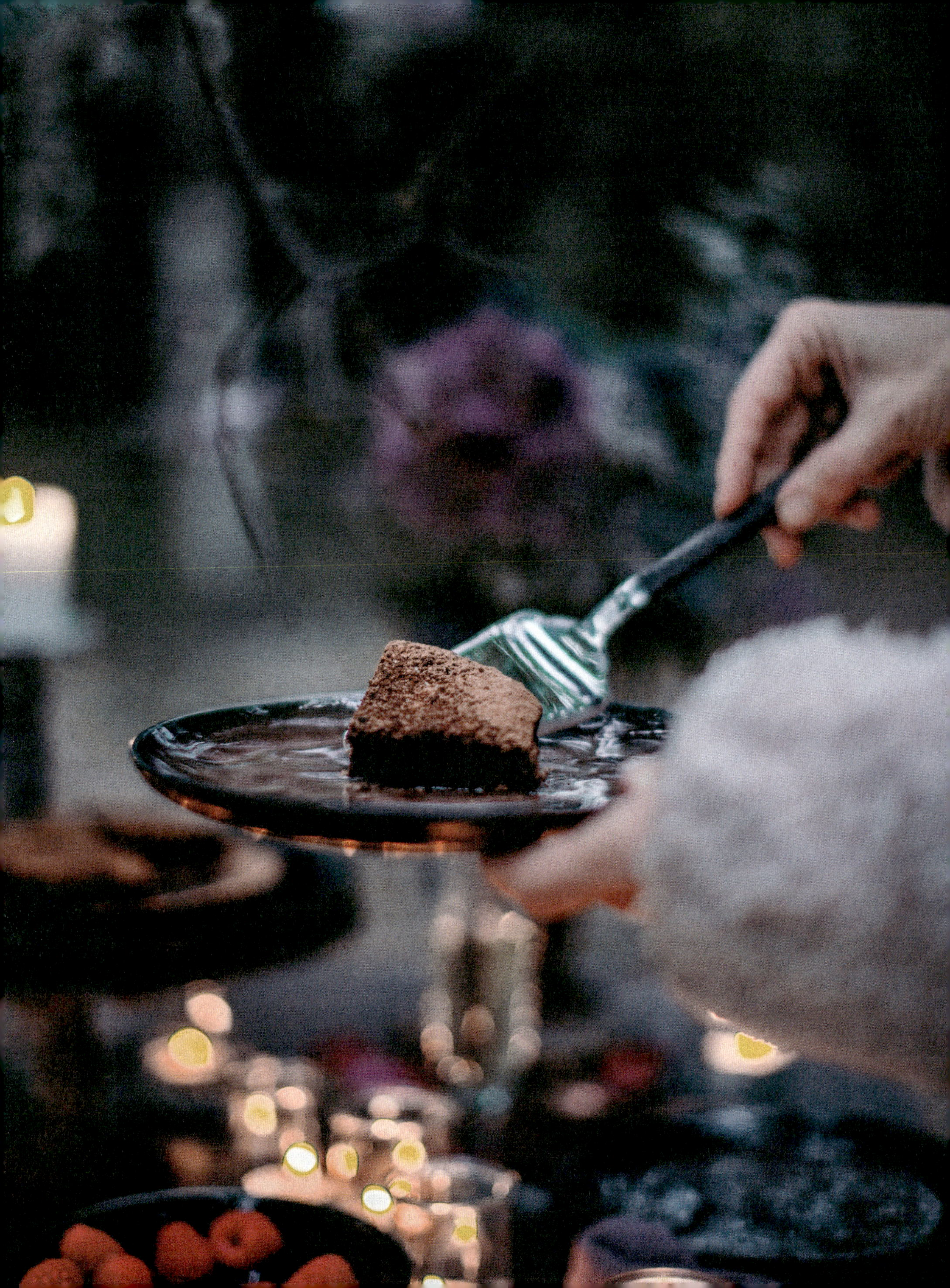

quick desserts

I find preparing desserts to be an extra treat, which means I often devote even more love and attention to it because I know it's something extra for those special moments. I believe there's no harm in the occasional dessert. If you are following a keto diet, desserts with sugar are a definite "no-go", as you will immediately go out of the ketose state if you eat sugar. If you're following a low-carb diet, use as little sugar as possible, or no sugar at all. My gut feeling says that you should follow your personal rhythm and find your sense of balance. That's what works best in the long term. However, if you've been off-balance for a while, now would be a good time to draw in the reins in a bit. And that's fine, it's all part of the rhythm of life. Find your own rhythm, your own balance, find whatever feels comfortable for you, anytime, anywhere. And above all, remember to savor it!

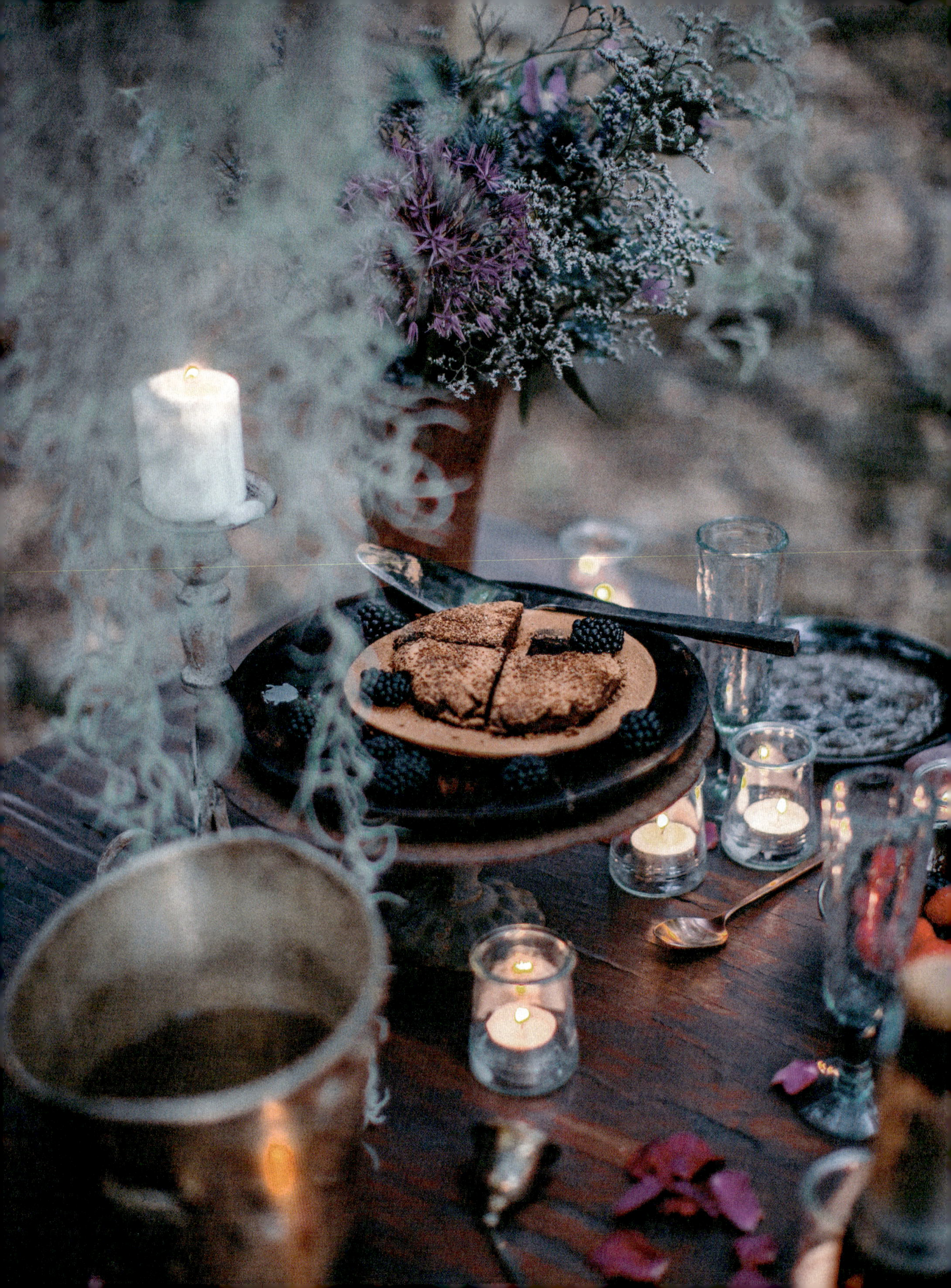

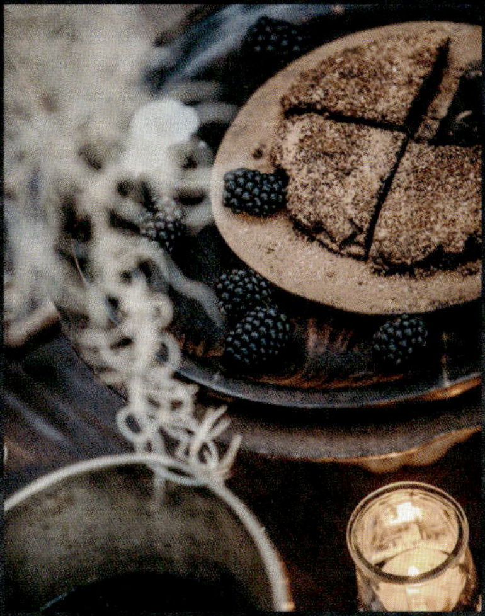

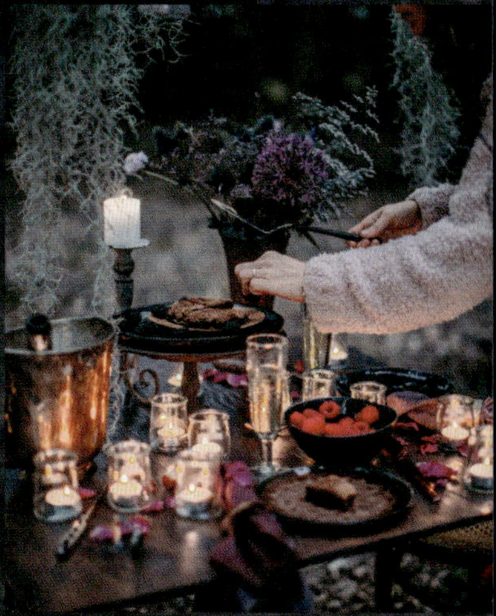

chocolate cake

Ingredients for 2 to 4 people:

- **1½ oz (40 g) dark chocolate**
- **2 oz (50 g) nut flour**
- **1 oz (25 g) cocoa powder + a little extra**
- **1 egg**

- 2 oz (60 g) butter -
- 1 oz (30 g) sugar -

extra: parchment paper

Preheat the oven to 350 °F (180 °C). Melt the chocolate together with the butter (see tip). Set some sugar and cocoa powder aside for later. Combine the nut flour with the egg and remaining cocoa powder and sugar. Stir in the melted buttery chocolate mixture. Pour the batter into a cake tin lined with parchment paper. Sprinkle some sugar and plenty of cocoa powder over the top and bake in the oven for about 15 minutes.

TIP: MELTING CHOCOLATE
I put the chocolate and butter in a bowl and place it in the oven at 160 °F (70 °C). The mixture is completely melted after about 7 minutes. It's a lot less work than using a double boiler or bain marie.

TIP: CAKE TIN
People often ask me: which cake tin? Just have a look and see which cake tins or baking dishes you have in your cupboard. I like to use my small baking dishes for this cake, they are 15 cm in diameter.

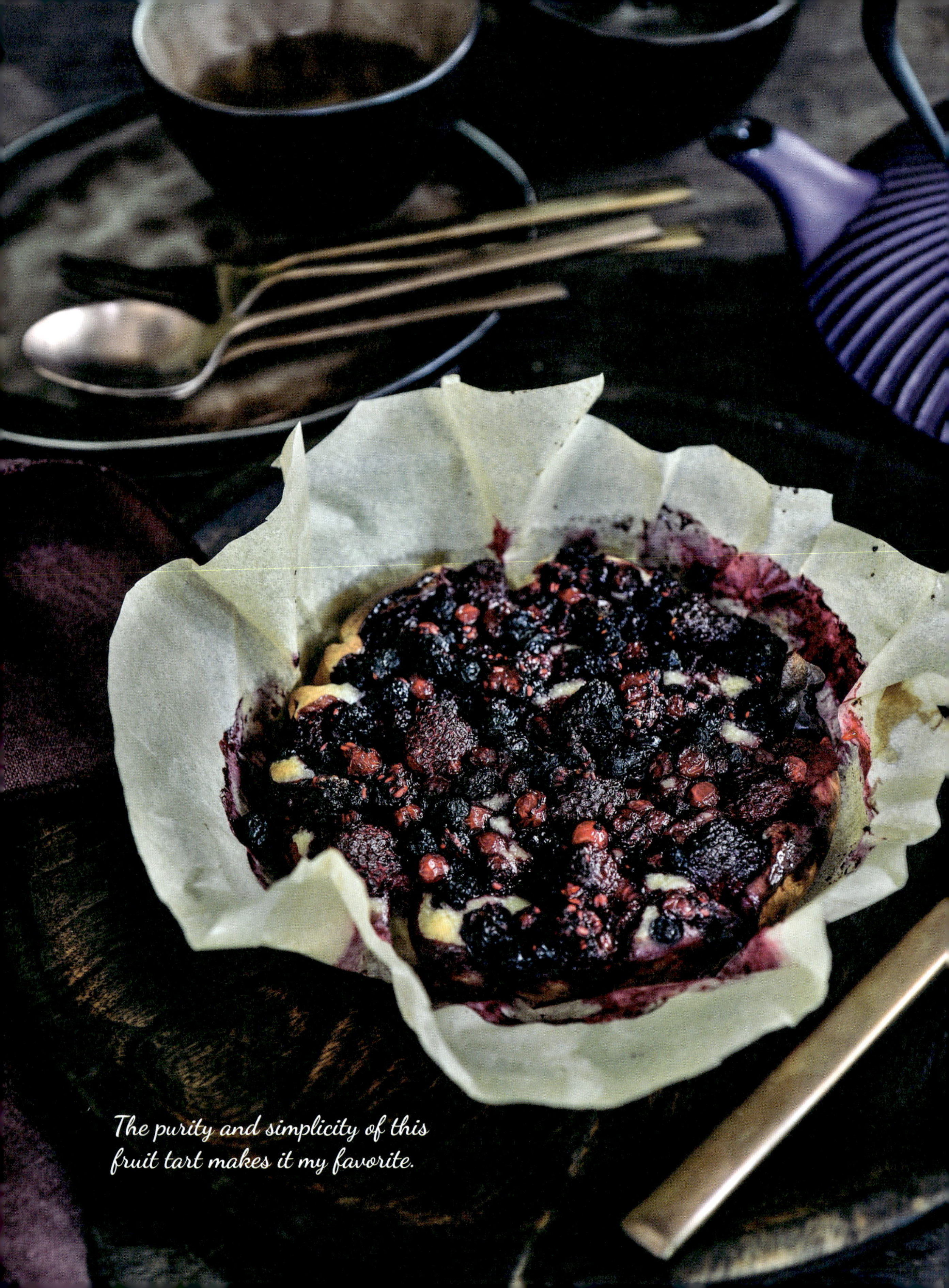

The purity and simplicity of this fruit tart makes it my favorite.

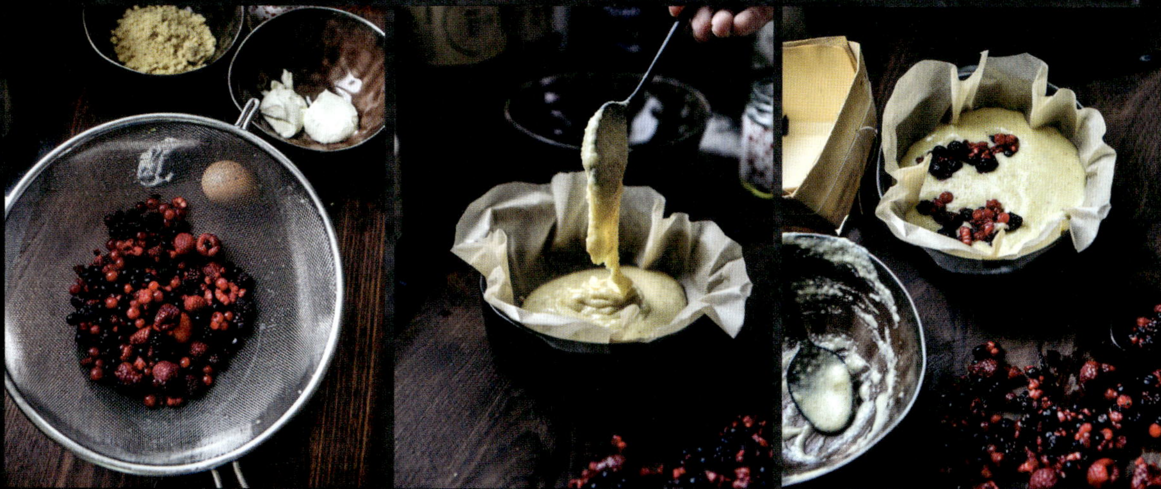

heavenly fruit tart

- **5 oz (150 g) frozen berries (or fresh)**
- **2 oz (50 g) mascarpone**
- **1 egg**
- **3 oz (70 g) nut flour**

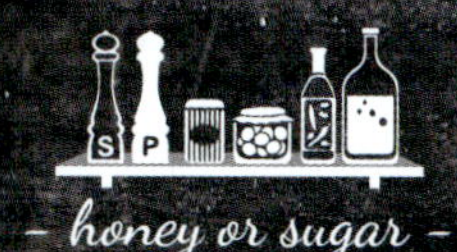

extra: parchment paper

Preheat the oven to 350 °F (180 °C). Combine the nut flour with the egg and mascarpone. I always heat up the mascarpone a little beforehand, which makes it easier to mix in with the other ingredients. Stir in 2 tablespoons of honey or sugar. Line a baking dish with parchment paper and spoon the batter into the dish. Place the fruit on top and drizzle another tablespoon of honey over the top. Bake in the oven for 20 minutes.

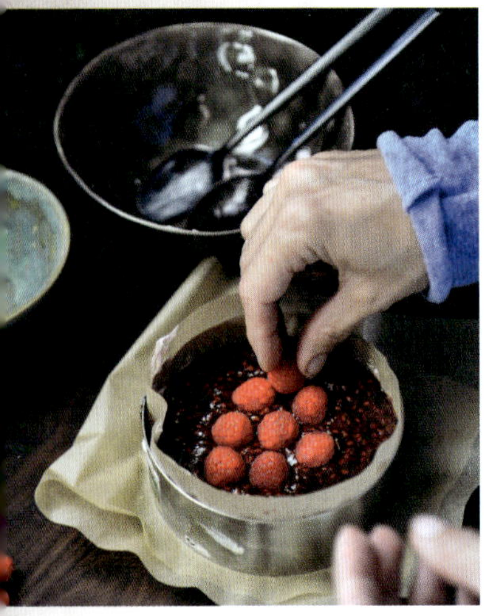

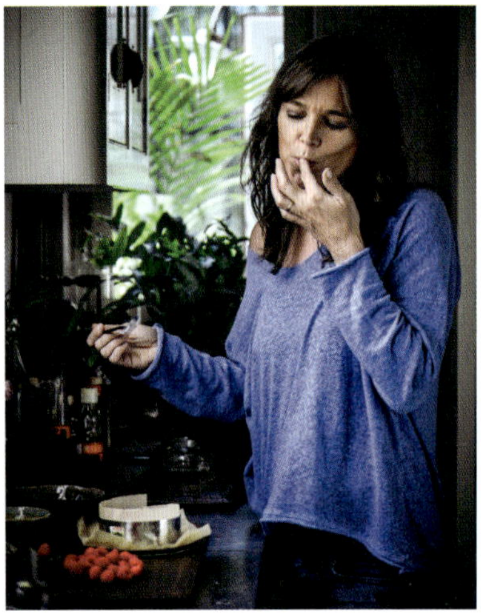

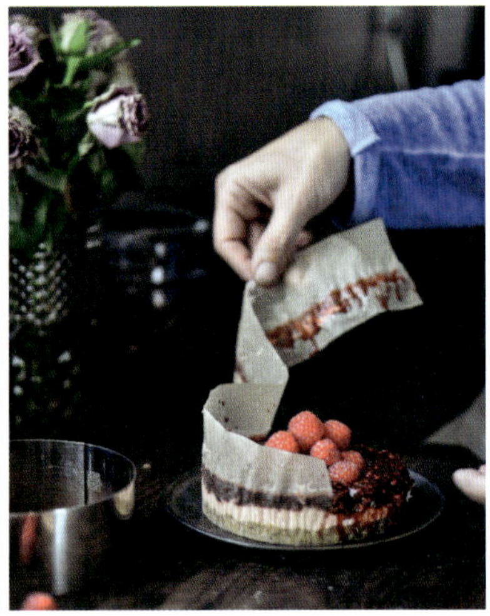

cheesecake
with raspberries

- **3½ oz (100 g) soft goat cheese**
- **3 oz (80 g) hazelnut or almond flour**
- **4½ oz (125 g) raspberries**
- **5 dates**

- coconut sugar -

extra: parchment paper

Mix the pitted dates with the hazelnut flour. If necessary, add a few more dates or a little more hazelnut flour so you can press the mixture together to form a thick paste.
Take a large cooking ring or another mold and line the bottom and sides with parchment paper. Spoon the date paste into the ring or mold and press down firmly. Combine the goat cheese with 5 raspberries to give the goat cheese a lovely pink color. Spoon the cheese over the date paste. Sauté the rest of the raspberries with a small amount of water to make a puree and add 3 teaspoons of coconut sugar to the puree. Cook for a little longer, then pour the puree over the cheesecake. Store the cake in the fridge until it's ready to be served, if you can wait that long.

TIP: SUGAR
A dessert doesn't have to be super sweet as far as I'm concerned, so add sugar to suit your own tastes. Remember that, on the whole, we tend to add more sugar than necessary.

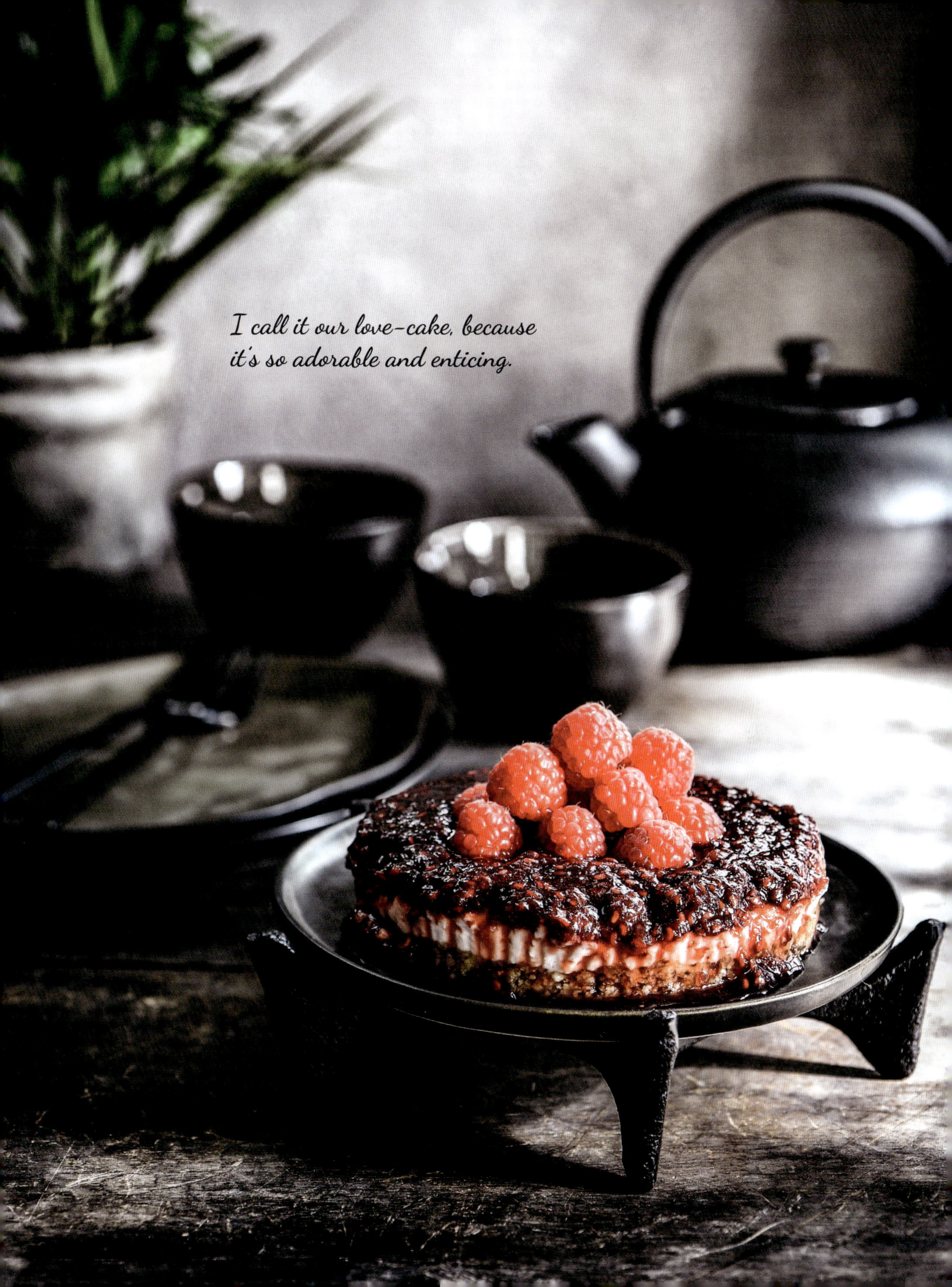
I call it our love-cake, because
it's so adorable and enticing.

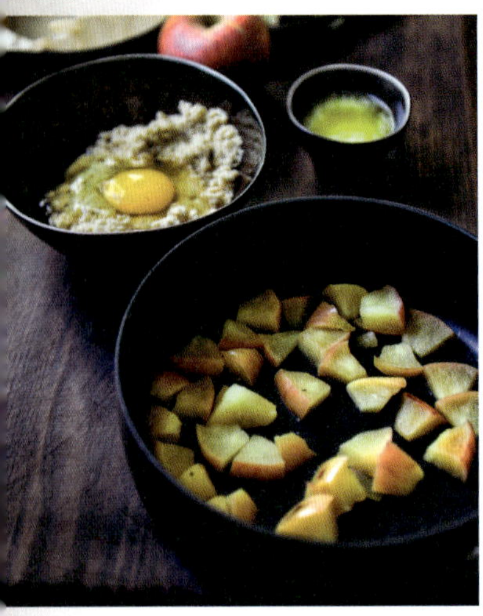
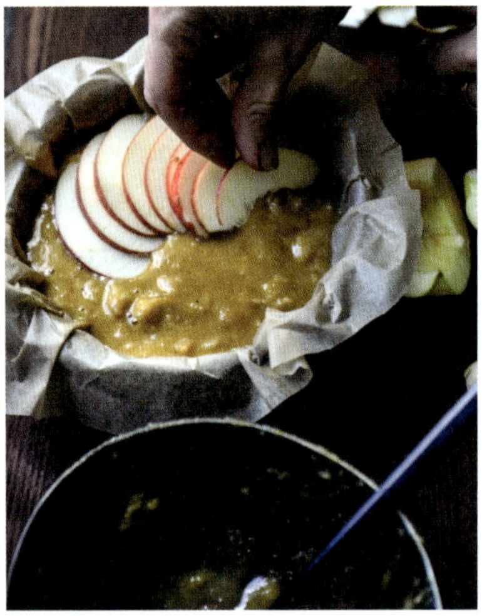

divine apple tart

- **2 apples**
- **3 oz (70 g) nut flour (see tip)**
- **1 egg**

- ¾ oz (20 g sugar) + a little extra -
- 1½ oz (40 g) butter + a little extra -

extra: parchment paper

Preheat the oven to 350 °F (180 °C). Core and dice one apple, leaving the skin on. Sauté the diced apple with a small glass of water to make apple sauce. Melt the butter and combine it with the nut flour, sugar and egg. Mash the cooked apple with a fork and mix it into the dough.
Line a baking dish with parchment paper and pour the dough into the dish. Slice the second apple and arrange the slices so they overlap slightly on the tart shell. Sprinkle some sugar over the tart and drizzle another 2 to 3 tablespoons of melted butter over the top. Bake in the oven for 15 to 20 minutes.

TIP: NUT FLOUR
There are various types of nut flours on the market today. I particularly like hazelnut flour. Nut flour is actually not a flour or a powder, it's simply ground nuts. You can easily make your own using your favorite types of nuts.

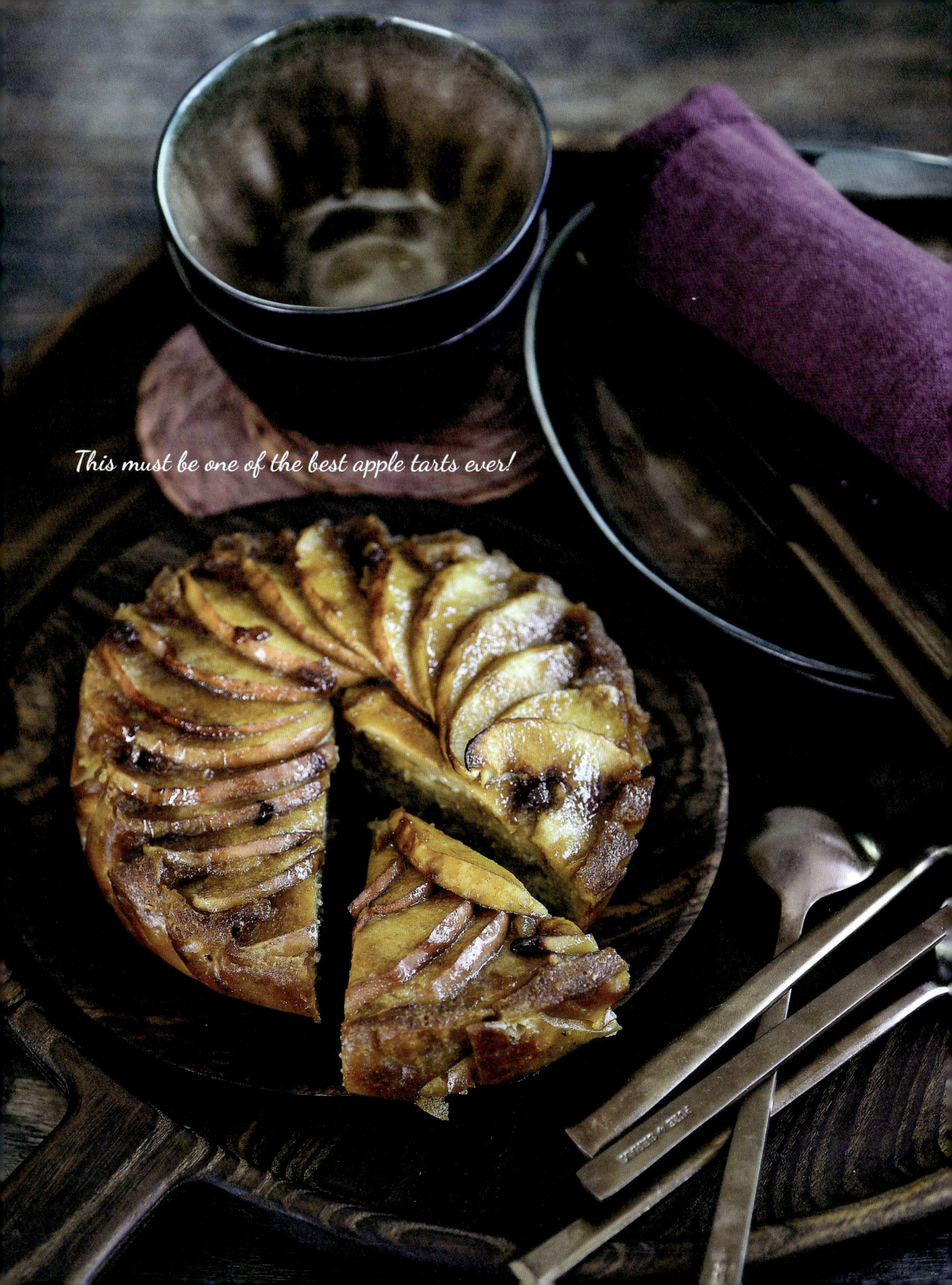

This must be one of the best apple tarts ever!

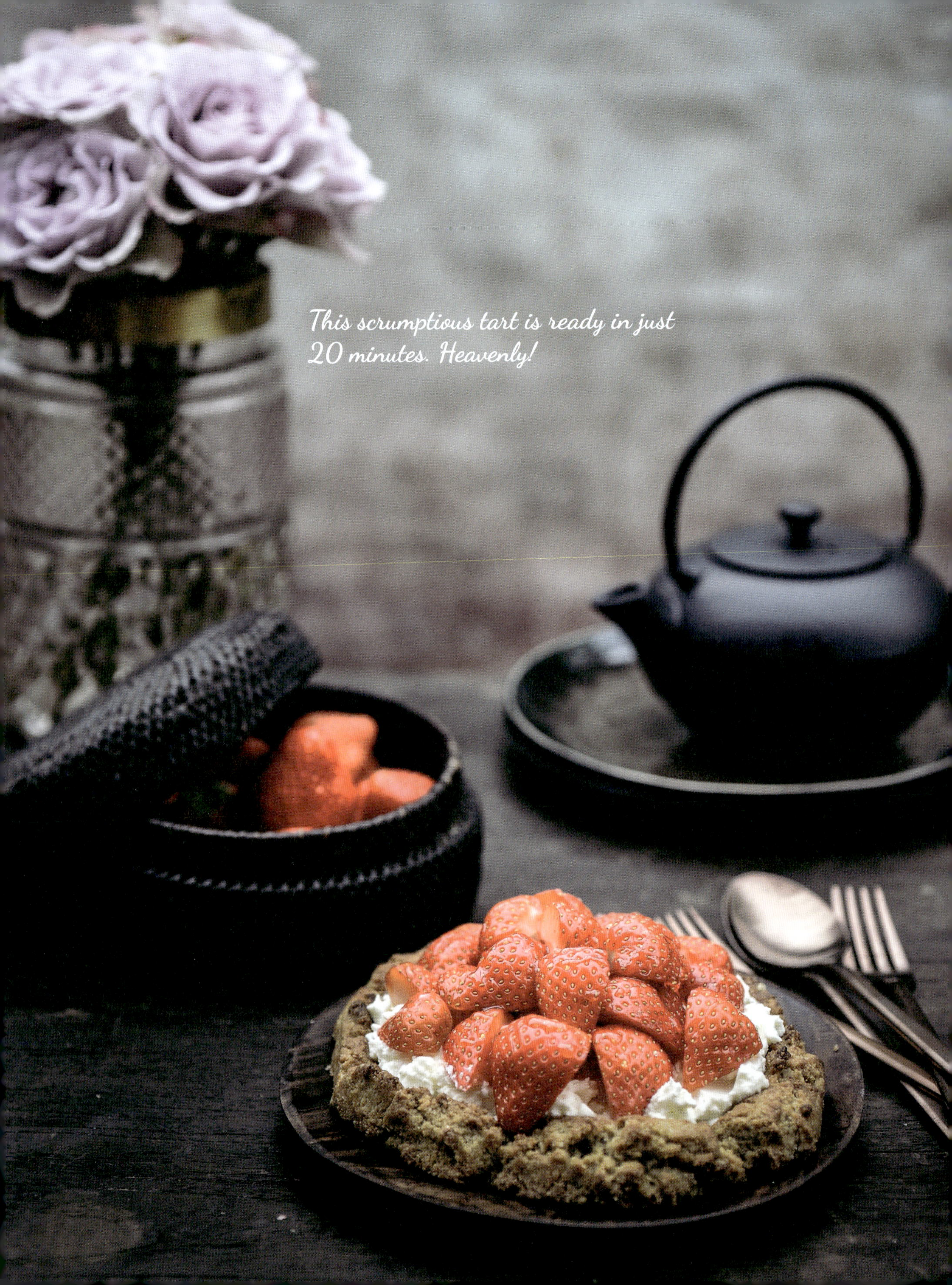

This scrumptious tart is ready in just 20 minutes. Heavenly!

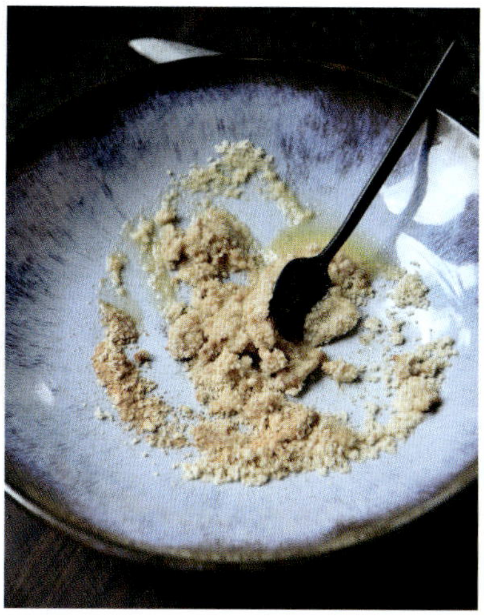
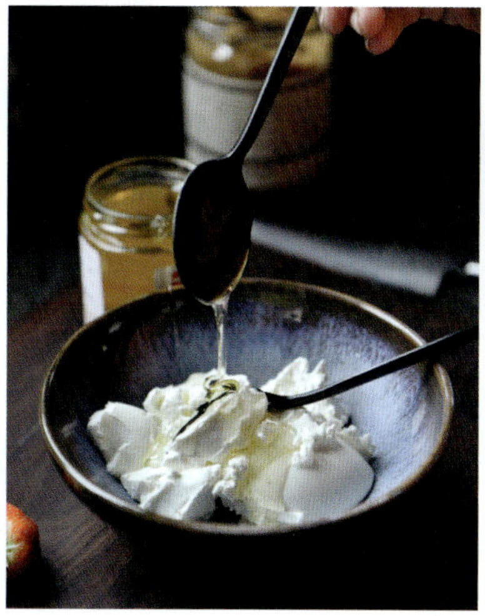
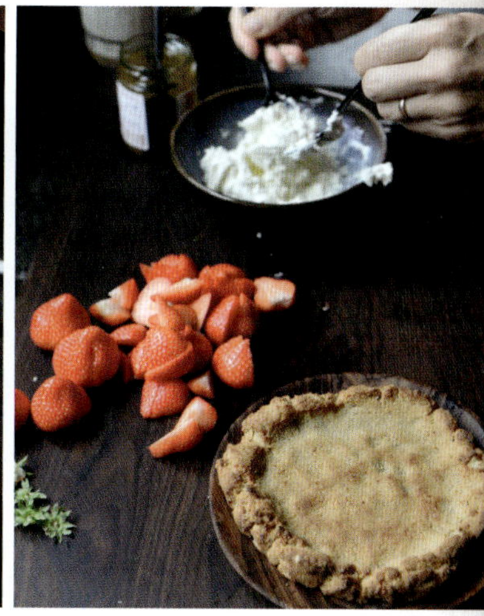

tart

with nuts, mascarpone and strawberries

- **a handful of strawberries**
- **4½ oz (120 g) hazelnut flour (see tip)**
- **1 egg white**
- **7 oz (200 g) mascarpone**

- butter -

- sugar (see tip) -

extra: parchment paper

Preheat the oven to 350 °F (180 °C). Combine the hazelnut flour with 2 oz (50 g) melted butter, ⅓ oz (10 g) sugar (or more to taste) and the egg white to form a thick dough. Place the dough on the parchment paper. Shape the dough into a round tart shell, making sure that the edges are slightly thicker. Bake for 10 minutes in the preheated oven. Meanwhile, combine the mascarpone with some sugar or honey and quarter the strawberries. Remove the tart shell from the oven and let it cool down a bit. Spoon the mascarpone into the shell, arrange the strawberries on top and garnish with a drizzle of honey, if you like.

TIP: HAZELNUT FLOUR
I think the word “flour” is a bit unfortunate, as it’s coarser than normal wheat flour. You could also use almond flour, but hazelnut flour is a delicious alternative. You can find it in the supermarket, or you can grind hazelnuts into a coarse flour yourself.

TIP: SUGAR
My favorite sugar is coconut sugar, because of its taste and the fact that it’s unprocessed. I prefer to use honey to sweeten mascarpone, as this doesn’t make the cheese turn brown.

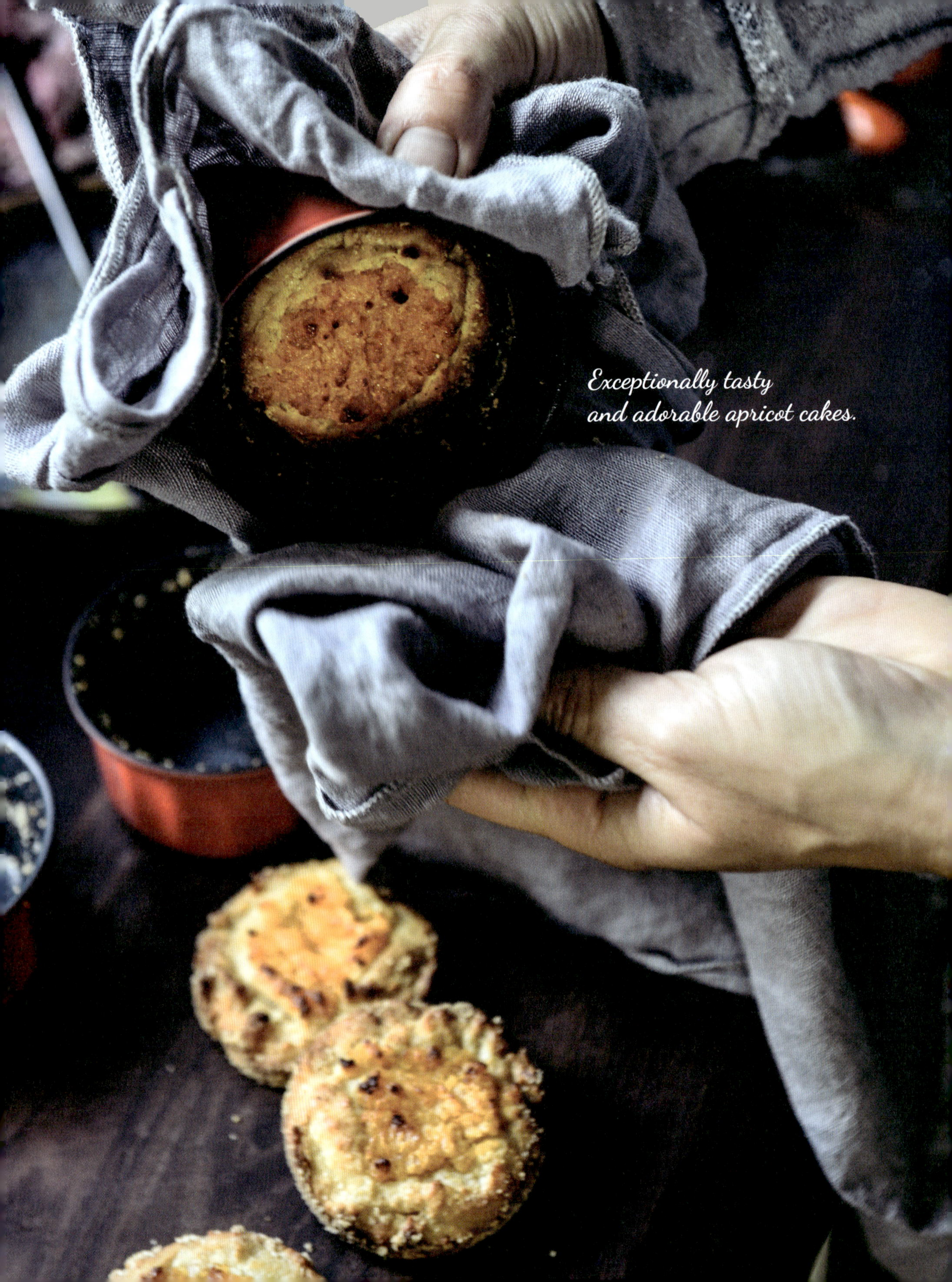

*Exceptionally tasty
and adorable apricot cakes.*

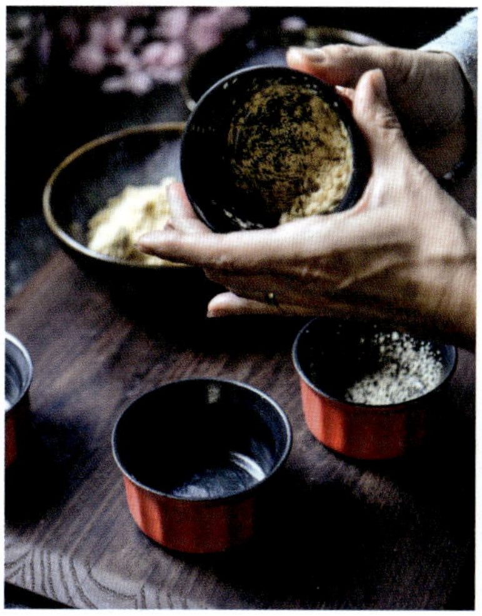

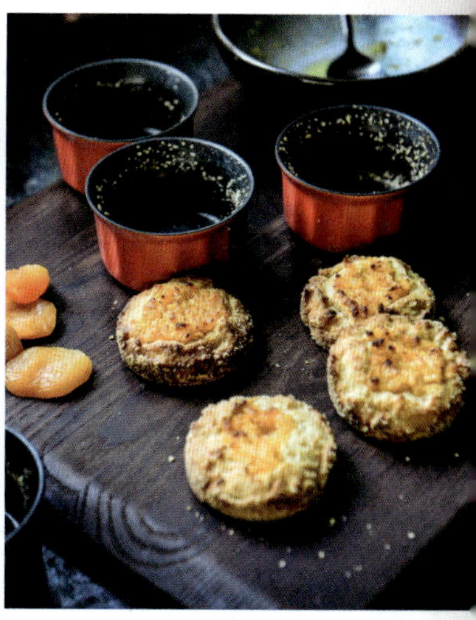

apricot cakes

- **3 oz (70 g) + a little extra hazelnut flour (see tip)**
- **3 oz (70 g) salted butter**
- **3 oz (70 g) dried apricots (see tip)**
- **1 egg**

Preheat the oven to 350 °F (180 °C). Melt the butter and combine with the apricots to form a sticky compote. Set 4 tablespoons of the compote aside and mix the rest with the hazelnut flour and egg. Grease four small cake tins with butter, coat the tins with extra hazelnut flour and divide the batter evenly between the four tins. Spoon some of the remaining compote in the middle of each cake. Bake for 12 to 14 minutes in the preheated oven.

TIP: HAZELNUT FLOUR
I love the fact that there are different nut flours available these days. We don't always have to use almond flour, which has a specific taste. I think the word "flour" is a bit unfortunate, as it's more of a coarse meal. You can also grind the nuts yourself to make a coarse flour.

TIP: SOFT DRIED APRICOTS
The apricots are dried, but they still contain moisture, making them very soft. You can find them in the supermarket. You can also make these cakes with dried apricots, but the cakes will come out drier.

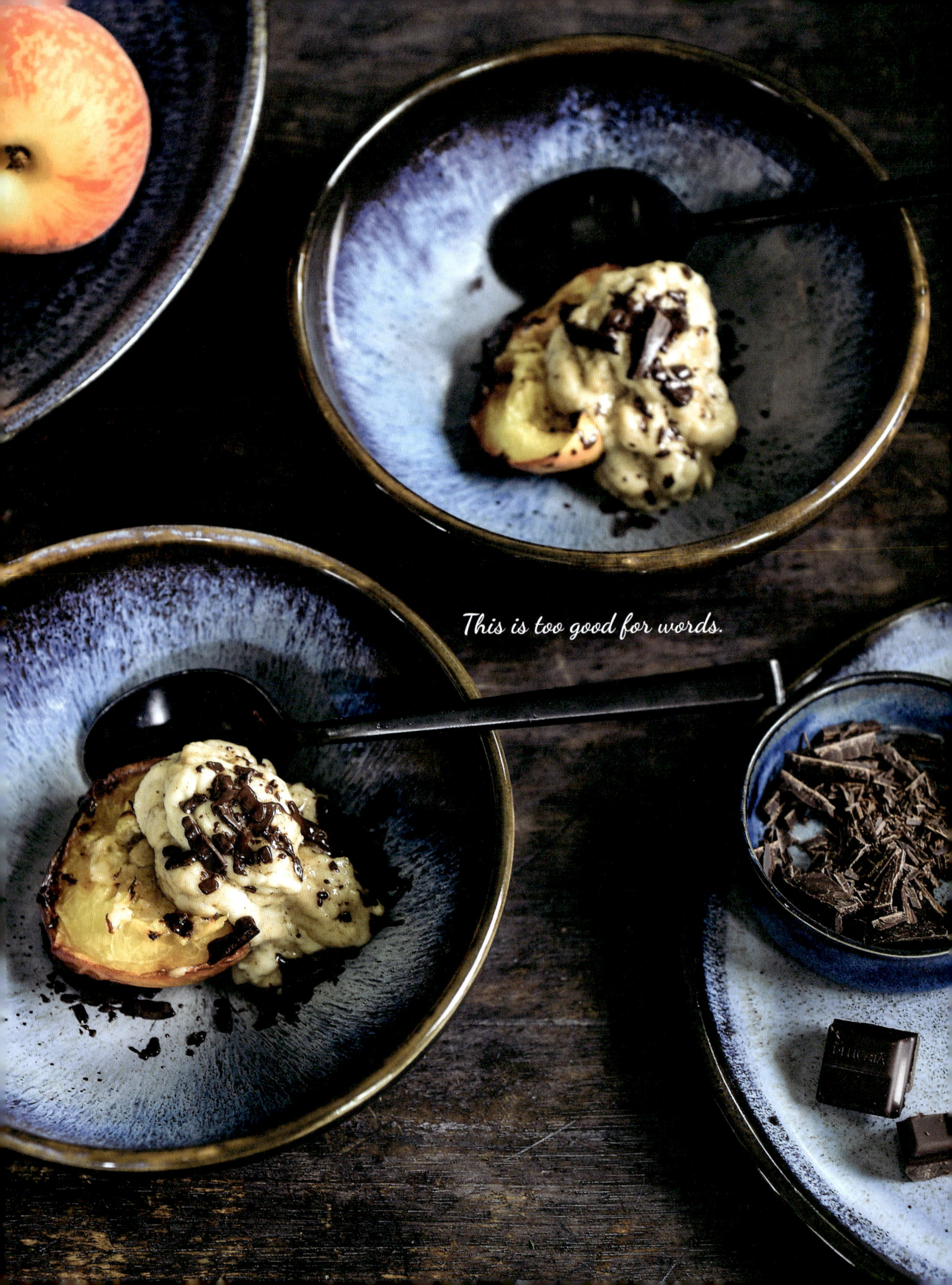

This is too good for words.

oven-baked yellow peaches

- **1 ripe peach**
- **3 tablespoons mascarpone**
- **1 tablespoon nut butter (peanut butter or another nut butter)**
- **¾ oz (20 g) dark chocolate**

– honey or sugar –

Preheat the oven to 350 °F (180 °C). Cut the peach in half and remove the stone. Place the peach halves, cut side up, in a baking dish and bake in the oven for 20 minutes.
Towards the end of the cooking time, combine the mascarpone and nut butter in a pan and heat slightly, stirring well. Chop the chocolate into small pieces. Remove the peaches from the oven and place them in a bowl. Spoon the sauce over the peaches and garnish with the chopped chocolate.

TIP: SUGAR
I don't need any sugar with this dish. As you will discover, this dessert is rich enough in flavor as it is.

TIP: STRAWBERRIES
If you are short on time, you can replace the cooked peaches with finely chopped uncooked fresh strawberries.

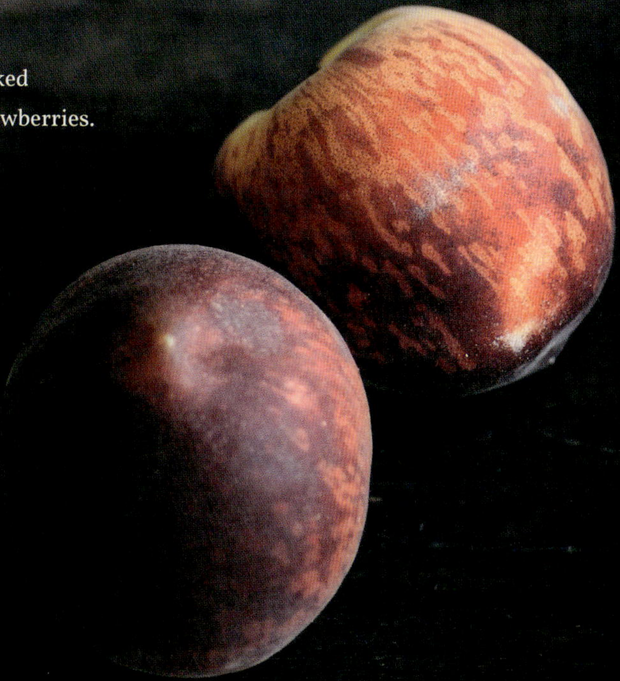

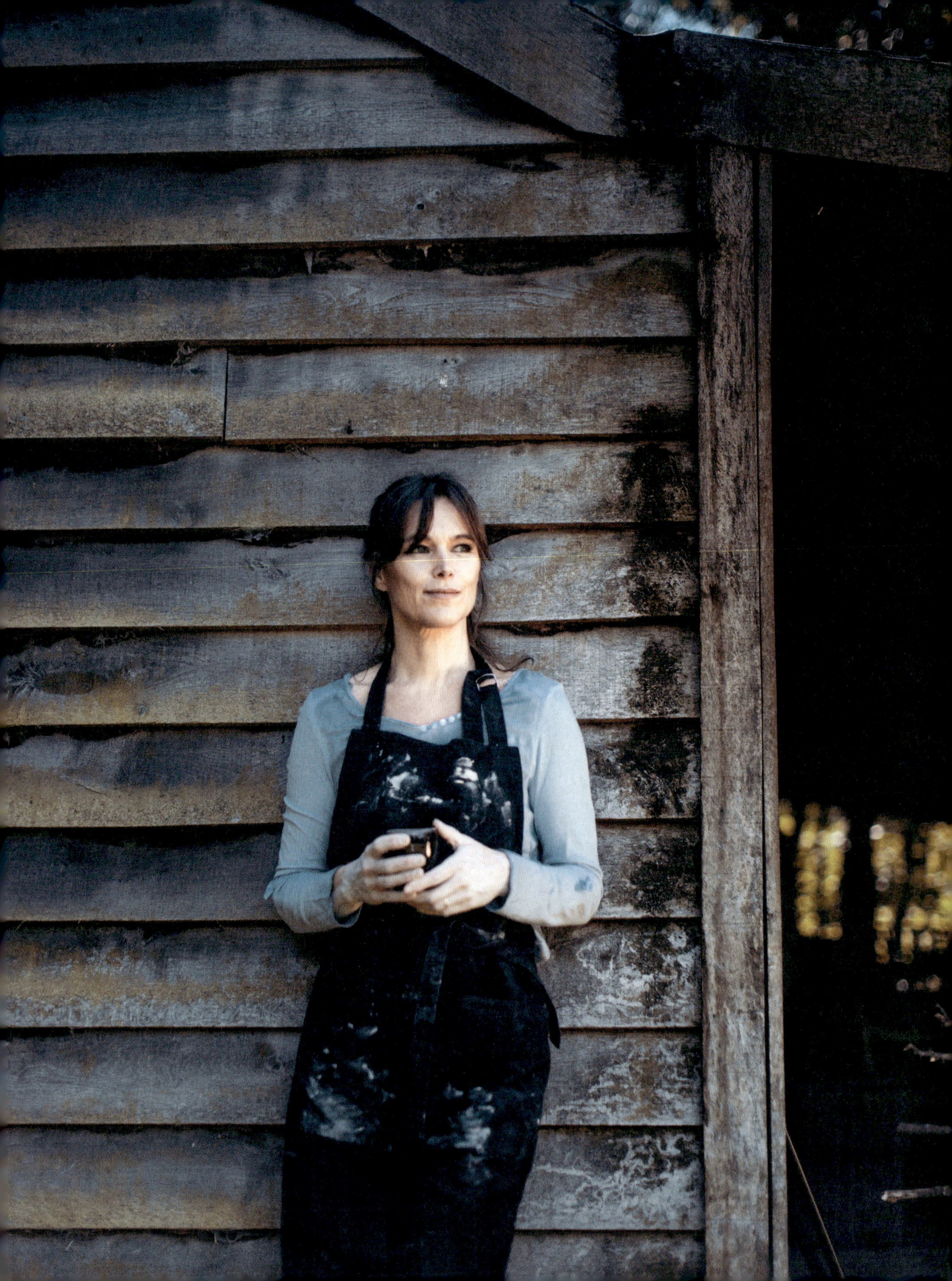

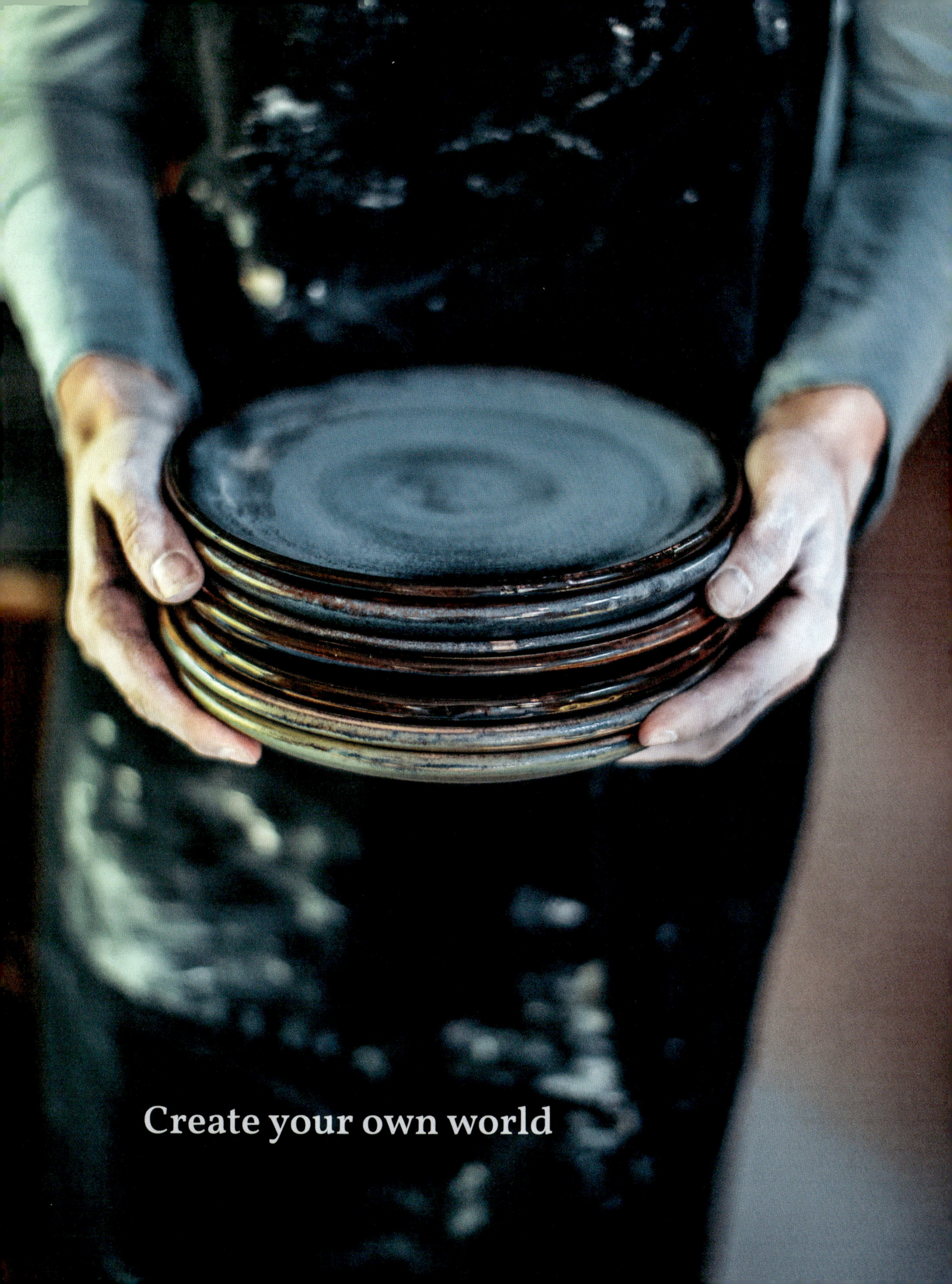
Create your own world

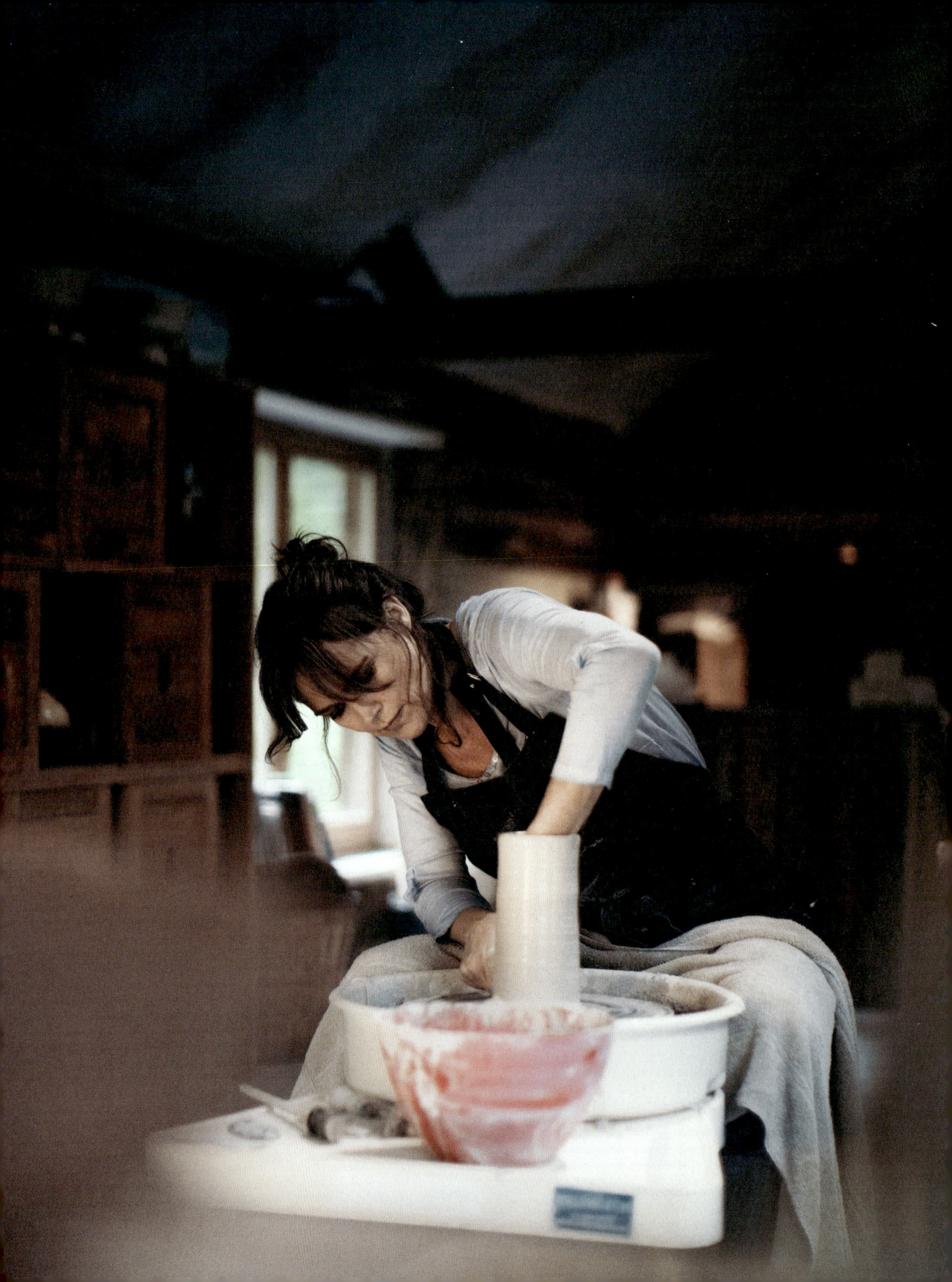

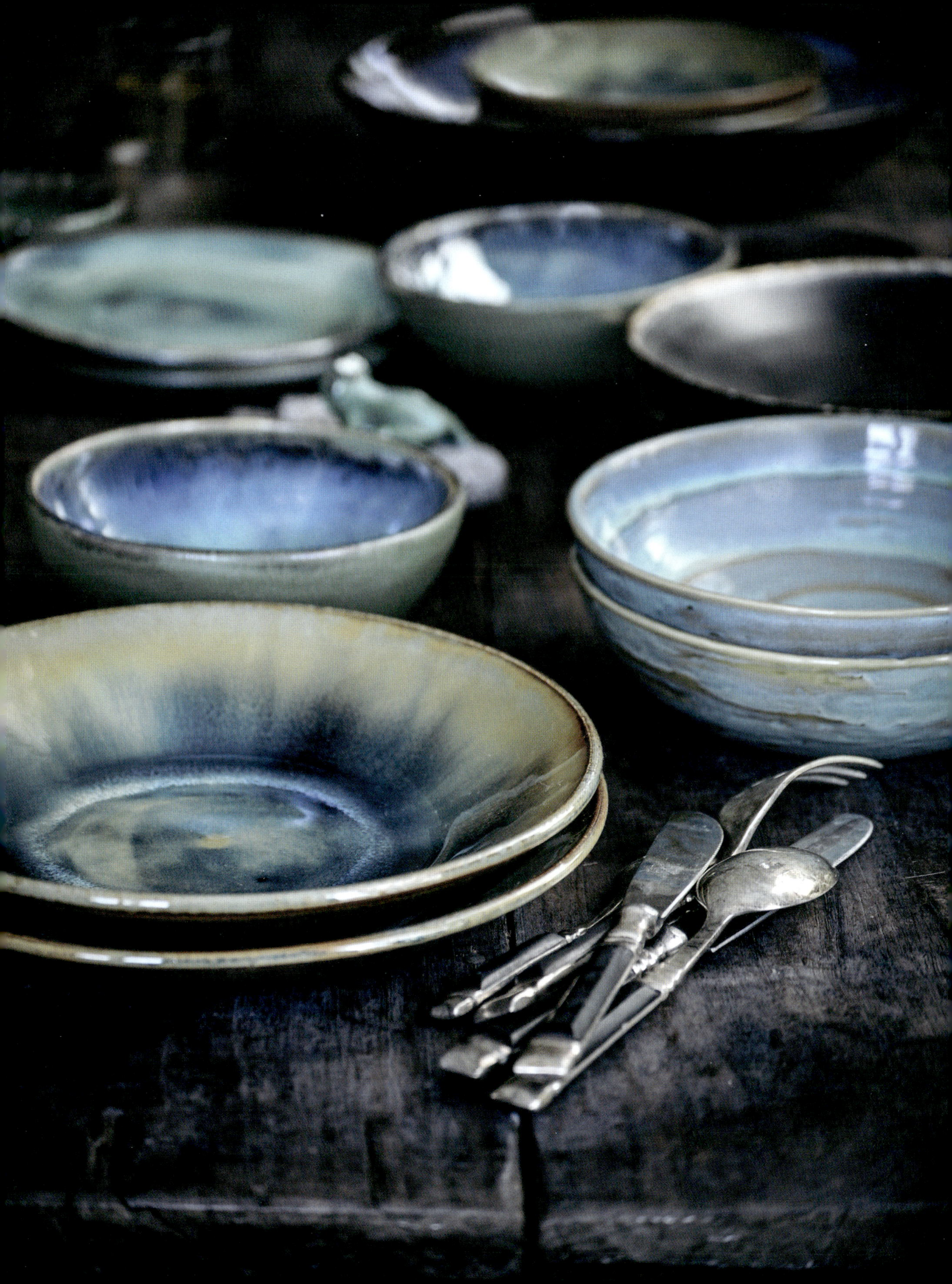

Make your gut happy

If you can keep your two to four pounds of gut bacteria happy, you'll be happier too. Your guts are the place where hormones, including your happiness hormone, are produced, and you need those to remain resilient and positive in life. Healthy intestinal flora is associated with good moods and great health.

Gut bacteria are living organisms who need food to survive, just like you do. They thrive especially well on fiber. But the consumption of fiber in our western diet has decreased significantly and lies far below the recommended amount. The most important reason is our change in lifestyle, where we eat fewer "real" and natural foods and more processed "fast" foods, from which the fiber has often been removed. We especially like eating starchy and sugary foods which are digested so quickly and easily that they don't even reach the large intestine; these include white bread, French fries, pasta, cookies, soft drinks ... The bacteria in your large intestine don't get the nutrition they need; we are literally starving them, causing some of them to disappear. Eat carbs that will make it to your large intestine. Those are fiber-rich, unprocessed carbs. I call them "large-intestine carbs".

The lack of fiber-rich foods in our diet is becoming disastrous for our health. Fiber is associated with a reduction in cholesterol levels, working proactively to reduce cardiovascular disease, type 2 diabetes and certain forms of cancer, as well as reducing the risk of infections and inflammatory diseases. Last but certainly not least: they stimulate our bowels. And regular toilet-goers tend to be happier people on the whole ☺.

Thankfully, our gut bacteria are flexible. According to Sonnenburg, a researcher who studied the Hadza, a native tribe in Tanzania, you can stimulate the regrowth of gut bacteria by eating more fiber. The Hadza consume ten times the amount of fiber that a normal person in the western world consumes. And they don't eat fiber-enriched foods or whole-wheat bread, they eat "real" food, straight from nature: berries, fruits, seeds, fiber-rich root vegetables, honey and game.(1) (2)

What is fiber?

Fiber is a carbohydrate found exclusively in plant-based foods. Animals have bones to keep them upright, plants have fiber. It's found in vegetables, fruit, nuts, seeds, pulses and whole grains. People who follow my way of eating effortlessly consume the recommended quantity of the (Belgian) Health Council of 1 ounce per day.

(1) https://science.sciencemag.org/content/357/6353/802.
(2) https://www.bbc.com/news/magazine-40686373

Fiber comes in a several varieties:

Non-fermentable fiber (insoluble fiber)
As the word suggests, this kind of fiber is not broken down in our digestive system or by our gut bacteria. It adds bulk to our waste products and makes the passage of bowel movements easier. Although it's very useful for cleaning the gut and stimulating bowel movements, this type of fiber is less interesting to our gut bacteria.

Fermentable fiber (soluble fiber)
Fruit is one of the best sources of soluble fiber, which enter the large intestine via the stomach and small intestine almost completely intact. This is because we don't have the enzymes to break down this kind of fiber; it forms a pulp which is consumed by our gut bacteria. In other words, this type of fiber is a kind of prebiotic: food for our gut bacteria. During this digestion process, short-chain fatty acids are produced, which in turn provide energy to the cells lining the large intestine. And this lets them do what they need to do: keep our gut healthy and prevent any leakage, which then strengthens our immune system. Soluble fiber has other health benefits too: it lowers cholesterol levels, slows down the intake of sugars in the body, and give you that full feeling. Soluble fiber is found in fruit, linseed, chia seed, oats, avocado, beans, broccoli ...
If possible, eat the skin of the fruit as well, as it contains the most fiber. This is why it's best to eat untreated (organic) fruits and vegetables.

Resistant starch (RS)
RS is a relatively newly acknowledged source of fiber that is almost completely fermented (read: broken down) by the bacteria in our large intestine, creating plenty of healthy short-chain fatty acids. The process works similarly to what happens to soluble fibers. RS is therefore another form of carb/fiber which cannot be broken down by our own enzymes. It's resistant to enzymes and therefore reaches our digestive system completely intact. As soon as this kind of starch reaches the large intestine, it becomes food for the gut bacteria (prebiotics), producing short-chain fatty acids. It is hard to determine exactly how much resistant starch a product contains. The amount changes with aging (reduces the level of RS), heating (reduces the level of RS), cooling (increases the level of RS) and storing (increases the level of RS). RS can be found in onions, leeks, artichokes, beans ... One of the richest sources of RS are green bananas. That's why I sometimes mix a green banana into my breakfast fruit, and it tastes quite good. I love the texture.

You could say that resistant starch and soluble fiber are our gut bacteria's best friends.

Food	Starch	RS	Glycemic Index (12)
Potatoes, fried	94%	<1%	93
White bread	88%	1%	70
Black beans, cooked	60%	5%	30
Pinto beans, cooked	61%	5%	39

Table: Harvard, Legumes and Resistant starch Dr. Guy Crosby (RS = Resistant Starch)

Harvard promotes pulses as a source of RS. The reason for this is that pulses don't cause your blood sugar levels to spike (as shown in the low value of the glycemic index) because they contain less starch and plenty of fiber. Raw potatoes are a good source of RS, but they're not that interesting because they need to be cooked before we eat them (I wouldn't recommend eating raw potatoes). They lose a lot of RS during the cooking process. You need to let them cool down for at least 24 hours for them to regain RS, and you need to eat them cold. In Belgium, we eat French fries and not cold potatoes. French fries, cooked potatoes and fried potatoes are not a good source of RS. Moreover, potatoes contain a lot of starch (see table) that is converted to glucose and taken up in the blood in the small intestine.

The trick is to choose plant-based foods that will give you fiber, resistant starch, vitamins, minerals, and healthy fats, but which will not cause your blood sugar levels to spike; in other words, plant-based foods that do not contain too much starch (= sugar).
That leaves you with vegetables, fruits, nuts, seeds and sometimes pulses.

Whole-wheat bread is not the only source of fiber, as some would have you believe.
What's more, whole-wheat bread isn't even the best source of fiber. It's recommended for people with a restricted diet who don't eat much "real" food, as a way to boost fiber intake. But, if you want to avoid (fast) carbs like I do, by eating "real" food and taking in plenty of healthy fiber, there is plenty of choice, such as the nutritional approach I recommend in this book.

Note: Today, "fiber" is considered a magic word. That's why you see lots of processed foods in stores which are supplemented with fiber or resistant starch powders. But that's not "real" food that you can cook. I believe that's the kind of food that will make you unhappy; I call it pill-food. Moreover, research has shown that processed foods, even when supplemented with fiber, are not a healthy alternative. It's a combination of all the components that determines what makes real food healthy and processed food unhealthy, whether it has added fiber or not.

Give me real, fresh food that I can smell, feel, choose, and use to make beautiful creations. Food that I can share, that will bring happiness to me and my loved ones. And once again, it all comes down to: buy fresh, cook your own meals and eat together.

Most plant-based foods contain a combination of soluble and insoluble fibers and resistant starch.

Fiber, in grams, per 100 grams (Source: voedingswaardetabel.nl
nice-info.be/nutrinews/voedingsvezel-de-feiten-op-een-rij)

Cocoa powder	34	Miso	7,3
Chia seed, dried	34,4	Avocado	6,7
Poppy seed	20,5	Blueberries	6,6
Jerusalem artichoke	18	Raspberries	6,5
Salsify (oyster plant)	16,96	Whole-wheat bread	6,4
Prunes, dried	16,1	Seaweed, mixed	6
Apricots, dried	14,4	Artichoke	5,4
Soybeans, cooked	13,2	Fresh dates	5
Chocolate, dark	10,9	Celeriac	4,9
Almonds	10,6	Peas	4,7
Chickpeas	9,5	Sunflower seeds	4,5
Brown beans (kidney beans), cooked	8,9	Mushrooms	4,0
Currants	7,9	Pomegranate	4,0
Brussels sprouts	8,15	String beans	4
Nuts, mixed	8,3	Persimmon	3,7
Walnuts	8	Carrots	2,8
Lentils	7,9	Quinoa	2,8
Peanuts	7,7	Coconut milk	2, 0
Sesame seeds	7,5	Strawberries	2,0
Oatmeal	7,5	White bread	1,0

Important note:
Not everyone benefits from a high fiber intake. Some people react to certain kinds of dietary fiber. They may experience symptoms such as stomach aches, diarrhea, constipation or a bloated sensation caused by a build-up of gas. This is also known as irritable bowel syndrome (IBS). In that case, I recommend you seek guidance from a professional.

https://rahadiandimas.staff.uns.ac.id/files/2013/05/Journal-Resistant-starch-as-functional-ingredient-A-review.pdf

What is a keto diet?

Keto is a term you come across increasingly often. What is it and what similarities does it have with my approach to food? This text will help you gain more insight.

My way of eating is moderately low-carb. You can spend your whole life eating like this without missing out on anything. Since my very first cookbook, I've always included a number of recipes that contain even fewer carbs. That's what we call "keto" today. In practice, keto means that you eat fewer than 2 ounces (50 grams) of carbs each day and eat more fat instead. All of my books contain a combination of low-carb and keto recipes. For those of you who really want to go "keto", or want to try it out for a while, from now on I will mark all my keto recipes with this symbol: ✓ keto, so you can make your own choice.

With a keto diet, your body starts to burn fats because of the absence of carbs (sugars). This way of eating works exceptionally well for people who want to lose a lot of weight without feeling hungry all the time, and for people with type 2 diabetes who want to turn their diabetes around. But that often works with a moderately low-carb diet as well.

Is it easy to stick to?

For some, it is. For others, it isn't. It also depends on what you want to achieve, of course. Some people, such as those who suffer from epilepsy, see it as a long-term lifestyle change. While others, such as those who want to lose lots of weight fast, see it more as the start of a diet for a limited period of time, a period which may last from a few months to a few years. I think that most people temporarily follow a keto diet to tackle weight or other health problems, after which they switch over to a moderately low-carb diet as outlined in my books.

In my books, you'll find many keto recipes that are integrated into my way of eating. My recipes vary naturally between low-carb and keto.

Our western way of eating is rich in carbs. Carbs became readily available with the rise of agriculture. Before then, carbs, and certainly fast carbs, were relatively scarce; fruit and honey were the only sources. When few or no carbs were available, people would naturally switch over to a keto diet until enough carbs were available. This switching between the two most important sources of energy, fat and glucose, was a regular and natural occurrence. It was the availability of food that determined which system the body would use to store energy. But, because our diet today includes a daily overdose of carbs, there is no longer the need for the body to switch over to burning fat.

I eat carbs mostly in the morning with my breakfast fruit. An average of 1 pound of low-carb fruit contains a little less than 2 ounces (45 grams) of carbs. During the rest of the day I eat the way I describe in my books, which means mostly dishes with few carbs and plenty of healthy fats. This means that my body is not in a permanent state of ketosis. But because I eat few carbs, especially on days when I have eggs for breakfast, my body automatically switches from burning sugars to burning fats. And to me, that seems a natural state where you have the best of both worlds.

The advantages of a keto diet:

A keto diet can also be a powerful way to battle various diseases:

Obesity: people lose weight quickly because the body switches to burning fat.
Epilepsy: the brain uses a different source of energy during a keto diet. This reduces the chance of seizures in epilepsy patients.
Type 2 diabetes: many people drive their type 2 diabetes into remission when they follow a keto diet. Depending on how far the disease has progressed, this can also be achieved with a moderately low-carb diet as described in my books.
Cancer: there are currently many promising studies looking into the link between a keto diet and cancer. A keto diet doesn't cure cancer, but it does help increase the effectiveness of traditional cancer treatments. To put it simply: cancer cells need plenty of glucose to survive and they cannot switch to ketones as a source of energy. With no glucose to feed them, they become weak and more vulnerable to classic treatments such as chemotherapy.
Ketones as super fuel for our bodies: Athletes who not only train to burn glucose, but also to burn fats, benefit from this approach. This is especially true for endurance athletes. Burning fat occurs when you train and have eaten few or no carbohydrates. When that happens, your body draws its energy from body fat.
There has been a lot of commotion recently around the use of ketones as a super fuel, and there has even been talk of doping. A research team from KU Leuven has discovered that the use of ketones can increase physical performance by up to 15 percent. It should be noted that they are referring to using ketones as a supplement, which is entirely different from what we described earlier. Professor Hespel called the results unprecedented.

Controversy

Although the keto diet has been shown to have many health benefits, the diet remains controversial. There are few reliable long-term studies. The biggest risk is for diabetes patients taking medication, as their medication may react negatively to this way of eating. Therefore, diabetes patients who wish to follow a keto diet should always seek out the guidance of a health or nutrition professional. Other controversial topics linked to keto are saturated fats, cholesterol, grains, red meat, etc.
It provides us with food for thought and further research.

Keto in detail

This text was written by Professor Hanno Pijl of Leiden University.

When we eat keto, our body produces what we call keto acids. Keto acids are produced when we break down, or burn, fats in the body. When a lot of fats are burned, the body cannot process all the keto acids that are released and they enter the bloodstream, where they are eventually passed via our urine. This is what we call the ketose state.

Glucose and fats are the most important fuels for our body. The hormone insulin is very important for regulating our metabolism. On the one hand, it stimulates the intake of glucose and fats into our tissues through our blood. On the other hand, insulin slows down the breaking down of fats. This means that when there is not much insulin in your blood, more fat will be broken down.
Glucose is the most important trigger for the production of insulin in the pancreas. Fat stimulates hardly any insulin production in the body, if it does so at all. When you eat sugar or starch, your digestive system converts that to glucose, which then enters your bloodstream via the gut lining. The pancreas starts to produce more insulin to transport the glucose from the blood to the tissues, but that also inhibits the breakdown of fats. Which makes sense, because when that happens, there is more than enough glucose available to fuel the body.

When you limit the amount of sugar and starch in your food, the glucose levels in your blood decrease, which in turn decreases the production of insulin. You start to burn more fat and produce keto acids. However, you will only reach ketosis if you severely limit your intake of sugar and starch; only a small amount of insulin is needed to inhibit the breakdown of fats. Moreover, you shouldn't be eating too much protein because amino acids also stimulate the production of insulin. How much sugar and starch you should be eating to reach ketosis varies per person, but on the whole the limit is around 1 to 1½ ounces (25 to 50 grams) per day. In theory, you are allowed to eat plenty of fat as fats do not stimulate insulin production. A common misconception about keto diets is that they must be high in fat. That doesn't have to be the case at all. The key to this diet is that it contains very little sugar and starch.

How about proteins in a keto diet?
Proteins are made up of amino acids, of which there are 22. Some amino acids can also stimulate the production of insulin. Therefore, some people say that you should be careful with proteins if you want to reach ketosis. This point, however, is still up for debate. There are indications that amino acids have less influence on insulin production when the diet contains very little sugar and starch. As of yet, there is no substantial evidence regarding the role of protein in a keto diet.

Eating keto, how do you do that?
Stay away from processed foods (they almost always contain sugar). Eat unprocessed foods as often as possible. Be sparing with (or avoid altogether) starchy foods such as bread, rice, pasta and potatoes. Eat mostly vegetables, nuts and seeds in every imaginable combination. Consume a moderate amount of meat, fish, eggs, and (full-fat) dairy products. Be careful with fruits, as these are also relatively rich in sugars.

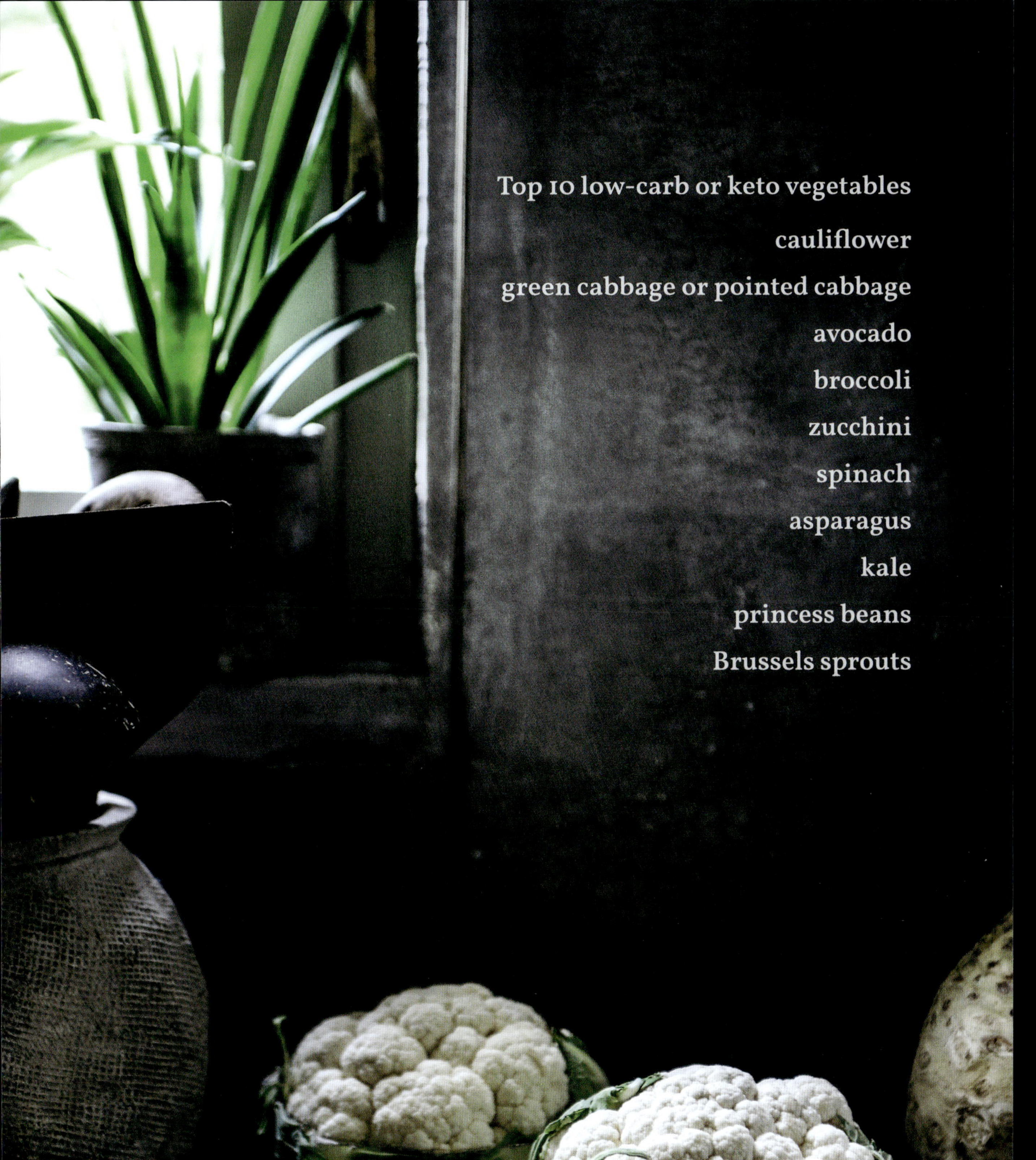

Top 10 low-carb or keto vegetables

cauliflower

green cabbage or pointed cabbage

avocado

broccoli

zucchini

spinach

asparagus

kale

princess beans

Brussels sprouts

Intermittent fasting

Intermittent fasting is another one of those terms you may be hearing a lot more often these days. What is it exactly and is it something worth looking into for you personally? The text below will help you gain more insight.

There was a time when we were advised to eat many small meals during the day to keep our metabolism going. New scientific insights now show that we should be doing the opposite. Sometimes skipping a meal and going to bed with an empty stomach seems to be beneficial for your health. This is something we've secretly known for quite some time, because fasting has been a common practice throughout the ages and across cultures. Centuries ago, people had to go without food for long periods of time because food just wasn't available. They were obliged to fast. Sick people were advised to eat nothing and stay in bed. This is something we also see in the animal kingdom. Sick animals rest and sleep, but they do not eat. Not eating triggers a healing process in the body.

Why would someone fast from time to time?

Overweight and type 2 diabetes: When you fast occasionally, you don't only lose weight because you eat less, but you also improve your sensitivity to insulin, which in turn stimulates the fat metabolism in your cells. Lowering insulin levels is especially beneficial for patients with diabetes.

Fasting reduces the risk of certain diseases such as some forms of cancer, Alzheimer's and cardiovascular diseases, and it promotes the recovery of cells in the body and genes. You will find an explanation of how that works under "Why is fasting so healthy?".

Anti-aging

Tests on animals have shown that restricting the intake of calories and periodically fasting has a positive influence on health and is linked to a longer, healthier life.

Is intermittent fasting a good choice for everyone?

I don't think so. I have learned from personal experience that anyone who is sensitive to eating disorders, who regularly binges, suffers from a yo-yoing weight and tends towards orthorexia, bulimia or anorexia should first try to bring balance to their eating habits and stick to three meals a day without snacks, unless they're really hungry. The problem is that, for some people, fasting can trigger extreme hunger cravings, after which they'll eat anything they can get their hands on, especially the unhealthier foods. And that defeats the purpose of intermittent fasting.
First try working on the basics, turning the large dials in your diet by focusing on natural, high-quality foods and finding the right balance for you.
As soon as you have that down, you can tweak the small dials in your diet and, if you wish, start to explore intermittent fasting. The easiest and least disruptive way to do so is to skip breakfast, as Professor Hanno Pijl explains in the following text.

Intermittent fasting: Why is fasting so healthy?

This text was written by Professor Hanno Pijl of Leiden University.

Some people think that we need to eat every day, because in the society we live in, eating every day is the norm. However, eating every day has only become common since the Industrial Revolution, which started a mere 250 years ago in the United Kingdom. Before then, over the course of evolutionary history, most people didn't have regular access to food. Our bodies are made to survive these periods of scarcity. Nature has given us very powerful biological mechanisms to do so. People can survive, on average, 60 (!) days without food (but not without water). It's obviously better not to fast for 60 days but, if you had to, you would probably be able to survive. Needing food every day is a myth. What's more, it turns out that fasting once in a while can be very good for you.

We are what we eat, so if we fast too long, we will run out of building blocks (body mass) and fuel. But alternating between eating every day with shorter periods in which you eat much less or nothing at all (intermittent fasting) does have health benefits. Intermittent fasting can be done in many different ways. The following are the most thoroughly researched, although it should be said that these studies have been carried out primarily on animals:

Fasting every other day

Living on water one day, eating whatever you want the next day (as healthily as possible, of course).

5-2 fasting

Living on water two days in a row, and then eating what you want the other five days.

Time-restricted eating

Eating only during a limited set of hours in the day, for example between 12 noon and 8 o'clock in the evening. You fast 16 hours a day. You can also choose a shorter fasting period.

Periodic fasting

Fasting for five consecutive days every couple of weeks (or months). With this type of fasting, people often choose modified fasting. This means that you do eat, but only foods which will give you the necessary nutrients, but not much fuel and few "building blocks". Sugar and starch are the most important sources of glucose in our blood, and glucose is our most important fuel. That's why the "fasting mimicking diet" used with periodic fasting contains practically no sugar or starch. And because protein is the most important building block for our body, such a diet also contains very little protein. This diet consists mostly of healthy fats and fiber-rich carbs.

Why is fasting so healthy? As mentioned earlier, we are made to survive periods when there is no food available. Our body understands that it's getting no fuel or building materials. The body reacts by doing three things: 1) It starts using its damaged cell structures as fuel, cleaning up the cells in the process; this is called "autophagy". 2) It stops using energy to grow and reproduce. Instead, the energy is used to maintain and repair existing cells. 3) The body starts protecting itself from all forms of stress (such as nutrient shortages, but also radiation, toxins, heat, etc.). Because the body needs time to get all these processes going, we suspect that periodic fasting (alternative 4) may be the most effective.

An important point to note here is that most of the available information on the effects of intermittent fasting comes from testing performed on animals. Current research is focused on human testing. Preliminary results suggest that intermittent fasting has the same beneficial effects for humans as for animals, but we are not certain yet. However, there is no reason to assume that people will react differently than animals, because human cells react the same way to food shortage as animal cells.

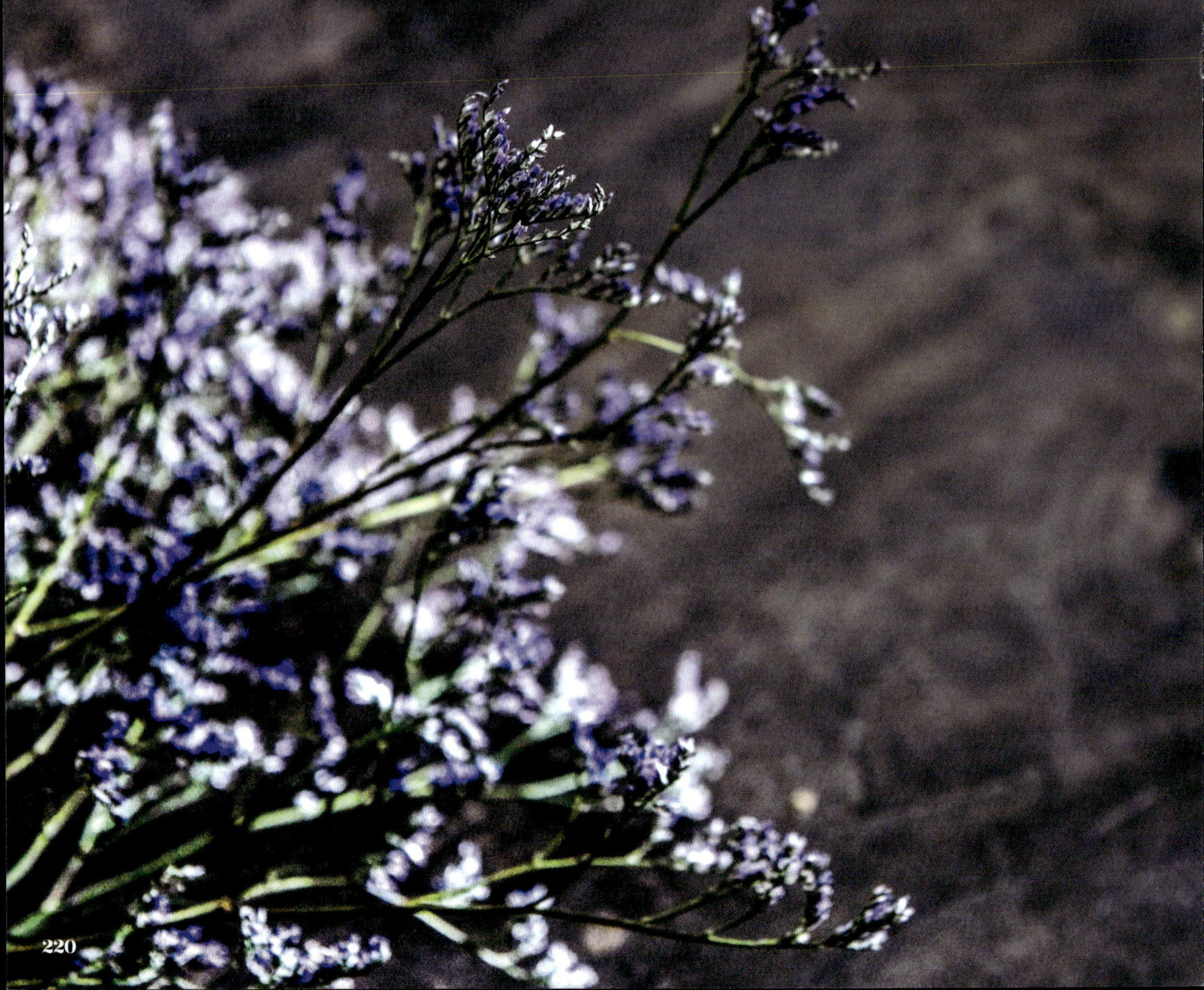

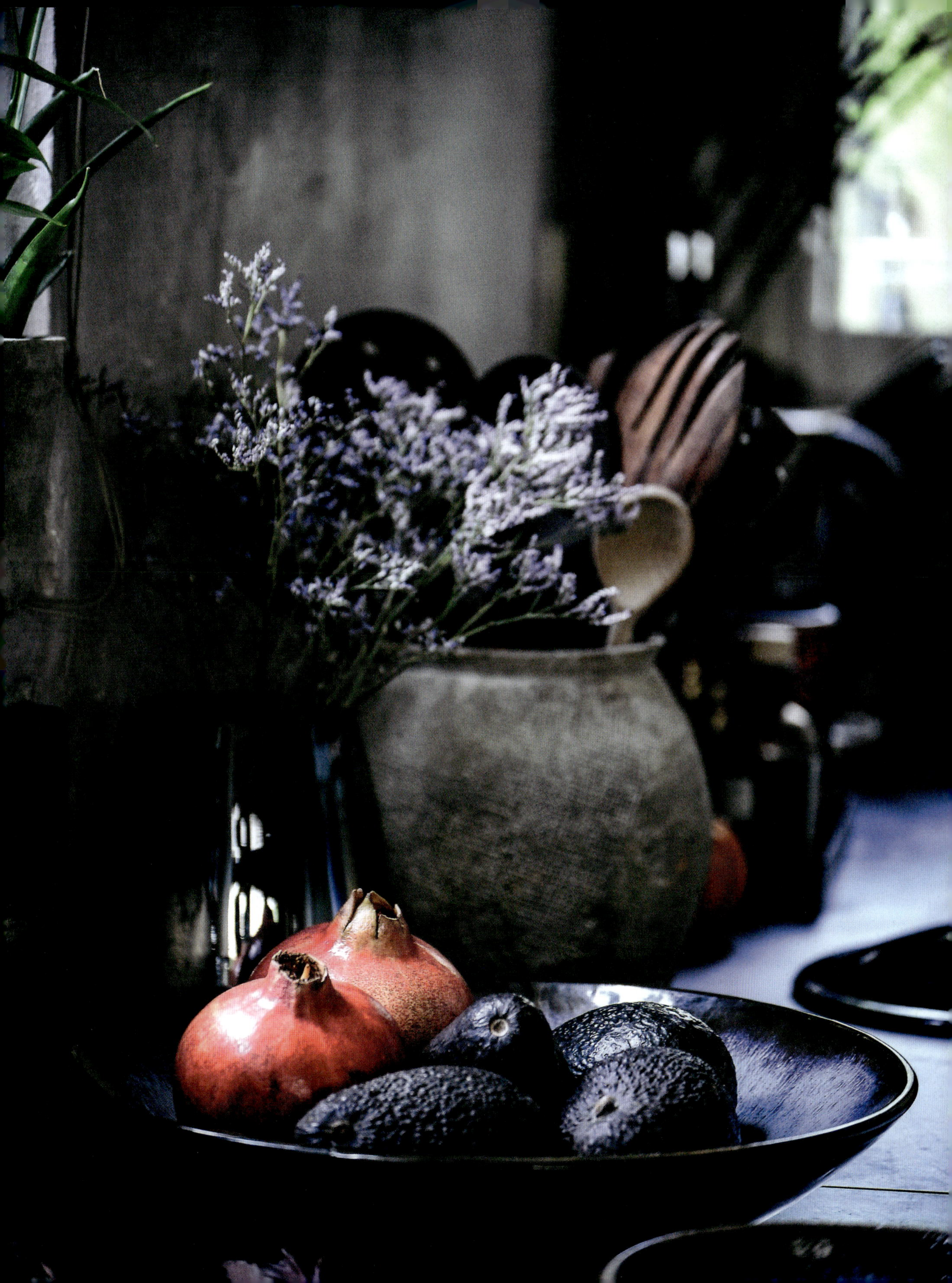

index

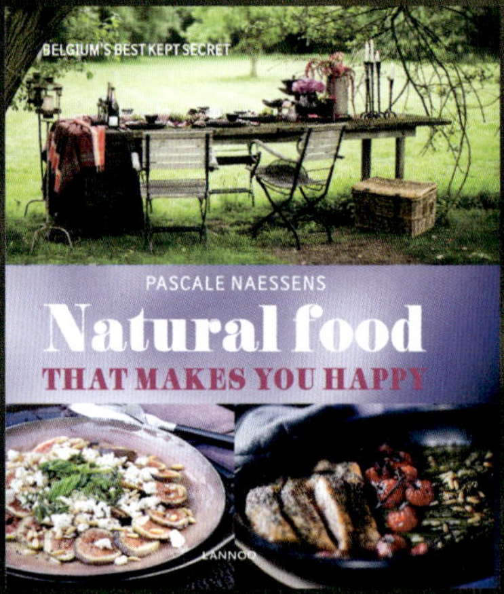

ISBN: 978 94 014 1983 3

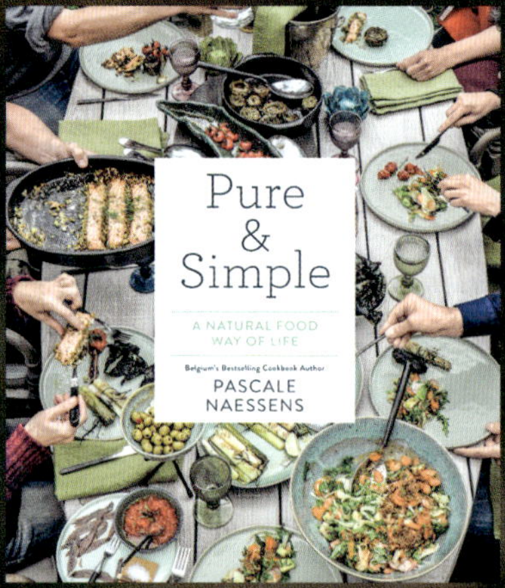

ISBN: 978 1 4197 2617 0

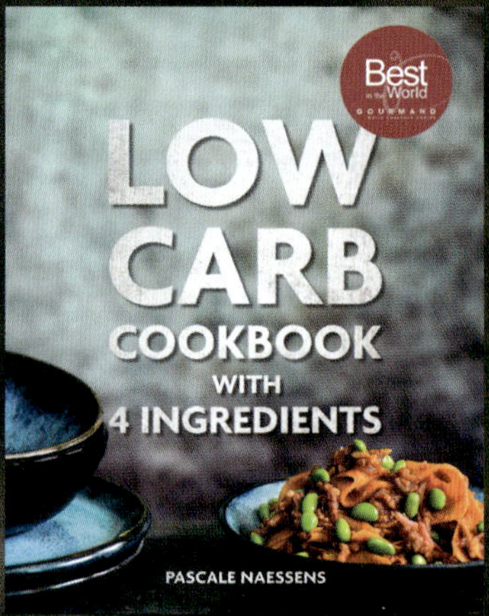

ISBN: 978 9 4014 6148 1

www.lannoo.com

www.purepascale.com

Would you like further information?
Contact publisher: Uitgeverij Lannoo, gunther.spriet@lannoo.be, www.lannoo.com
Contact author: Pascale Naessens, info@purepascale.com, www.purepascale.com

RECIPES, TEXTS, STYLING AND CONCEPT: Pascale Naessens
PHOTOGRAPHY: Roos Mestdagh, James Wood, Charis Boel, Arno De Pooter, Ramon de Llano
DESIGN AND LAYOUT: Kris Torfs - Gemex Publishing bvba
ENGLISH TRANSLATION AND LAYOUT: Textcase, Deventer

The ideas and recipes in this book serve as a source of inspiration and as part of a varied menu for healthy people. Anyone suffering from a condition should consult a doctor or health professional at all times. The information in the book should not be used as medication or as a substitute for any form of medical treatment.

If you have any comments or questions, please do not hesitate to contact the publisher: redactielifestyle@lannoo.be

D/2020/45/159 – NUR 440-441
ISBN: 978 94 014 6841 1

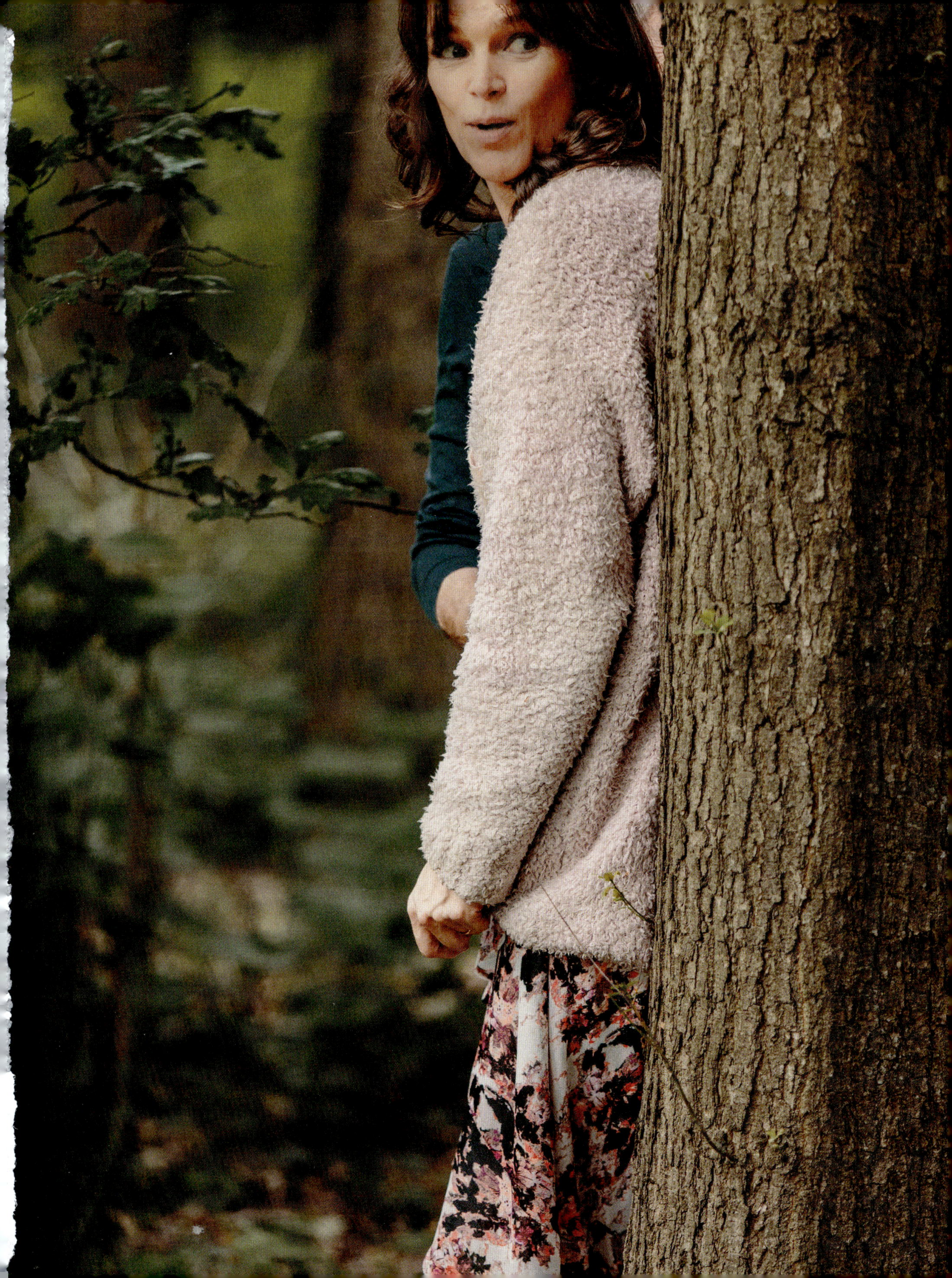

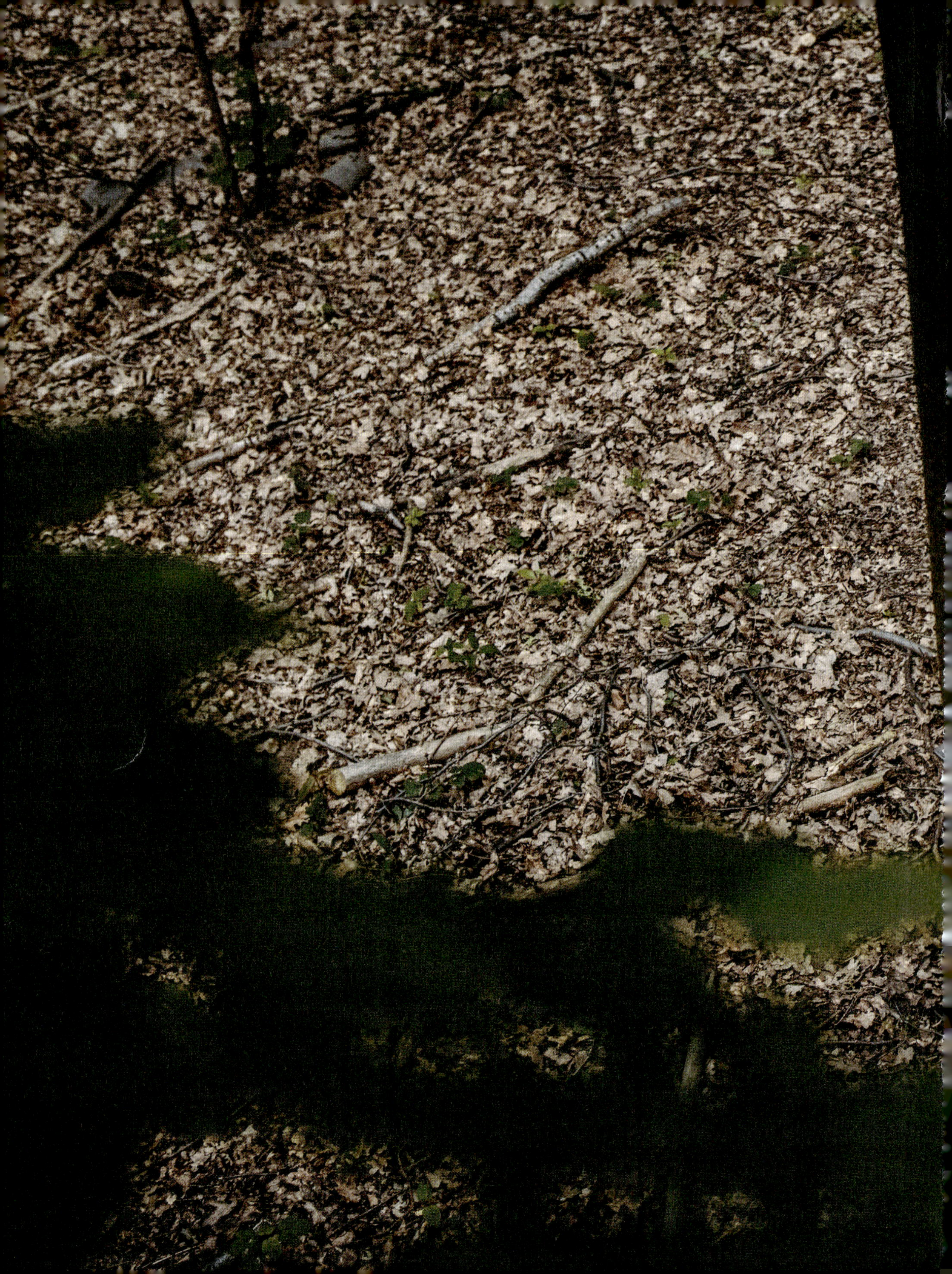